Acyclovir Therapy for Herpesvirus Infections

INFECTIOUS DISEASE AND THERAPY

Series Editors

Brian E. Scully, M.B., B.Ch.

College of Physicians
and Surgeons
Columbia University
New York, New York

Harold C. Neu, M.D.

College of Physicians
and Surgeons
Columbia University
New York, New York

Additional Volumes in Preparation

Acyclovir Therapy for Herpesvirus Infections

edited by

DAVID A. BAKER
Health Sciences Center
State University of New York
Stony Brook, New York

MARCEL DEKKER, INC.   New York and Basel

Library of Congress Cataloging-in-Publication Data

Acyclovir therapy for herpesvirus infections / edited by David A.
Baker.
        p.   cm. -- (Infectious disease and therapy ; v. 4)
    Includes bibliographical references.
    ISBN 0-8247-8091-4 (alk. paper)
    1. Herpesvirus diseases--Chemotherapy.   2. Acyclovir.   I. Baker,
David A.   II. Series.
    [DNLM: 1. Acyclovir--therapeutic use.   2. Herpesvirus Infections-
-drug therapy.   W1 IN406HMN v. 4 / WC 571 A189]
RC147.H6A28   1989
616.9'25--dc20
DNLM/DLC
for Library of Congress   89-17175
                                                                    CIP

This book is printed on acid-free paper.

MARCEL DEKKER, INC.
270 Madison Avenue, New York, New York 10016

Current printing (last digit):
10 9 8 7 6 5 4 3 2 1

PRINTED IN THE UNITED STATES OF AMERICA

Foreword

The '70s and '80s have been years of great change in science and technology. The tremendous accomplishments in the area of cancer treatment are indicative of scientific innovation coupled with perseverance. Intimate knowledge of cellular growth and metabolism, molecular biology, and the application of classical approaches in defining pharmacologic and pharmacokinetic properties has been combined to make the majority of cancers treatable, and a great many of them curable.

Many spin-off areas of investigation have come from the field of cancer research. One of the most important of these is the antiviral research field. Like cancer research, the antiviral research story is full of false starts, frustrations, and failures. However, these difficulties are as important as the so-called advances—as Thomas Henry Huxley has been quoted, "Next to being right in this world, the best of all things is to be clearly and definitely wrong."

The principle of "selective toxicity" has emerged as the common denominator to the successes of antiviral as well as anticancer chemotherapy. In the case of acyclovir, this is apparent as a drug activity against the virus in the virally infected cell which spares the adjacent, otherwise normal cells from the toxic effects of the agent.

This mechanism was eloquently and completely defined by Dr. G. Elion and co-workers at Burroughs Wellcome Company. Acyclovir is selectively activated in the herpes-infected cell and selectively binds to and inhibits viral DNA polymerase. This results in a wide ratio of therapeutic versus toxic potential. Unlike most other drugs, acyclovir was developed with early knowledge of its mechanism of action. This knowledge has resulted in a greater level of confidence in the in vitro, animal and human studies alike, as well as more targeted research planning.

A great number of animal models that were designed as surrogates for human infections have been validated or reconfirmed during the course of the development of acyclovir. Examples include the rabbit model for ocular herpes infection, genital herpes in the guinea pig and mouse, herpes encephalitis in the mouse, and the Delta-herpes model in the patas monkey (as a varicella-like infection). Many of these animal model studies were done in collaboration with the National Institute of Allergy and Infectious Diseases.

Acyclovir has advanced and legitimized the antiviral field by building upon the research programs associated with idoxuridine (Stoxil®), vidarabine (Vira-A®), and trifluridine (Viroptic®). It has also been identified by the FDA as an example of useful cooperation and collaboration with the agency and as a benchmark for the development of new antivirals.

The first acyclovir symposium in September 1981 defined preclinical, antiviral, and toxicologic parameters, and outlined pharmacologic and pharmacokinetic properties in man. That forum also described results of phase II studies which formed the beginnings of a clinical database that has subsequently been expanded many orders of magnitude.

The reviews and discussions in this compendium will bring the reader up to date on newer data to help assess contemporary efficacy and safety issues of this important agent.

Daniel H. King, Ph.D.
Vice President
Research and Development
Oclassen Pharmaceuticals
Corte Madera, California

Preface

Viral infections causing significant morbidity and mortality are clearly increasing in humans. Over the past decade, careful scientific studies have increased our knowledge and understanding of one important group of viruses, the herpesviruses. Varicella-zoster virus and herpes simplex virus have been extensively investigated. The incidence, epidemiology, and clinical presentations of these agents have been demonstrated skillfully. With our increased understanding of the biology of these viruses, research has enabled the development of an antiviral agent that has been shown to be both safe and highly effective in the treatment of herpes simplex and varicella-zoster viral infections.

The development and testing of acyclovir is a breakthrough in the field of antiviral chemotherapy. Acyclovir, because of its unique properties, is considered a prototype drug. In addition, the extensive and carefully controlled preclinical and clinical studies using this drug have set new standards for the medical community.

The authors of this book are the scientists and clinicians who developed and tested acyclovir. They bring their expertise in presenting a clear and current status of the clinical application and cautions in the use of acyclovir.

The initial chapters of the book deal with the molecular biology and toxicology of acyclovir. The majority of the book then focuses on herpes simplex virus infections. These particular chapters are arranged by site of infection in the body. Therapy of varicella-zoster viral infections is then discussed, and Epstein-Barr viral infection is then presented. The concluding chapters are on therapy in the immunocompromised host.

Herpesvirus infections are observed and treated by a wide range of clinical specialties, ophthalmology, dentistry, infectious disease (internal medicine), dermatology, pediatrics, obstetrics, and gynecology. This book will be invaluable to all health care workers involved in the examination and treatment of patients with these viral infections.

David A. Baker

Contents

Contributors

Ann M. Arvin, M.D. Associate Professor, Department of Pediatrics, Infectious Diseases Division, Stanford University School of Medicine, Stanford, California

Steven T. Baldwin, M.D. Professor of Pediatrics and Microbiology, Department of Pediatrics, School of Medicine, University of Alabama at Birmingham, Birmingham, Alabama

Zane A. Brown, M.D. Professor, Division of Maternal/Fetal Medicine, Department of Obstetrics and Gynecology, University of Washington, Seattle, Washington

L. M. T. Collum, F.R.C.S., F.R.C.S.I., F.C.Ophth. Professor of Ophthalmology, Department of Ophthalmology, Royal College of Surgeons in Ireland and Royal Victoria Eye and Ear Hospital, Dublin, Ireland

Marcus A. Conant, M.D. Clinical Professor, Department of Dermatology, University of California, San Francisco, California

Lawrence Corey, M.D. Head, Virology Division, Departments of Laboratory Medicine, Medicine, and Microbiology, Children's Orthopedic Hospital and Medical Center, University of Washington, Seattle, Washington

Joan L. Drucker, M.D. Medical Advisor, Department of Clinical Microbiology and Immunology, Burroughs Wellcome Co., Research Triangle Park, and Clinical Associate in Medicine, Duke University Medical Center, Durham, North Carolina

Sandor Feldman, M.D. Professor of Pediatrics, Chief, Pediatric Infectious Diseases, Department of Pediatrics, University of Mississippi Medical Center, Jackson, Mississippi

Cynthia L. Fowler, M.D.* Senior Fellow, Division of Infectious Diseases, Department of Medicine, University of New Mexico School of Medicine, Albuquerque, New Mexico

Phillip Furman, Ph.D. Associate Division Director, Division of Virology, Burroughs Wellcome Co., Research Triangle Park, North Carolina

M. John Gill, M.B., F.R.C.P. (C) Assistant Professor, Departments of Microbiology and Infectious Diseases, and Medicine, Faculty of Medicine, University of Calgary, Calgary, Alberta, Canada

Stuart M. Goldsmith, M.D. Fellow, Department of Pediatrics, School of Medicine, University of Alabama at Birmingham, Birmingham, Alabama

Sam Hopkins, Ph.D. Senior Research Scientist, Division of Virology, Burroughs Wellcome Co., Research Triangle Park, North Carolina

J. Clark Huff, M.D. Associate Professor, Department of Dermatology, University of Colorado School of Medicine, Denver, Colorado

Clifton C. Jones, M.D.[†] Senior Fellow, Division of Infectious Diseases, Department of Medicine, University of New Mexico School of Medicine, Albuquerque, New Mexico

Andria G. M. Langenberg, M.D.[‡] Fellow, Virology, Departments of Laboratory Medicine, Medicine, and Microbiology, University of Washington, Seattle, Washington

H. Reid Mattison, M.D. Assistant Professor, Infectious Diseases Unit, Department of Medicine, University of Rochester School of Medicine and Dentistry, Rochester, New York

Gregory J. Mertz, M.D. Assistant Professor, Division of Infectious Diseases, Department of Medicine, University of New Mexico School of Medicine, Albuquerque, New Mexico

G. Wayne Raborn, D.D.S., M.S. Clinical Professor, Faculty of Dentistry, Department of Dentistry, University of Alberta Hospitals, Edmonton, Alberta, Canada

Present affiliations:
*Senior Staff Fellow, Clinical Pathology Department, National Institutes of Health, Bethesda, Maryland
[†]Internal Medicine, Professional Association, Topeka, Kansas
[‡]Dermatology Resident, Department of Dermatology, University of California, San Francisco, California

Richard C. Reichman, M.D.   Associate Professor of Medicine, Infectious Diseases Unit, Department of Medicine, University of Rochester School of Medicine and Dentistry, Rochester, New York

Stephen E. Straus, M.D.   Head, Medical Virology Section, Laboratory of Clinical Investigation, National Institute of Allergy and Infectious Diseases, National Institutes of Health, Bethesda, Maryland

George M. Szczech, D.V.M., Ph.D.   Senior Toxicologic Pathologist, Division of Toxicology and Pathology, Burroughs Wellcome Co., Research Triangle Park, North Carolina

Walter E. Tucker, Jr., D.V.M.   Director, Division of Toxicology and Pathology, Burroughs Wellcome Co., Research Triangle Park, North Carolina

Richard J. Whitley, M.D.   Professor of Pediatrics, Microbiology, and Medicine, Department of Pediatrics, School of Medicine, University of Alabama at Birmingham, Birmingham, Alabama

1
Molecular Basis for the Antiviral Activity of Acyclovir

Sam Hopkins and Phillip Furman   *Burroughs Wellcome Co., Research Triangle Park, North Carolina*

INTRODUCTION

During the past 20 years our ability to develop antiherpetic agents has benefited greatly from an increased understanding of the basic biochemical processes involved in the replication of herpesvirus DNA. Of particular importance is the discovery that viral DNA replication is critically dependent on virally encoded thymidine kinase, DNA polymerase, deoxyribonuclease, and ribonucleotide reductase, which are enzymatically distinct from their isofunctional cellular counterparts (1-5). The substrate specificity, binding affinities for various inhibitors, allosteric regulation, and cofactor requirements of these virally induced enzymes form the bases for the development of a new generation of safe and effective antiviral drugs directed against herpesvirus infections. To date acyclovir represents the most extensively studied of these agents.

In general, antiherpetic nucleosides such as 5-iodo-2'-deoxyuridine, trifluorothymidine, and arabinosyl adenine require phosphorylation to their respective nucleoside triphosphates which are the species that inhibit virus replication by competing with the natural substrates for binding to the virus-encoded DNA polymerase and by disrupting replicative events by their incorporation into newly synthesized viral DNA (6-9). Since these compounds are converted into their corresponding triphosphates by cellular kinases, they have met with limited success, because they demonstrate little or no selectivity for their activation pathway. Furthermore, these triphosphates inhibit cellular and viral DNA polymerases as well as other cellular enzymes (6-9). The discovery of acyclovir constitutes the development of a new generation of analogs that exhibit enhanced antiviral activity by virtue of their highly selective pathway for activation and their preferential ability to inhibit viral rather than cellular enzymes.

SELECTIVE ACTIVATION

In contrast to uninfected cells, virally infected cells rapidly anabolize acyclovir to the nucleotide level (10,11). For example, acyclovir triphosphate levels in HSV-1-infected Vero cells or WI38 cells are 40-fold or 200,000-fold higher than in the respective uninfected cells (Table 1). Further studies on viral anabolism of acyclovir demonstrate that HSV-1 and HSV-2, which are most susceptible to inhibition by acyclovir, induce cells to form high levels of acyclovir triphosphate. In contrast, vaccinia virus and human cytomegalovirus (HCMV), which are relatively insensitive to

TABLE 1 Phosphorylation of Acyclovir in Uninfected and HSV-1-Infected Vero and WI38 Cells[a]

| Cell | Concn (pmol/10^6 cells) in: | |
	Uninfected[b] cells	Infected[c] cells
WI38		
Monophosphate	<0.01	147
Diphosphate	<0.01	269
Triphosphate	<0.01	2,084
Total	<0.03	2,500
Vero		
Monophosphate	0.1	2.0, 2.9 (3.6, 6.4)
Diphosphate	1.2	2.1, 3,3 (11.4, 8.7)
Triphosphate	1.4	20.1, 14.4 (61.0, 79.2)
Total	2.7	24.2, 20.6 (76.0, 94.3)

[a]Cells were infected with the H29 strain of HSV-1 at a multiplicity of infection of 5 to 10 plaque-forming units per cell. Infected cells were treated with 100 μM acyclovir 1 h after absorption. Cells were harvested 7 h after drug treatment, and nucleotides were extracted as described in the text.
[b]Uninfected Vero cells were from the stock of Vero cells obtained from the ATCC and maintained at Wellcome Research Laboratories.
[c]Infected Vero cells were from two different stocks, one maintained at Wellcome Research Laboratories and the other maintained at Sidney Farber Cancer Institute. (Values in parentheses.)

acyclovir inhibition, induce little or no acyclovir triphosphate formation (10,12,13). This varied ability to metabolize acyclovir is attributed to virally induced thymidine kinase that phosphorylates acyclovir and initiates the process of triphosphate formation. Although HCMV is a member of the herpesvirus group, it does not code for a thymidine kinase (14). Vaccinia virus, which is not a herpesvirus member, codes for a thymidine kinase that lacks the ability to use acyclovir as a substrate (15).

A large body of evidence now exists that supports the hypothesis that HSV-1 infection induces a novel thymidine kinase activity that is essential for the first step in the selective activation of acyclovir. This evidence includes (a) thymidine prevents the antiviral activity of acyclovir; (b) acyclovir phosphorylating activity and thymidine kinase increase upon viral infection; (c) acyclovir phosphorylating activity and thymidine kinase activity copurify on thymidine agarose; (d) acyclovir and thymidine exhibit mutually exclusive binding to the purified activity; and (e) thymidine kinase-deficient viruses are resistant to acyclovir. Evidence that the host cell thymidine kinase does not play a significant role in the conversion of acyclovir to acyclovir monophosphate includes (a) acyclovir is a weak inhibitor of purified thymidine kinase and is not a detectable substrate; (b) the trace phosphorylation of acyclovir in uninfected cells is not prevented by thymidine; and (c) host cells deficient in thymidine kinase phosphorylate acyclovir. Acyclovir monophosphate is generated in uninfected cells by cellular cytoplasmic 5′-nucleotidase (16). Normally this enzyme catalyzes the cleavage of purine nucleoside phosphate esters (Fig. 1). Apparently acyclovir competes with water for binding to the enzyme phosphoryl intermediate and substitutes for water as the phosphate acceptor. Although

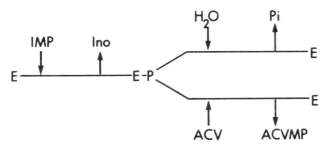

FIGURE 1 Acyclovir phosphorylation by the cytoplasmic 5′ nucleotidase.

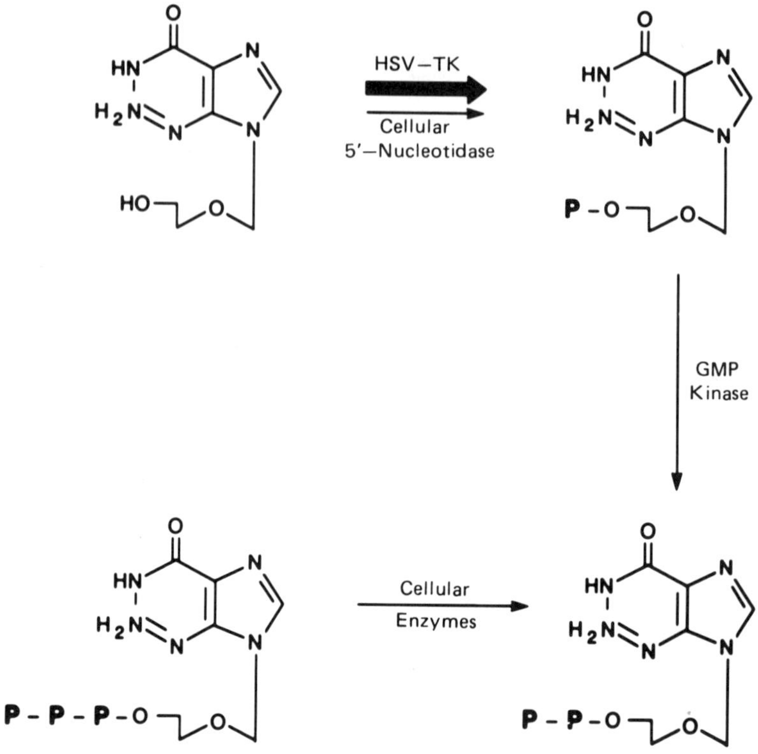

FIGURE 2 Enzymatic phosphorylation of acyclovir to its mono-, di-, and tri-phosphate derivatives.

acyclovir is a relatively inefficient phosphate acceptor for this enzyme, its reactivity is sufficient to account for the amount of acyclovir monophosphate that accumulates in uninfected cells. At the present time it is not known if any other cellular enzymes phosphorylate acyclovir.

Acyclovir monophosphate is converted to the diphosphate by a cellular guanylate kinase (Fig. 2) (17). The levels of guanylate kinase pre- and postinfection are equivalent. The conversion of acyclovir diphosphate to the triphosphate is catalyzed by several cellular kinases and phosphotransferases (18). Based on cellular enzyme levels and kinetic studies, phosphoglycerate kinase is postulated as the principal enzyme responsible for triphosphate synthesis (18).

SELECTIVE INHIBITION OF THE HSV-ENCODED
DNA POLYMERASE

Early studies examining the effects of acyclovir treatment on Vero cells infected with HSV-1 indicate that viral DNA synthesis is much more sensitive to inhibition by acyclovir than host cell DNA synthesis (19). The synthesis of viral DNA in the presence of acyclovir was measured at various time points by cRNA-DNA hybridization. Following a 24-h incubation with either 0.1 μM or 1.0 μM acyclovir, viral DNA synthesis was inhibited 20% and 55%, respectively. Acyclovir 10 μM completely inhibited viral DNA synthesis. DNA synthesis in actively growing uninfected Vero cells is not inhibited by 50 μM acyclovir. In addition, this study demonstrates that acyclovir triphosphate selectively inhibits viral DNA polymerase. The apparent K_i value for acyclovir triphosphate for the viral DNA polymerase is threefold to 50-fold lower than the apparent K_i values obtained for alpha-type polymerases.

Selective inhibition of virally induced DNA polymerase by acyclovir triphosphate is the principal route by which HSV replication is inhibited in vivo. The mechanism of inhibition of the HSV-1 DNA polymerase involves elements of chain termination, competitive inhibition, and apparent suicide inactivation (20). Because of the absence of an extendible 3′ hydroxyl group on the acyclic sugar moiety of acyclovir triphosphate, the incorporation of acyclovir monophosphate into a growing DNA strand should cause immediate cessation of DNA synthesis. Pulse chase experiments show that tritium-labeled DNA fragments synthesized in infected cells in the presence of acyclovir remain near the top of alkaline sucrose gradients (21). The sedimentation characteristics of the labeled fragments do not change after chasing in isotope-free medium, which is consistent with the hypothesis that incorporation of acyclovir monophosphate into a growing DNA strand causes chain termination. Despite the presence of an associated 3′,5′-exonuclease with the HSV-1 DNA polymerase, acyclovir monophosphate is not released from acyclovir monophosphate-terminated DNA (22). As a result, reactivation of DNA synthesis is not observed. The inability of the exonuclease to remove acyclo-GMP residues from DNA suggests the possibility that acyclo-GMP-terminated DNA may function as an inhibitor of the HSV-1 DNA polymerase. Studies with enzymatically prepared acyclo-GMP-terminated DNA suggest that this polymer may inhibit the enzyme (22). However, the low levels of acyclo-GMP contained in the DNA template make it difficult to state conclusively that this species contributes significantly to the inhibition of the polymerase.

Acyclovir triphosphate is a potent inhibitor of the purified HSV-1 DNA polymerase (10,19,20,22). The inhibition is competitive with respect to dGTP with a K_i of 3 nM (20,22). The ratio of the K_m for dGTP to the K_i of acyclovir triphosphate is 50. In contrast, purified human DNA polymerase alpha is inhibited relatively poorly by acyclovir triphosphate (10, 19,20,22). The K_i is 0.18 μM, and the ratio of K_m to K_i is 8. The mechanism of inhibition of the viral polymerase is complicated by the apparently irreversible inactivation of the enzyme during turnover in the presence of acyclovir triphosphate (20). Acyclovir triphosphate causes a time-dependent progressive inhibition of the HSV-1 DNA polymerase in the presence of activated DNA, saturating amounts of dATP, dCTP, TTP, and 5 μM dGTP (Fig. 3). The inhibition of DNA synthesis is reversed only by the

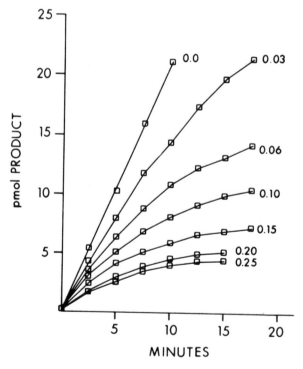

FIGURE 3 Time-dependent progressive inhibition of the HSV DNA polymerase by increasing concentration by ACVTP in the presence of 5 μM dGTP.

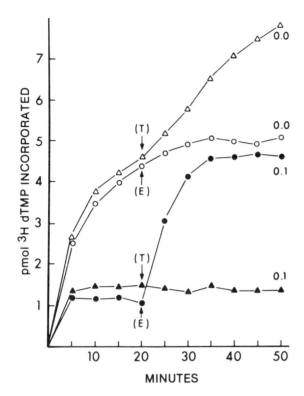

FIGURE 4   Determination of the functionality of enzyme and template follow-ing inhibition by ACVTP. After preincubating at 37 °C for 20 min, excess dGTP and fresh enzyme (E) or fresh template (T) were added to the indicated reaction mixtures. △ , ○ , Control reaction mixtures lacking ACVTP; ▲ , ● , reaction mixtures containing ACVTP.

addition of a bolus of fresh enzyme to the spent reaction mixture, which argues against the production of a reversible inhibitor and indicates that enzyme inactivation may be occurring (Fig. 4).

Preincubation studies have shown that acyclovir triphosphate does not directly inactivate either template primer or enzyme, and inactivation is only observed when acyclovir triphosphate is being processed as an alternate substrate (20). The time-dependent decrease of enzyme activity during turnover in the presence of acyclovir triphosphate is a pseudo-first-order process that depends on the concentration of acyclovir triphosphate.

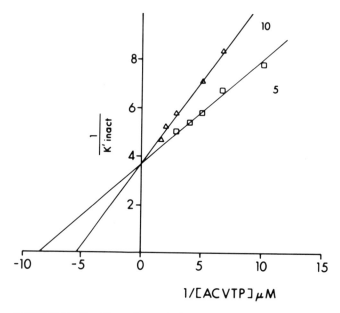

FIGURE 5   Double reciprocal plot of the pseudo-first-order rate constants for inactivation with varied ACVTP.

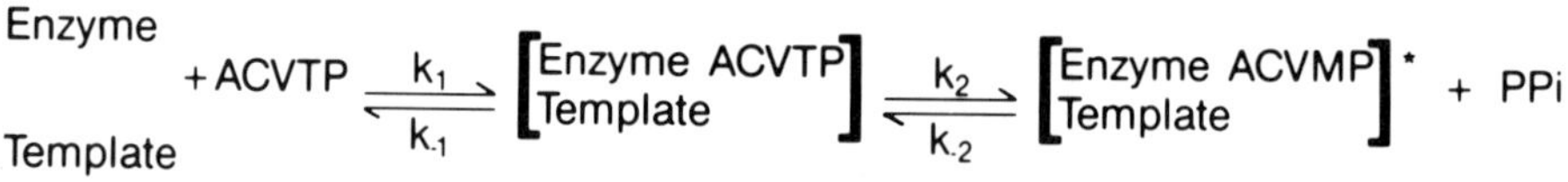

Enzyme
   $+$ ACVTP $\xrightarrow[k_{-1}]{k_1}$ $\left[\begin{array}{l}\text{Enzyme ACVTP}\\\text{Template}\end{array}\right]$ $\xrightarrow[k_{-2}]{k_2}$ $\left[\begin{array}{l}\text{Enzyme ACVMP}\\\text{Template}\end{array}\right]^*$ $+$ PPi
Template

FIGURE 6   A postulated scheme for the inactivation of the HSV DNA polymerase by ACVTP is depicted by the following equation where $K_D = k_1/k_1$. [ ] Encloses the reversible Michaelis-type complex; [ ]* encloses the apparently irreversible complex. k_2 = First-order rate constant for enzyme inactivation; k_2 = rate constant for the reversion of the inactivated complex to the reversible Michaelis-type complex.

The existence of a positive y-axis intercept in a plot of $1/k'_{inact}$ (the pseudo-first-order rate constant for the inactivation process) versus $1/[ACVTP]$ is consistent with the formation of a Michaelis-type complex prior to inactivation (Fig. 5). Enzyme activity is not regenerated by rapid Sephadex G-25 gel filtration which resolves free acyclovir triphosphate from inactivated enzyme complex (20). This result and the demonstration of the lack of product inhibition support the hypothesis that the inactivation process is irreversible. Although not unique, Figure 6 describes the inactivation of the HSV-1 DNA polymerase by acyclovir triphosphate where brackets enclose the reversible Michaelis complex and brackets with an asterisk enclose the apparently irreversible complex.

DISCUSSION

The discovery of acyclovir represents the development of a new generation of antiviral drugs that are both safe and effective by virtue of their ability to exert toxic effects primarily against virally infected cells. Herpes simplex virus infection induces the synthesis of a viral thymidine kinase that, in contrast to cellular thymidine kinase, readily phosphorylates acyclovir. Trace amounts of acyclovir monophosphate are formed in uninfected cells by cytoplasmic 5'-nucleotidase. The principal mode of action of acyclovir resides in the ability of acyclovir triphosphate to selectively inhibit the virally encoded DNA polymerase. Whereas purified host cell DNA polymerase alpha is only weakly inhibited by acyclovir triphosphate (K_m/K_i ratio of 8), the HSV-1 encoded DNA polymerase is inhibited to a much greater extent (K_m/K_i ratio of 50). In addition, the HSV-1 DNA polymerase, in contrast to DNA polymerase alpha, is apparently inactivated by turnover in the presence of acyclovir triphosphate. The DNA polymerases encoded by human cytomegalovirus, varicella zoster virus, and Epstein-Barr virus are more sensitive to inhibition by acyclovir triphosphate than cellular DNA polymerases; however, no evidence of enzyme inactivation in the presence of acyclovir triphosphate has been reported for any of these enzymes (12,13,23). Polymerase beta is not inhibited by 50 μM acylcovir triphosphate at 1.0 μM dGTP and therefore appears to be insensitive to the effects of this analog. The selectivity and low degree of toxicity observed with acyclovir therapy result from the physical differences that exist between viral and cellular enzymes. Selective phosphorylation of acyclovir by the virally encoded thymidine kinase ensures that only infected cells will accumulate acyclovir triphosphate to an appreciable extent. Selective inactivation of the viral DNA polymerase ensures that only viral DNA synthesis will terminate, while the essential host cell functions of DNA replication and repair will proceed to allow for the survival of the cell.

Although the mechanism of inhibition of the HSV-1 DNA polymerase has been referred to as suicide inactivation, it should be noted that this mechanism has been derived primarily on the basis of kinetic evidence. To determine the exact nature of the inactivation event it will be necessary to perform a rigorous physical study of the process.

The importance of virally induced enzymes in the mechanism of action of acyclovir has been confirmed by genetic studies (24-26). Complimentation and recombination experiments performed with laboratory isolates of acyclovir-resistant herpes simplex type 1 viruses indicate that resistance-confirming mutations map exclusively to either the thymidine kinase locus or the DNA polymerase locus (24-26). Phenotypically these mutants express either low levels of thymidine kinase, thymidine kinase with an altered substrate specificity, or DNA polymerase with a decreased sensitivity to acyclovir triphosphate (26-29).

In the absence of any definitive information that could explain why acyclic nucleotides bind preferentially to viral polymerases, it is interesting to note that several researchers have postulated that present-day genetic material may have evolved from a polymer constructed from flexible, acyclic, prochiral nucleotide analogs that were readily synthesized on primitive earth (30). If this is true, then one might consider that viruses may have evolved in a world that made exclusive use of acyclic sugars as components of their genetic material. The continued survival of viruses depended on their ability to adapt to a world that later evolved toward the exclusive use of RNA/DNA genetic systems. Throughout this evolutionary process viruses may have retained their ability to bind acyclics. Today, evidence of this evolutionary pathway may be reflected by the selective inhibition of herpesvirus DNA polymerase by acyclic nucleotide analogs.

ACKNOWLEDGMENTS

The authors thank Dr. D. Porter for helpful discussion in the preparation of this manuscript.

REFERENCES

1. Kier, H. M., and Gold, E. (1963). Deocyribonucleic acid nucleotidyltransferase and deoxyribonuclease from cultured cells infected with herpes simplex virus. *Biochim. Biophys. Acta* 72:263-276.

2. Kit, S., and Dubbs, D. R. (1963). Acquisition of thymidine kinase activity by herpes simplex virus infected mouse fibroblast cells. *Biochem. Biophys. Res. Commun.* 11:55-59.

3. Ponce de Leon, M., Eisenberg, R. J., and Cohen, G. H. (1977). Ribonucleotide reductase from herpes simplex virus (types 1 and 2) infected and uninfected KB cells: Properties of the partially purified enzymes. *J. Gen. Virol.* 36:163-173.

4. Chen, M.S., and Prusoff, W. H. (1978). Association of thymidylate kinase activity with pyrimidine deoxyribonucleoside kinase induced by herpes simplex virus. *J. Biol. Chem.* 253:1325-1327.

5. Knopf, K. W. (1979). Properties of herpes simplex virus DNA polymerase and characterization of its associated exonuclease activity. *Eur. J. Biochem.* 98:231-244.

6. Sugar, J., and Kaufman, H. E. (1973). Halogenated pyrimidines in antiviral therapy. In Carter, W. A. (ed.): *Selective Inhibitors of Viral Functions.* Cleveland, CRC Press, pp. 295-311.

7. Heidelberger, C., and King, D. (1979). Trifluorothymidine. *Pharmacol. Ther.* 6:427-442.

8. Drach, J. C. (1984). Purine nucleoside analogs as antiviral agents. In DeClercq, E., and Walker, R. T. (eds.): *Targets for the Design of Antiviral Agents.* New York, Plenum Press, pp. 221-258.

9. Shannon, W. M. (1984). Mechanism of antiviral action. In Galasso, G. J., Merigan, T. C., and Buchanan, R. A. (eds.): *Antiviral Agents and Viral Diseases in Man.* New York, Raven Press, pp. 55-121.

10. Elion, G. B., Furman, P. A., Fyfe, J. A., DeMiranda, P., Beauchamp, L., and Schaeffer, H. J. (1977). Selectivity of action of an antiherpetic agent, 9-(2-hydroxyethoxymethyl)guanine. *Proc. Natl. Acad. Sci. USA* 74:5716-5720.

11. Furman, P. A., DeMiranda, P., St. Clair, M. H., and Elion, G. B. (1981). Metabolism of acyclovir in virus-infected and uninfected cells. *Antimicrob. Agents Chemother.* 20:518-524.

12. Biron, K. K., Stenbuck, P. J., and Sorrell, J. B. (1984). Inhibition of DNA polymerases of varicella zoster virus and human cytomegalovirus by the nucleoside analogs 9-(2-hydroxyethoxymethyl)guanine (ACU) and 9-{[2-hydroxy-1-(hydroxymethyl)ethoxy]methyl}guanine (BW759U). In Rapp, F. (ed.): *Herpesvirus.* New York, Alan R. Liss, pp. 677-685.

13. Biron, K. K., Stanat, S. C., Sorrell, S. B., Fyfe, J. A., Keller, P. M., Lambe, C. U., and Nelson, D. J. (1985). Metabolic activation of the nucleoside analog 9-{[2-hydroxy-1-(hydroxymethyl)ethoxy]methyl}guanine in human diploid fibroblasts infected with human cytomegalovirus. *Proc. Natl. Acad. Sci. USA* 82:2473-2477.

14. Estes, J. E., and Huang, E. S. (1977). Stimulation of cellular thymidine kinases by human cytomegalovirus. *J. Virol.* 24:13-21.

15. Fyfe, J. A., Keller, P. M., Furman, P. A., Miller, R. L., and Elion, G. B. (1978). Thymidine kinase for herpes simplex virus phosphorylates the new

antiviral compound, 9-(2-hydroxyethoxymethyl)guanine. *J. Biol. Chem.* 253: 8721-8727.

16. Keller, P. M., McKee, S. A., and Fyfe, J. A. (1985). Cytoplasmic 5'-nucleotidase catalyzes acyclovir phosphorylation. *J. Biol. Chem.* 260:8664-8667.

17. Miller, W. H., and Miller, R. L. (12980). Phosphorylation of acyclovir (acycloguanosine)monophossphate by GMP kinase. *J. Biol. Chem.* 255:7204-7207.

18. Miller, W. H., and Miller, R. L. (1982). Phosphorylation of acyclovir disphosphate by cellular enzymes. *Biochem. Pharmacol.* 31:3879-3884.

19. Furman, P. A., St. Clair, M. H., Fyfe, J. A., Rideout, J. L., Keller, P. M., and Elion, G. B. (1979). Inhibition of herpes simplex virus-induced DNA polymerase activity and viral DNA replication by 9-(2-hydroxyethoxymethyl)-guanine and its triphosphate. *J. Virol.* 32:72-77.

20. Furman, P. A., St. Clair, M. H., and Spector, T. (1984). Acyclovir triphosphate is a suicide inactivator of the herpes simplex virus DNA polymerase. *J. Biol. Chem.* 259:9575-9579.

21. McGuirt, P. V., Shaw, J. E., Elion, G. B., and Furman, P. A. (1984). Identification of small DNA fragments synthesized in herpes simplex virus-infected cells in the presence of acyclovir. *Antimicrob. Agents Chemother.* 25:507-509.

22. Derse, D., Cheng, Y.-C., Furman, P. A., St. Clair, M. H., and Elion, G. B. (1981). Inhibition of purified human and herpes simplex virus-induced DNA polymerases by 9-(2-hydroxy-ethoxymethyl)guanine triphosphate. Effects on primer-template function. *J. Biol. Chem.* 256:11447-11541.

23. Datta, A. K., Colby, B. M., Shaw, J. E., and Pagano, J. S. (1980). Acyclovir inhibition of Epstein-Barr virus replication. *Proc. Natl. Acad. Sci. USA* 77: 5163-5166.

24. Coen, D. M., and Schaffer, P. A. (1980). Two distinct loci confer resistance to acycloquanosine in herpes simplex virus type 1. *Proc. Natl. Acad. Sci. USA* 77:2265-2269.

25. Schnipper, L. E., and Crumpacker, C. S. (1980). Resistance of herpes simplex virus to acycloguanosine: The role of viral thymidine kinase and DNA polymerase loci. *Proc. Natl. Acad. Sci. USA* 77:2270-2273.

26. Furman, P. A., Coen, D. M., St. Clair, M. H., and Schaffer, P. A. (1981). Acyclovir-resistant mutants of herpes simplex virus type 1 express altered DNA polymerase or reduced acyclovir phosphorylating activities. *J. Virol.* 40:936-941.

27. Larder, B. A., Derse, D., Cheng, Y.-C., and Darby, G. (1983). Properties of purified enzymes induced by pathogenic drug-resistant mutants of herpes simplex virus—evidence for virus variants expressing normal DNA polymerase and altered thymidine kinase. *J. Biol. Chem.* 258:2027-2033.

28. Fyfe, J. A., McKee, S. A., and Keller, P. M. (1983). Altered thymidine-thymidylate kinases from strains of herpes simplex virus with modified drug sensitivities to acyclovir and (E)-5-(2-bromovinyl)-2'-deoxyuridine. *Mol. Pharmacol.* 24:316-323.

29. St. Clair, M. H., Miller, W. H., Miller, R. L., Lambe, C. U., and Furman, P. A. (1984). Inhibition of cellular αDNA polymerase and herpes simplex virus-induced DNA polymerases by the triphosphate of BW759U. *Antimicrob. Agents Chemother.* 25:191-194.
30. Joyce, G. F., Schwartz, A. W., Miller, S. L., and Orgel, L. E. (1987). The case for an ancestral genetic system involving simple analogues of the nucleotides. *Proc. Natl. Acad. Sci. USA* 84:4398-4402.

2
Safety Studies of Acyclovir: Preclinical and Clinical

Joan L. Drucker *Burroughs Wellcome Co., Research Triangle Park, and Duke University Medical Center, Durham, North Carolina*

Walter E. Tucker, Jr. and George M. Szczech *Burroughs Wellcome Co., Research Triangle Park, North Carolina*

INTRODUCTION

Early in the development of acyclovir, wide separation between antiviral and cytotoxic concentrations was observed in tissue culture systems, and the mechanism explaining this separation was defined (1,2). In ensuing preclinical and clinical safety studies this selectivity of action has continued to be apparent. Considerable experience to date indicates that the drug has a low order of toxicity in animals and humans. This is contrasted with the relatively high toxicity of other nucleoside analogs, some of which are either no longer used or used only sparingly (3-5,29,30).

Because of the perception of nucleoside analogs as being intrinsically very toxic, the preclinical and clinical safety evaluation of acyclovir was particularly exhaustive, and development of the drug proceeded in a cautious and conservative manner. The details of the preclinical and clinical safety assessment of acyclovir are described in a number of published reports and will be referenced but not redescribed here. Rather, this chapter will attempt to summarize information thought to be important to physicians who treat patients with acyclovir.

PRECLINICAL SAFETY EVALUATION

Safety assessment is a continuous process that starts after the discovery of a potentially useful therapeutic property of a chemical entity, continues during clinical trials, and takes the form of postmarketing surveillance. The preclinical part of the process provides an integrated base of biological information that gives some guidance to the conduct of clinical trials.

The preclinical toxicologic assessment of acyclovir was diverse and extensive because of several main considerations: the four proposed routes of administration (dermal, ophthalmic, intravenous, and oral); the diverse potential patient population (the healthy general population, including pregnant women, in addition to neonates and the immunocompromised); the likelihood of chronic intermittent or continuous therapy in humans; and, as mentioned above, the relatively high level of general concern about the toxicity of nucleoside analogs.

In addition to standard toxicity tests, the disposition and pharmacokinetics of the drug were determined in animals and correlated with toxic effects (6,7,9-12). Also, there was heavy emphasis on studies designed to determine the potential for acyclovir to adversely affect reproductive processes (10,17-20), the immune system (14), the genetic integrity of animals (12,21,24,25), and its potential to induce tumor formation (11,12). For the reader unfamiliar with types of in vitro and in vivo techniques used in preclinical studies, Table 1 lists the main experiments with acyclovir. The details of most of these experiments have been described in a series of reports that are further referenced in Table 1 and will only be broadly summarized.

Acyclovir was shown to be well distributed in body tissues and excreted largely unchanged via the kidney. Primary cytotoxic effects in animals occurred mainly with parenteral administration, resulting in very high drug concentrations in plasma (manyfold higher than human plasma levels after therapeutic doses). Target tissues were those with rapid cell turnover (e.g., bone marrow, gastrointestinal tract, lymphoid tissues, thymus, testicles, stratum germinativum). Signs of toxicosis were related to the underlying morphological and functional disturbances associated with the cytostatic effect of acyclovir in high doses (e.g., diarrhea, anemia, infections, nail loss in dogs, and death).

A secondary type of toxicity, observed in dogs and rats, was related to precipitation of acyclovir crystals in renal tubules and collecting ducts after rapid intravenous bolus injection of relatively high doses. This led to transient renal impairment and, with repeated dosing, obstructive nephropathy. This secondary toxicity was a function of the relatively low solu-

TABLE 1   List of Preclinical Safety Evaluation Studies Performed with Acyclovir

Species	Study type/route
I. In vivo studies	
	Acute studies (8)
Rat, mouse	LD_{50}/PO, IV, IP
	Subchronic studies (8,9,15,16)
Rat	3 wk/IV (8)
Rat	1 mo/IP (8)
Dog	1 mo/IV (8)
Mouse	1 mo/PO (8)
Guinea pig	Primary skin irritation and systemic toxicity/ topical (9)
Guinea pig	Skin sensitization/ID (9)
Domestic white pig	Epidermal wound healing/topical (15)
Rabbit	Ocular irritation/topical (9)
Rabbit	Corneal wound healing/topical (16)
	Chronic toxicity and carinogenicity studies (11)
Dog	6 mo/PO
Dog	12 mo/PO
Rat	6 mo/IP
Rat	12 mo/PO
Rat	2-yr carcinogenicity bioassay/PO
Mouse	2-yr carcinogenicity bioassay/PO
	Reproductive and developmental toxicity studies (10,17-20)
Rat	Teratology/SC (10,18)
Rabbit	Teratology/SC (10)
Rabbit	Teratology/IV (20)
Rat	Neonatal-perinatal/SC (19)
Rat	Neonatal/SC (10)
Mouse	2-Generation reproduction-fertility/PO (10)
Rat	Reproduction-fertility/SC (17)
II. Special in vitro and in vivo studies (genetic and immunological)	
	Genetic toxicology studies (12,21,24-26)

A. Microbial
   1. Ames plate
   2. Ames preincubation
   3. *E. coli*, polA
   4. *S. cerevisiae*, D4

Table 1 continues

TABLE 1 Continued

B. Cultured mammalian cells: Mutagenicity and clastogenicity
1. Mouse lymphoma L5178Y/OUA^R
2. Mouse lymphoma L5178Y/HGPRT
3. Mouse lymphoma L5178Y/TK
4. CHO/OUA^R
5. CHO/HGPRT
6. CHO/APRT
7. Human lymphocyte cytogenetics
C. Cultured mammalian cells: Neoplastic transformation
1. C3H/10T1/2
2. BALB/c-3T3
D. In vivo, mammalian
1. Mouse dominant lethal [two studies in male mice (12,24) and one in female mice (25)]
2. Chinese hamster bone marrow cytogenetics (12)
3. Rat bone marrow cytogenetics (12)
4. Mouse micronucleus bone marrow assay (21)

Immunotoxicological studies (14)

A. In vitro tests
1. Lymphocyte-mediated cytotoxicity
2. Neutrophil chemotaxis
3. Rosette formation
4. In vitro human lymphocyte function
5. Division of fibroblasts
6. Inhibition of thymidine incorporation by peripheral blood
7. Inhibition of T cell proliferation without apparent effect on release of lymphokines or monocyte function
B. In vivo mouse tests
1. Complement-dependent cellular cytotoxicity
2. Complement-independent cellular cytotoxicity
3. Delayed hypersensitivity
4. Graft vs. host reaction
5. Circulating antibody and Jerne plaque-forming cell
6. Potentiation by acyclovir of immunosuppressive effect of azathioprine on antibody function
C. Bone marrow stem cell assays
1. In vitro study—granulocyte progenitor cells (26)
2. In vitro/in vivo study—hematopoietic progenitor cells of mice (27)
3. In vitro study—hematopoietic progenitor cells of humans (28)

bility of acyclovir in urine. It was particularly pronounced in the rat (a water-conserving species), which, in comparison to dogs and humans, has urine of higher specific gravity and osmolality. Kimes et al. (13) performed detailed studies on the kidneys of dogs given intravenous acyclovir and confirmed that the drug decreased the ability of the kidney to concentrate urine but did not find other important nephrotoxic effects.

Dermal and ophthalmic formulations of acyclovir were well tolerated. No primary skin irritation, interference with dermal or corneal wound healing, sensitizing potential or systemic toxic effects were associated with the application of these materials (8,9,15,16).

To investigate the potential immunotoxicity of acyclovir, a large battery of in vitro and in vivo assays was performed (14). No effects on either humoral or cell-mediated immunity were seen at clinically relevant doses.

Since bone marrow toxicity was observed with 5-iodo-2'-deoxyuridine and cytosine arabinoside, the effect of acyclovir on granulocyte-monocyte colony-forming cells was studied in vitro. Little effect was seen at concentrations of acyclovir as high as 220 μM (26). Similarly, acyclovir had minimal effect on hematopoietic progenitor cells in mice given a single LD_{50} dose of 400 mg/kg IV (27) and in an in vitro clonogenic assay using normal human hematopoietic progenitor cells (28).

In a comprehensive series of whole-animal studies done at maximum tolerated doses and designed to detect potential adverse effects of acyclovir upon reproductive and developmental processes, there were no significant effects. Reproductive processes and prenatal, perinatal, and postnatal development of offspring were normal in rats, rabbits, and mice (10,17-20). In an experimental setting, teratogenic effects were observed in rat embryos cultured in vitro (22). These effects were later correlated with similar effects in nonstandard rat teratology studies in which pregnant rats were given 300 mg/kg (100 $\times$ 3) acyclovir by SC injection on gestation day 10 (23). This dose far exceeds the maximum tolerated dose which is 50 mg/kg/day (25 $\times$ 2) given SC to pregnant rats.

In studies using extremely high parenteral doses administered subchronically (dogs, rats) and chronically (rats), reversible testicular hypoplasia was observed (Table 2). At these doses there were also more severe toxic effects in other organ systems and even deaths. When acyclovir was given orally to dogs for 1 year at 60 mg/kg/day and to rats and mice for 2 years at 450 mg/kg/day, no testicular effects were observed. None of the reproductive toxicity studies in mice and rats, including those that examined for second-generation effects, gave evidence of adverse effects on testicular function (Table 3).

Overall, acyclovir does not appear to differ from the natural nucleosides in its mutagenic activity (12). Positive results occurred in two of 11 in

TABLE 2 Summary of Preclinical Studies in Which There Was Evidence of Gonadal Toxicity[a]

Species	Top dose[b] (mg/kg/day)	Dose route	Dose duration	Animal plasma level (µg/ml)	Human plasma multiple formulations[c]			Other toxicity
					IV	PO	Topical	
Rat	320	IP	4 weeks	ND	NA	NA	NA	Renal Hematopoietic Death
Rat	80	IP	26 weeks	26	1-3	16-39	163	Renal Hematopoietic Death
Dog	100	IV	4 weeks	84	4-8	53-125	525	Renal Gastrointestinal Hematopoietic Death

ND = not done; NA = not applicable.

[a]Reversibility was under way at 4 weeks postdose when the 4-week rat IP study was terminated and was demonstrated in the 26-week rat IP study, and, although few dogs survived, in the 4-week dog IV study there was histopathologic confirmation that testicular germ cells were intact.

[b]In the three studies showing gonadal toxicity it was only seen at the top dose except that very ill dogs at the mid dose (100 mg/kg/day) in the 4-week IV study had gonadal atrophy.

[c]Human plasma level values used to calculate approximate multiples.
Ointment = 0.16 µg/ml (product label); IV powder = 10.13 µg/ml (product label), 20.70 µg/ml (10 mg/kg 1 h infusion; ref. 24); capsule = 0.67-0.90 µg/ml (product label), 1.35-1.58 µg/ml (unpublished data for 800 mg once/day—of interest for suppression).

TABLE 3 Summary of Reproductive Toxicity Studies

Species	Study	Top dose and route (mg/kg/day)	Duration	Adverse effect	Animal plasma level[a] (μg/ml)	Multiple of human plasma level[b]		
						IV	PO	Topical
Mouse[c]	Two-generation fertility	450 PO	9 weeks	None	14.2	1	9-21	89
Rat[c]	Fertility	50 SC	9 weeks	None	16.4	1-2	10-24	103
Rat	Teratology	50 SC	Days 6-15	None	16.4	1-2	10-24	103
Rat[c]	Teratology	50 SC	Days 7-17	None	16.4	1-2	10-24	103
Rat	Teratology	50 SC	Days 6-15	None	16.4	1-2	10-24	103
Rat (23)	Teratology	300 SC	Day 10	Head and tail malformations	99.1	5-10	63-148	619
Rabbit	Teratology	50 SC	Days 6-18	None	16.4	1-2	10-24	103
Rabbit	Teratology	50 IV	Days 6-18	None	146	7-14	92-218	913
Rat[c]	Perinatal	50 SC	Day 17 to weaning	None	16.4	1-2	10-24	103

[a]Approximate peak plasma levels, measured by radioimmunoassay either in the studies shown or in separate pharmacokinetic studies.
[b]See Table 2.
[c]Studies in which offspring were tested for behavioral deficits.

vitro mutagenicity assays (12). These involved chromsomal damage at extremely high drug concentrations. In contrast, no evidence of chromosomal damage occurred in four out of four in vivo assays at nontoxic and maximum tolerated dosage levels under conditions more relevant to clinical use of the drug (12,24,25). At extremely toxic doses—5 and 10 times the maximum tolerated dose—chromosomal damage was seen in Chinese hamster bone marrow (12). Lethal doses induced micronuclei in male mice (21). While one of two cell transformation assays gave positive results, no oncogenic potential for acyclovir was indicated by lifetime oral carcinogenicity bioassays in rats and mice (11).

CLINICAL SAFETY EVALUATION

The first clinical trials of a new drug involve establishing the safety of a dosage in the anticipated therapeutic range. Initial studies of intravenous acyclovir tested dosage regimens increasing progressively from 0.5 mg/kg to 15 mg/kg tid given by infusion over 1 hour (31). Similarly, acyclovir capsules underwent pharmacokinetic trials at doses from 200 to 5000 mg per day (32). Acyclovir was well tolerated at all doses used in these trials.

Because of the diversity of both the herpes infections and the host populations, an extensive series of rigorously controlled clinical trials using topical, oral, and intravenous formulations was conducted. Acyclovir demonstrated a wide margin of safety. Although side effects were infrequent, certain adverse experiences are well described.

Renal impairment has been associated with the use of intravenous acyclovir. Transient increases in serum creatinine and urea nitrogen have been observed in patients receiving high doses or bolus injections. In a retrospective review article, Brigden et al. noted elevated plasma urea concentrations in 46 of 354 patients with life-threatening infections treated with bolus injections (33). In 27 of 46 patients, the abnormality was associated with the use of acyclovir, and plasma urea concentrations returned to baseline when the drug was discontinued. In the remainder there were other, more likely etiologies; for example, seven patients had preexisting renal impairment. In these patients the dosage had not been adjusted for underlying renal dysfunction. In all but one, who died of a cerebrovascular accident during the study, the abnormality was transient.

Renal toxicity occurs when the solubility of acyclovir in urine (1.3 mg/ml) is exceeded. This results in precipitation of acyclovir crystals in the lower renal tubules. It is recommended that patients be well hydrated to keep the urine output at 500 ml per gram of drug infused to avert complications. It is emphasized that slow (1 hour) intravenous infusion is re-

TABLE 4 Dose Adjustments in Renal Failure

Creatinine clearance (ml/min/1.73 M²)	Acyclovir dose (mg/kg)	Dosing interval (hours)
>50	5	8
25-50	5	12
10-25	5	24
0-10	2.5	24

commended and that bolus doses are to be avoided. Additionally, patients receiving intravenous doses of 10 mg/kg for serious infections such as encephalitis should have the dosage adjusted for ideal body weight. Recommended dose modifications for patients with renal impairment are shown in Table 4. Note that the adjustment is based on creatinine clearance.

Impairment of renal function has not been described with acyclovir capsules. Limited bioavailability of oral acyclovir prevents the development of high serum concentrations. Fletcher et al. studied the pharmacokinetics of acyclovir tablets (800 mg investigational formulation) in 12 renal transplant recipients for 12 weeks posttransplant. Doses were increased from 800 mg to 3200 mg per day as renal function recovered. Nine patients maintained a serum creatinine concentration of approximately 2 mg/dl. Creatinine greater than 2 mg/dl occurred in two patients who had acute graft rejection. In the last patient, creatinine fluctuated between 1.8 and 3.7 mg/dl and stabilized at 2.5 mg/dl. Subsequent challenges with increased doses of acyclovir did not affect creatinine. The investigators concluded that oral doses of up to 3.2 g per day were well tolerated (48).

Acyclovir crosses the blood-brain barrier well. Concentrations in cerebrospinal fluid are approximately 50% of serum levels. Neurologic toxicity has been reported anecdotally (39-43,47) and has been described in 1% of patients in clinical trials of high intravenous doses of acyclovir (unpublished data, Burroughs Wellcome Co.).

Wade and Meyers first reported possible acyclovir-associated neurologic symptoms in six of 143 patients who had undergone bone marrow transplantation and had received, in aggregate, 187 courses of IV acyclovir. Acyclovir doses ranged from 250 mg/m² for localized HSV to 3000 mg/m² per day for cytomegalovirus infections. The latter dose is 4-5 times the dose recommended for treatment of HSV. All patients had been treated with intrathecal methotrexate, and three of six had received human alpha interferon. The symptoms consisted of lethargy or agitation in five, tremor in five, disorientation in one, and transient paresthesia and slurred speech in one. They began 2-18 days after initiation of therapy and resolved 4-15 days after cessation. All six patients had normal renal function. Peak plasma levels of acyclovir ranged from 10 to 67 μg/ml (45).

Tomson et al. (46) reported reversible psychiatric side effects in three dialysis patients receiving 8-10 mg/kg daily. Hallucinations or confusion developed within 12-24 h. There were no focal neurologic deficits, and symptoms resolved after discontinuation of acyclovir.

Phlebitis has been observed in rare instances after extravasation of intravenous acyclovir (58). This appears to result from the alkalinity (pH 10-11) of the solution. No specific therapy is required. Other dermatologic reactions include a burning sensation after use of 5% acyclovir ointment, which has been attributed to polyethylene glycol in the vehicle. Rash has been reported with equal frequency (about 5%) in patients receiving either acyclovir capsules or placebo daily for 2 years. There are no documented cases of hypersensitivity.

Nausea and emesis have been reported with nearly equal frequency in studies of oral acyclovir. In an ongoing study of patients who have received 400 mg of acyclovir twice daily for 2 years, the incidence of gastrointestinal symptoms declined from 4% in the first 3 months to 1% in the last 3-month period (50).

Since acyclovir became available by prescription, Burroughs Wellcome Co. has developed an epidemiologic surveillance program to evaluate reports of adverse drug experiences. Although exact incidence values cannot be determined from such systems, the data are consistent with the fact that adverse experiences are infrequent. In patients treated with acyclovir capsules, the following adverse experiences have been reported in approximately one patient per 1000 treatments: nausea, vomiting, headache, diarrhea, rash.

SPECIAL POPULATIONS

New drugs are tested in a variety of patient populations to elucidate responses that may be unique for physiologic or pathophysiologic reasons. Because of adverse experiences with earlier nucleoside analogs, acyclovir was first tested in patients at high risk of morbidity or mortality from HSV infections. Although efficacy may be readily demonstrated in such populations, safety may be more difficult to assess. Every abnormality could be related to either the drug or the underlying disease.

Infants and Children

Acyclovir was first tested in immunocompromised children who met the eligibility criteria for ongoing trials in adults (59). As the safety profile of acyclovir expanded, the rationale for treating healthier children evolved. Since children often metabolize drugs differently from adults, separate pharmacokinetic studies were undertaken.

Yeager treated nine infants with CMV or HSV with intravenous acyclovir, 5-15 mg/kg tid, for 5-10 days (37). The infants' ages ranged from 4 to 60 days, and five were premature. No renal toxicity was observed, and hematologic abnormalities at entry resolved during the study. In a continuation of that trial, Hintz et al. reported that no toxicity was observed even when the infants who were treated at the low dose continued treatment with higher doses (38).

As a result of these studies, doses of 250 or 500 mg/m^2 were recommended for subsequent studies. Prober et al. (54) studied intravenous acyclovir, 500 mg/m^2, in 20 immunocompromised children with varicella who were a subset of a larger multicenter adult trial. One child had a transient rash on the first day of treatment; otherwise there were no significant adverse experiences.

The major usage in infants has arisen from an ongoing trial comparing acyclovir and vidarabine in the treatment of neonatal herpes. Whitley et al. (53) reported that no significant clinical or laboratory abnormalities were seen.

Studies of an oral regimen for young children have been hampered by the lack of an easily administered form of acyclovir, which is insoluble in the usual elixirs. Clinical development of a suspension of acyclovir has begun. Sullender et al. conducted a pharmacokinetic study in 18 children (3 weeks to 9 years old) with HSV or VZV, who were given acyclovir suspension, 300 mg/m^2 or 600 mg/m^2 qid, for 7 days. Mild adverse experiences were reported in three patients (diarrhea, vomiting, diaphoresis) and resolved despite continued drug administration (51).

Controlled trials are under way in immunocompetent children to determine the role of acyclovir for treatment of the common viral diseases, gingivostomatitis, and chickenpox.

Elderly

The elderly may exhibit subtle differences in responses to drugs because of renal senescence, organic brain syndrome affecting compliance with treatment, or medications for concurrent diseases.

Pharmacokinetic studies in uninfected elderly patients have not been conducted. Older patients may be found in the highest proportion in studies of herpes zoster. Bean and Aeppli reported transient renal insufficiency in 11 of 23 outpatients treated with intravenous acyclovir, 1500 mg/m^2/day (36). The authors speculated that the patients may not have been adequately hydrated. It should be noted that the dose used in this study was higher than the dose subsequently shown to be useful for zoster in immunocompetent adults. No adverse effects were observed in a lower-dose study (15 mg/kg/day) in which the mean age of treated patients was 66 years (69).

Patients over 60 years old were enrolled in a British study of oral acyclovir in herpes zoster. No clinically important adverse experiences were observed with doses of 4000 mg daily (52).

A multicenter study of herpes zoster in the United States was designed to evaluate the potential risk of acyclovir to the elderly. The randomization of patients to acyclovir or placebo was stratified by age. The incidence of adverse experiences did not increase in patients over 50 years old. The most frequent complaint was nausea in four of 93 patients who received acyclovir, compared to 10 of 94 who received placebo (66).

Young Adults

Treatment of genital herpes entails the use of acyclovir during the peak reproductive years. Clinical investigations have excluded women who were pregnant or who were not adequately protected against conception. Thus the safety of acyclovir during pregnancy has not been established. Although plasma levels achieved in humans treated at recommended doses with the intravenous formulation are still well below levels required to produce malformations in rats (23), there is a need for caution with IV therapy in women. Acyclovir has been used when the risk from infection has outweighed potential drug toxicity.

A few published anecdotes describe successful outcomes in pregnant women treated for disseminated herpes or varicella (61-63). A registry has been established by the manufacturer to evaluate acyclovir in pregnancy as one aspect of an extensive epidemiology study (34). The program was established, despite the lack of evidence of preclinical reproductive toxicity, because of the possibility of inadvertent drug exposure during the first trimester. The paucity of data at this time does not support any conclusions regarding safety. This topic is discussed in greater detail in Chapter 9.

Young, sexually active men using oral acyclovir daily may also be concerned about future fertility. To evaluate the effect of acyclovir on sperm production, a placebo-controlled study was performed in men with frequently recurrent genital herpes. No clinically significant effect was observed on sperm count, motility, or morphology in 31 men receiving drug or placebo for 6 months (35). Another study showed no increase, as compared to controls, in chromosomal aberrations after daily or intermittent use of acyclovir for 12 months (68).

Transplant Recipients

Transplant recipients are at high risk of acquiring or reactivating herpes infections. The fragility of recent transplants and their complicated management provide the setting for altered metabolism or increased toxicity of new drugs. In a small controlled study of HSV in bone marrow transplant recipients, Saral et al. observed that recovery of granulocytes, reticulocytes, and platelets was similar in acyclovir and placebo recipients (60).

Renal function was evaluated in three placebo-controlled studies of intravenous acyclovir (59,60,64). The combined data showed that two of 72 acyclovir recipients and three of 61 placebo recipients developed renal insufficiency. Shepp et al. (65) raised the question of a drug interaction between acyclovir and cyclosporine in bone marrow transplant recipients. A subsequent study by Johnson et al. (66) showed no evidence of nephrotoxicity from the combination in renal allograft recipients. There were no significant changes in serum creatinine values or inulin, albumin and B-2 microglobulin clearances. It is nevertheless recommended that patients be kept well hydrated and that cyclosporine levels be monitored carefully.

DISCUSSION

Herpes simplex infections may range from mild nuisances to life-threatening illnesses. A therapeutic index (ratio of benefit to risk) must be established for each. Side effects in a patient with encephalitis may be considered more acceptable than in the healthy young adult with mild genital herpes. Because the viral infection becomes latent and subsequently recurs, an effective therapeutic regimen not only must be safe initially but must not exhibit cumulative toxicity after repeated or chronic use. Also, antiviral drugs should not enhance the acknowledged oncogenic potential of herpesviruses.

The safety of acyclovir has been demonstrated in a comprehensive series of preclinical tests and a variety of well-controlled clinical trials that have recently been reviewed by Dorsky and Crumpacker (55). These studies defined acceptable, reversible, and manageable effects on the kidney when certain IV dose regimens are given to certain patients. Impairment of renal function has usually been readily reversible. Careful administration of fluids, slow infusion, and attention to the venous cannula should minimize the risk of complications. Less than 1% of patients receiving IV acyclovir have manifested reversible encephalopathic changes characterized by lethargy, obtundation, confusion, hallucinations, or seizures. Many of these patients had prior neurologic reactions to cytotoxic drugs or had underlying renal insufficiency resulting in high serum concentrations of acyclovir. All preclinical studies were negative for adverse effects relating to the central nervous system.

Organ systems in which cytostatic effects were seen in animals at high parenteral doses have received close attention in clinical studies. Although nausea and vomiting have been reported, gastrointestinal, bone marrow, lymphoid, and gonadal toxicity are not characteristic of acyclovir.

Clinical trials have also demonstrated that the topical application of acyclovir is useful to manage HSV skin infections. There were no significant differences between groups treated with 5% acyclovir ointment or placebo ointment in the rate or type of adverse reactions reported. This correlates well with the negative results in preclinical tests for skin and eye irritation and sensitization.

There are still unanswered questions about the safety of acyclovir. The optimal therapeutic regimen for several infections has yet to be determined. It is not known whether higher doses or longer duration could improve the outcome of patients with life-threatening infections. As a general rule, immunocompromised patients are treated with twice the dose used in immunologically intact patients. The rationale is that compromised patients should have treatment tailored to the ID_{90} rather than the ID_{50} of the virus (the concentration of drug necessary to inhibit 90% or 50% of virus in vitro). The need for higher doses of acyclovir has not been proved in a controlled manner for different degrees of immunosuppression. These issues are further complicated by the fact that inhibitory concentrations in vitro do not correlate well with either serum concentrations or clinical outcome.

The maximum duration of treatment to be recommended has not been established. Oral acyclovir has been administered daily for over 3 years (71) without evidence of toxicity. In cases where the frequency of a patient's recurrences were to decrease over time, a periodic drug holiday may be considered for patients receiving continuous suppressive therapy.

Experience with acyclovir during pregnancy is limited. The decision to treat pregnant women must be individualized. Whether treatment of genital herpes could obviate the need for cesarean delivery remains to be determined. Prophylaxis for neonatal herpes has not been evaluated in either the mother or the infant.

Therapeutically useful antiviral drugs, acyclovir being the most successful, have been available for only 10-15 years. The safety, utility, and high therapeutic ratio of acyclovir have all been demonstrated in extensive preclinical testing and in well-controlled clinical trials. As the first selective, specific, and safe antiherpes agent, acyclovir has encouraged the development of other specific antivirals for other virus infections. Galasso (5), among others, has given the reasons one should not expect broad spectrum or "penicillinlike" antivirals to emerge in the near future.

However, we can focus on extending the usefulness of acyclovir to treat new diseases, patients who are currently therapeutic orphans, or patients for whom prophylaxis is important. Ultimately, it would be desirable to show that treatment of herpes infections prevents viral transmission to susceptible individuals. Since virus shedding continues during the first few days of therapy, patients should be counseled about means of limiting transmission. Attempts to block transmission are complicated further by asymptomatic viral shedding, which can now be diagnosed (70). Answers to the preceding questions are important. However, one might expect that the answers will only slightly modify the rapidly accumulating body of safety data.

ACKNOWLEDGMENT

The authors thank Mrs. Dena Bottomly for skillful help in the preparation of this manuscript.

REFERENCES

1. Elion, G. B. (1982). Mechanism of action and selectivity of acyclovir. *Am. J. Med.* 73(1A):7-13.
2. Elion, G. B. (1986). History, mechanism of action, spectrum and selectivity of nucleoside analogs. In Mills, J., and Corey, L. (eds.): *Antiviral Chemotherapy: New Directions for Clinical Application and Research.* New York, Elsevier, pp. 118-137.
3. Szczech, G. M. (1986). The toxicity of nucleoside analogs. In Mills, J., and Corey, L. (eds.): *Antiviral Chemotherapy: New Directions for Clinical Application and Research.* New York, Elsevier, pp. 204-225.

4. Shannon, W. M. (1984). Mechanisms of action and pharmacology: Chemical agents. In Galasso, J. G., Merigan, T. C., and Buchanan, R. A. (eds.): *Antiviral Agents and Viral Diseases of Man*, Second Edition. New York, Raven Press, pp. 55-121.

5. Galasso, G. J. (1984). Antiviral agents: Why not a "penicillin" for viral infections? In DeClercq, E., and Walker, R. T. (eds.): *Targets for the Design of Antiviral Agents*. New York, Plenum Press, pp. 337-362.

6. De Miranda, P., Krasny, H. C., Page, D. A., and Elion, G. B. (1982). Species differences in the disposition of acyclovir. *Am. J. Med.* 73(1A):31-35.

7. Good, S. S., and De Miranda, P. (1982). Metabolic disposition of acyclovir in the guinea pig, rabbit and monkey. *Am. J. Med.* 73(1A):91-95.

8. Tucker, W. E. Jr., Macklin, A. W., Szot, R. J., Johnston, R. E., Elion, G. B., De Miranda, P., and Szczech, G. M. (1983). Preclinical toxicology studies with acyclovir: Acute and subchronic tests. *Fundam. Appl. Toxicol.* 3: 573-578.

9. Tucker, W. E. Jr., Johnston, R. E., Macklin, A. W., Szot, R. J., Elion, G. B., De Miranda, P., and Szczech, G. M. (1983). Preclinical toxicology studies with acyclovir: Ophthalmic and cutaneous tests. *Fundam. Appl. Toxicol.* 3:569-572.

10. Moore, H. L. Jr., Szczech, G. M., Rodwell, D. E., Kapp, R. W. Jr., De Miranda, P., and Tucker, W. E. Jr. (1983). Preclinical toxicology studies with acyclovir: Teratologic, reproductive and neonatal tests. *Fundam. Appl. Toxicol.* 3:560-568.

11. Tucker, W. E. Jr., Krasny, H. C., De Miranda, P., Goldenthal, E. I., Elion, G. B., Hajian, G., and Szczech, G. M. (1983). Preclinical toxicology studies with acyclovir: Carcinogenicity bioassays and chronic toxicity tests. *Fundam. Appl. Toxicol.* 3: 579-586.

12. Clive, D., Turner, N. T., Hozier, J., Batson, A. G., and Tucker, W. E. Jr. (1983). Preclinical toxicology studies with acyclovir: Genetic toxicity tests. *Fundam. Appl. Toxicol.* 3:587-602.

13. Kimes, A., Holtzclaw, D., McCullough, K., Teller, D., Spector, D., Dobyan, G., and Kumor, K. (1985). Effects of acyclovir on canine renal function. *Kidney Int.* 27:232.

14. Quinn, R. P., Wolberg, G., Medzihradsky, J., and Elion, G. B. (1982). Effect of acyclovir on various murine in vivo and in vitro immunologic assay systems. *Am. J. Med.* 73(1A):62-66.

15. Spruance, S. L., and Krueger, G. G. (1981). Effect of topical acyclovir on epidermal wound healing in pig. *Clin. Res.* 29:82A (abstract).

16. Lass, J. H., Pavan-Langston, D., and Park, N. H. (1979). Aciclovir and corneal wound healing. *Am. J. Ophthalmol.* 88:102-108.

17. Wellcome Research Laboratories. (1982). Rat fertility study of acyclovir, administered subcutaneously. (Unpublished data.)

18. Wellcome Research Laboratories. (1982). Rat fetal toxicity study of acyclovir, administered subcutaneously. (Unpublished data.)

19. Wellcome Research Laboratories. (1982). Rat peri- and postnatal study of acyclovir, administered subcutaneously. (Unpublished data.)

20. Wellcome Research Laboratories. (1982). Rabbit fetal toxicity study of acyclovir, administered intravenously. (Unpublished data.)

21. Wellcome Research Laboratories. (1984). Micronucleus test of acyclovir with mice. (Unpublished data.)

22. Klug, S., Lewandowski, C., Blankenberg, G., Merker, H.-J., and Neubert, D. (1985). Effect of acyclovir on mammalian embryonic development in culture. *Arch. Toxicol.* 58:89-96.

23. Stahlmann, R., Klug, S., Lewandowski, C., Chahoud, I., Bochert, G., Merker, H.-J., and Neubert, D. (1987). Letter to the Editor: Teratogenicity of acyclovir in rats. *Infection* 15:261-262.

24. Wellcome Research Laboratories. (1987). A dominant lethal study in male mice given acyclovir by intraperitoneal injection (second study at top dose of 100 mg/kg). (Unpublished data.)

25. Wellcome Research Laboratories. (1988). A study to evaluate reproductive capacity in female mice given acyclovir by intraperitoneal injection prior to mating. (Unpublished data.)

26. McGuffin, R. W., Shiota, F. M., and Myers, J. D. (1980). Lack of toxicity of acyclovir to granulocyte progenitor cells in vitro. *Antimicrob. Agents Chemother.* 18:471-473.

27. Bogliolo, G. V., Lerza, R. A., Saviane, A., and Pannacciulli, I. M. (1986). Effects of acyclovir on hematopoietic progenitor cells in mice. *IRCS Med. Sci.* 14:1116-1117.

28. Sommadossi, J.-P., and Carlisle, R. (1987). Toxicity of 3'-azido-3'-deoxythymidine and 9-(1,3-dihydroxy-2-propoxymethyl) guanine for normal human hematopoietic progenitor cells in vitro. *Antimicrob. Agents Chemother.* 452-454.

29. Stevens, D. A., Jordan, G. W., Waddell, T. F., and Merigan, T. C. (1973). Adverse effect of cytosine arabinoside on disseminated zoster in a controlled trial. *N. Engl. J. Med.* 289:873-878.

30. Boston Interhopsital Virus Study Group and the NIAID-Sponsored Cooperative Antiviral Clinical Study. (1975). Failure of high dose 5-iodo-2'-deoxyuridine in the therapy of herpes simplex virus encephalitis. *N. Engl. J. Med.* 292:599-603.

31. Whitley, R. J., Blum, M. R., Barton, N., and De Miranda, P. (1982). Pharmacokinetics of acyclovir in humans following intravenous administration: A model for the development of parenteral antivirals. *Am. J. Med.* 73(1A):165-171.

32. Van Dyke, R. B., Connor, J. D., Wyborny, C., Hintz, M., and Keeney, R. E. (1982). Pharmacokinetics of orally administered acyclovir in patients with herpes progenitalis. *Am. J. Med.* 73(1A):172-175.

33. Brigden, D., Rosling, A. E., and Woods, N. C. (1982). Renal function after acyclovir intravenous injection. *Am. J. Med.* 73(1A):182-185.

34. Andrews, E. A., Tilson, H. H., Hurn, J. A. L., and Cordero, J. F. (1988). Acyclovir in pregnancy registry: An observational epidemiologic approach. *Am. J. Med.* 85(2A):123-128.

35. Douglas, J. M., Davis, L. G., Remington, M. L., Paulsen, C. A., Perrin, E. B., Goodman, P., Conner, J. D., King, D., and Corey, L. (1988). A double-blind placebo-controlled trial of the effect of chronic oral acyclovir on sperm production in men with frequently recurrent genital herpes. *J. Infect. Dis.* 157:588-593.

36. Bean, B., and Aeppli, D. (1985). Adverse effects of high-dose intravenous acyclovir in ambulatory patients with acute herpes zoster. *J. Infect. Dis.* 151: 362-365.

37. Yeager, A. S. (1982). Use of acyclovir in premature and term neonates. *Am. J. Med.* 73(1A):205-209.

38. Hintz, M., Connor, J. D., Spector, S. A., Blum, M. R., Keeney, R. E., and Yeager, A. S. (1982). Neonatal acyclovir pharmacokinetics in patients with herpes virus infections. *Am. J. Med.* 73(1A):210-214.

39. Vartian, C. V., and Shlaes, D. M. (1983). Intravenous acyclovir and neuro-logic effects. *Ann. Intern. Med.* 99:568.

40. Bataille, P., Devos, P., Noel, J. L., Dautrevaux, C., and Lokiec, F. (1985). Psychiatric side-effects with acyclovir. *Lancet* 2:724.

41. Cohen, S. M. Z., Minkove, J. A., Zebley, J. W. III, and Mulholland, J. H. (1984). Severe but reversible neurotoxicity from acyclovir. *Ann. Intern. Med.* 100:920.

42. Jones, P. G., and Beier-Hanratty, S. A. (1986). Acyclovir: Neurologic and renal toxicity. *Ann. Intern. Med.* 104:892.

43. Auwerx, J., Knockaert, D., and Hofkens, D. (1983). Acyclovir and neuro-logic manifestations. *Ann. Intern. Med.* 99(6):882-883.

44. Meyers, J. D., Flournoy, N., Wade, J. C., Hackman, R. C., McDougall, J. K., Neiman, P. E., and Thomas, E. D. (1983). Biology of interstitial pneu-monia after marrow transplantation. In Gale, R. P. (ed.): *Recent Advances in Bone Marrow Transplantation.* New York, Alan R. Liss, pp. 405-424.

45. Wade, J. C., and Meyers, J. D. (1983). Neurologic symptoms associated with parenteral acyclovir treatment after marrow transplantation. *Ann. Intern. Med.* 98:921-925.

46. Tomson, C. R., Goodship, T. H. J., and Rodgers, R. S. C. (1985). Psychia-tric side-effects of acyclovir in patients with chronic renal failure. *Lancet* 2: 385-386.

47. Feldman, S., Rodman, J., and Gregory, B. (1988). Excessive serum concen-trations of acyclovir and neurotoxicity. *J. Infect. Dis.* 157:385-387.

48. Fletcher, C., Chinnock, B., Chace, B., Vicary, C., Welo, P., and Balfour, H. Jr. (1986). Pharmacokinetics and safety of 800 mg oral acyclovir (ACV) tablets in renal allograft recipients (RTx). In *Program and Abstracts of the 26th Interscience Conference on Antimicrobial Agents and Chemotherapy.* New Orleans, American Society for Microbiology, p. 211.

49. Goldberg, L. H., Kaufman, R., Conant, M. A., Sperber, J., Allen, M. L., Illeman, M., and Chapman, S. (1986). Oral acyclovir for episodic treatment of recurrent genital herpes. *J. Am. Acad. Dermatol.* 15:256-264.

50. Mertz, G. J., Eron, L., Kaufman. R., Goldberg, L., Raab, B., Conant, M., Mills, J., Kurtz, T., Davis, L. G., and the Acyclovir Group (1988). Prolonged continuous versus intermittent oral acyclovir treatment in normal adults with frequently recurring genital herpes simplex virus infection. *Am. J. Med.* 85(2A):14-19.

51. Sullender, W. M., Arvin, A. M., Diaz, P. S., Connor, J. D., Straube, R., Dankner, W., Levin, M. J., Weller, S., Blum, M. R., and Chapman, S. (1987). Pharmacokinetics of acyclovir suspension in infants and children. *Antimicrob. Agents Chemother.* 31:1722-1726.

52. McKendrick, M. W., McGill, J. I., White, J. E., and Wood, M. J. (1986). Oral acyclovir in acute herpes zoster. *Br. Med. J.* 293:1529-1532.

53. Whitley, R. J., Arvin, A., Corey, L., Powell, D., Plotkin, S., Starr, S., Alford, C., Connor, J., Nahmias, A. J., and Soong, S. J. (1986). Vidarabine versus acyclovir therapy of neonatal herpes simplex virus, HSV, infection. *Pediatr. Res.* 20:A323 (abstract).

54. Prober, C. G., Kirk, L. E., and Keeney, R. E. (1982). Acyclovir therapy of chickenpox in immunosuppressed children—a collaborative study. *Am. J. Pediatr.* 101:622-625.

55. Dorsky, D. I., and Crumpacker, C. S. (1987). Drugs five years later: Acyclovir. *Ann. Intern. Med.* 107:859-874.

56. Keeney, R. E., Kirk, L. E., and Bridgen, D. (1982). Acyclovir tolerance in humans. *Am. J. Med.* 73(1A):176-181.

57. Blum, M. R., Liao, S. H., and De Miranda, P. (1982). Overview of acyclovir pharmacokinetic disposition in adults and children. *Am. J. Med.* 73(1A): 186-192.

58. Sylvester, R. K., Ogden, W. B., Draxler, C. A., and Lewis, F. B. (1986). Vesicular eruption: A local complication of concentrated acyclovir infusions. *JAMA* 255:385-386.

59. Mitchel, C. D., Gentry, S. R., Boen, J. R., Bean, B., Groth, K. E., and Balfour, H. H. Jr. (1981). Acyclovir for mucocutaneous herpes simplex infections in immunocompromised patients. *Lancet* 1:1389-1392.

60. Saral, R., Burns, W. H., Laskin, O. L., Santos, G. W., and Lietman, P. S. (1981). Acyclovir prophylaxis of herpes-simplex-virus infections. *N. Engl. J. Med.* 305:63-67.

61. Lagrew, D. C., Furlow, T. G., Hager, W. D., and Yarrish, R. L. (1984). Disseminated herpes simplex virus infection in pregnancy: Successful treatment with acyclovir. *JAMA* 252:2058-2059.

62. Landsberger, E. J., Hager, W. D., and Grossman, J. H. 3d. (1986). Successful management of varicella pneumonia complicating pregnancy: A report of three cases. *J. Reprod. Med.* 31:311-314.

63. Hankins, G. D., Gilstraple, L. C. III, and Patterson, A. R. (1987). Acyclovir treatment of varicella pneumoia in pregnancy. *Crit. Care Med.* 15:336-337.

64. Meyers, J. D., Wade, J. C., Mitchell, C. D., Saral, R., Lietman, P. S., Durack, D. T., Levin, M. J., Segreti, A. C., and Balfour, H. H. Jr. (1982). Multicenter collaborative trial of intravenous acyclovir for treatment of mucocutaneous herpes simplex virus infection in the immunocompromised host. *Am. J. Med.* 73(1A):229-235.
65. Shepp, D. H., Dandliker, P. S., and Meyers, J. D. (1986). Treatment of varicella-zoster virus infections in severely immunocompromised patients: A randomized comparison of acyclovir and vidarabine. *N. Engl. J. Med.* 314: 208-212.
66. Johnson, P. C., Kumor, K., Welsh, M. S., Woo, J., and Kahan, B. D. (1987). Effects of coadministration of cyclosporine and acyclovir on renal function of renal allograft recipients. *Transplantation* 44:329-331.
67. Huff, J. C., Bean, B., Balfour, H. H., Laskin, O., Connor, J. D., Corey, L., Bryson, Y. J., and McGuirt, P. (1988). Therapy of herpes zoster with oral acyclovir. *Am. J. Med.* 85(2A):84-89.
68. Clive, D., Hozier, J., and Davis, G. (1988). A double-blind, placebo controlled cytogenetic study in recurrent genital herpes patients following acute and chronic oral dosing with acyclovir. Unpublished data, Wellcome Research Laboratories.
69. Peterslund, N. A., Ipsen, J., Schonheyder, H., Seyer-Hansen, K., Esmann, V., and Juhl, H. (1981). Acyclovir in herpes zoster. *Lancet* 2:827-831.
70. Rooney, J. F., Felser, J. M., Ostrove, J. M., and Straus, S. E. (1986). Acquisition of genital herpes from an asymptomatic sexual partner. *N. Engl. J. Med.* 314:1561-1564.
71. Wellcome Research Laboratories. (1988). Unpublished data.

3

Acyclovir Therapy for Herpesvirus Infections of the Eye

L. M. T. Collum *Royal College of Surgeons in Ireland and Royal Victoria Eye and Ear Hospital, Dublin, Ireland*

INTRODUCTION

Ocular infection with the herpes simplex virus is a serious problem, constituting a major component of external eye disease clinics. It is a significant cause of ocular morbidity (1) and is responsible for a considerable loss of working days. It produces all degrees of ocular damage from mild to severe and, in certain circumstances, can be a blinding condition. For these reasons, exact diagnosis, management, and treatment are important. Acyclovir has contributed very significantly to reducing problems associated with the virus and to more effective therapy of severe manifestations of the disease.

As with all virus problems, there is no drug, or any form of therapy, yet available that will totally eliminate the causative agent. Treatment, even with acyclovir, still consists of the management of current attacks. This of course begs the question of recurrences, which is generally still the major problem with herpes simplex infections (2-4). For the future, research will be aimed toward producing a drug that will eliminate the virus, identify the latent virus, or be effective on a preventive basis. None of the antivirals available until the advent of acyclovir were readily suitable for use in prevention, with the possible exception of interferon (5,6). Acyclovir, however, has opened up the field of prevention, as it is relatively nontoxic to the corneal epithelium (7), can be used long term (8),

35

and can be given systemically (9). Systemic administration has significant advantages over local application, in that it avoids the problems of blurring of vision, smearing of the ointment on spectacles, and the general discomfort of foreign material in the eye (9). The oral preparation is also relatively nontoxic (9,10) and is therefore useful in those who are getting frequent attacks.

ACYCLOVIR

Acyclovir, a purine analog, has made a major contribution to the management of herpetic eye disease, both corneal and intraocular (7-9,11,12). Because it is not incorporated into normal cellular DNA (13,14), it does not damage normal corneal or conjunctival cells. It only interferes with virus-infected cells (13,14) and therefore does not have the problems and side effects well documented and associated with idoxuridine (15). It does not affect the puncta and is generally nonirritative, except in patients with tear film disorders (16). Because, therefore, of its activity and nontoxicity, it is an admirable drug in the management of corneal and conjunctival herpes simplex infections (7-9,17). Its other great advantage is that, given orally in doses of 400 mg, five times daily, it produces therapeutic levels in the tears, serum, and aqueous humor (9,11). This makes it an extremely useful drug in patients who would otherwise be unsuited to using the ointment.

This group of patients includes those with arthritis affecting the hands, which prevents them from instilling ointment properly; mentally defective persons; and individuals with conditions such as Parkinson's disease and other disabling problems (9). In addition, there is a group of patients who are unwilling to use ointments and whose compliance is therefore doubtful; these patients are eminently suitable for oral treatment.

It has also become apparent that in patients with tear film disorders it is probably better to avoid using local treatment, as the ointment tends to lodge in the lower fornix. With deficient lubrication the ointment is not washed away and produces a constant irritation. This irritation produces a punctate keratopathy and a spotty staining of the conjunctiva (16). This side effect has been reported in the past (7), but the significance of the association with tear film disorders has not been noted until recently. Nevertheless, because oral acyclovir is sufficiently absorbed (9), the clinician can still use acyclovir in these patients. The question arises as to whether enough of the drug is introduced to the virus if the tear film is deficient. However, it has been shown that deficient lubrication does not seem to effect the efficiency of systemic acyclovir (16).

The optimum treatment with the 3% ophthalmic ointment is five times daily applications, for approximately 10-14 days in dendritic ulceration. It has to be given for a longer period of time in geographic ulceration and often for months in stromal disease (12). However, in the longer-term conditions, it is usually possible to reduce the frequency of use, and, indeed, it can be combined with the oral preparation to make the treatment regimen more tolerable for patients in relation to their work and social life.

Herpes Simplex Primary Infection

Primary herpes simplex infections may occur in the region of the eye (Table 1). It is uncommon, however, to get primary infections in the cornea, and they usually occur in the skin and/or conjunctiva. Frequently the initial manifestations are minimal and of no great consequence as far as the patient is concerned, who may merely notice a slight rash on his eyelids. However, the primary infection can be severe, producing a fever and a local lymphadenopathy (Fig. 1, after page 46). This will usually, however, clear without any permanent sequelae. Primary infections in the conjunctiva produce a nonspecific conjunctivitis, but if the conjunctiva is stained with fluorescein, small dendritic figures will be seen, and a diagnosis can therefore be made. The condition is, unfortunately, frequently missed, owing to unawareness of this as a presenting feature of herpes simplex disease. When the condition settles, there are usually no particular problems, and many patients never have any further ocular symptoms. The virus becomes latent, however, and lies probably in the sensory ganglion of the trigeminal nerve. Activation of this virus will then produce

TABLE 1   Classification of Herpes Simplex Eye Disease

Herpes simplex primary infection
   Lids
   Conjunctiva
   Elsewhere
Recurrent herpes simplex infection
   Lids
   Conjunctiva
   Cornea
   Uveal Tract

recurrence of the disease, which will usually manifest as problems in the cornea or the uveal tract. These precipitating factors do not differ significantly from those described for other areas of the body. Fever and extremes of temperature are certainly important, but stress would also appear to be significant.

Primary infections occurring elsewhere, particularly on the nose and lips, may also subsequently manifest as recurrences in the eye. It does not follow, therefore, that the secondary attacks will be in the same area as the primary disease. In fact, most patients that present with herpetic corneal disease do not give a history of a primary infection anywhere around the eye. It should be stressed that many of the primary infections are subclinical, and there may not be any indications whatsoever to draw the patient's attention to the fact that he has had herpes.

Because most cases of primary infection are subclinical, or very mild, no treatment is necessary. However, if the patient is having significant symptoms, or if the condition is extensive, acyclovir skin cream can be used combined, if necessary, with acyclovir ointment to the conjunctival sac. This will usually clear up the condition within a few days. It is important to realize, however, that this will treat the actual attack, but it does not in any way prevent the problem of recurrence, though it is suggested that early administration of acyclovir may reduce the incidence of latency (18).

The diagnosis of herpetic lesions of the skin or conjunctiva is relatively simple clinically. The only condition that it may be confused with is herpes zoster. Zoster is not common in the younger age group and will tend to have a different clinical pattern. If there is any doubt, cultures may be taken, or electron microscopic studies carried out. Most of the laboratory tests are expensive, however, and not available in all centers. A simplier technique is immunocytochemical antigen antibody staining for herpes simplex particles (19,20), which can be readily carried out even in unsophisticated departments. This test should therefore be considered in any cases where the diagnosis is not obvious. It is important to be sure of the diagnosis, as inaccurate therapy will confuse the clinical picture for the future.

Herpetic Conjunctivitis

Herpetic conjunctivitis may be a primary manifestation of the condition. However, it may also be a feature of recurrences. It is a diagnosis that is frequently missed, owing to lack of awareness. Fluorescein staining will show dendrites on the conjunctiva, and simple laboratory investigations, such as immunoperoxidase staining, will confirm the diagnosis (19,20). These patients should be treated with an antiviral, so as to minimize damage to the conjunctiva and possible spread to the cornea. While antivirals, such as idoxuridine, adenine arabinoside, and trifluorothymidine may be used, acyclovir for many practitioners is the treatment of choice because of its relative nontoxicity. It is to be remembered that most of the other antivirals will be incorporated into normal cellular DNA and therefore will produce a punctate keratopathy, which can be troublesome for the patient and present diagnostic problems. Acyclovir, therefore, should be considered to be the treatment of choice. Application of the ointment five times a day for a week to 10 days will usually clear up the problem without after-effects. It does not eliminate the problem of recurrence.

Keratitis

Keratitis due to the herpes simplex virus is a serious disease, which manifests itself in a variety of ways (see Table 2).

Superficial Punctate Keratopathy

Superficial punctate keratopathy is a common clinical finding. In accident and emergency departments it is frequently taken to be synonymous with the herpes simplex virus. This is far from the truth, as most cases will be due to some other factor. Superficial punctate keratopathy is always pathological, and a methodical examination of the lids and lashes should be made to rule out local lid pathology—namely, entropion, ectropion, trichasis, and other lesions around the eyelids, such as papillomata and molluscum contagiosum. A very common cause of punctate keratopathy is tear film disease, and a careful assessment of the tears should be made in all cases. In addition, trauma should be kept in mind, and air pollution itself

---

TABLE 2 Herpetic Keratitis

1. Superficial punctate keratopathy
2. Dendritic ulceration
3. Geographic ulceration
4. Stromal keratitis
5. Endotheliitis
6. Keratouveitus
7. Complicated corneal ulceration (metaherpetic ulcers)

may be implicated. The occupation of the patient should be taken into consideration, because if he is working with chemicals he may be traumatizing his cornea directly or from the fumes. Another important cause is iatrogenic disease. For instance, a potent cause of punctate keratopathy is idoxuridine (15).

It must be appreciated therefore that punctate keratopathy, while it may be due to herpes simplex, is very much more often due to other causes, and a full history and ocular examination are mandatory.

In order to establish a definite diagnosis of herpes simplex as a cause of the keratopathy, immunocytochemical examination or other laboratory testing should be carried out, because it is only then that the correct therapy can be introduced. Inappropriate treatment simply aggravates the condition. Any of the antivirals may be used, but acyclovir is the treatment of choice, as it will not add to the epithelial cell damage.

Dendritic Ulceration

Dendritic ulceration is the classical lesion produced by herpes simplex (Fig. 2, after page 46). The typical dendritic pattern is found in no other condition. The lesions can be single or multiple, central or peripheral. The ulcers have an undermined edge, and the branching pattern is almost pathognomonic. Laboratory investigation is usually unnecessary, as the diagnosis is obvious. If it is necessary to make a laboratory diagnosis, cells may be taken from the edge of the ulcer and submitted to the required procedure.

The management of dendritic ulceration of the cornea is straightforward, though there is some debate as to which is the best form of treatment. There is no doubt that mechanical debridement is still very acceptable (21,22) and is particularly suitable for peripheral lesions, though recurrences is a problem (23). It is not suitable for multiple lesions.

Mechanical debridement, as well as being therapeutic, may be used diagnostically. In addition, debridement may be combined with an antiviral (24), and this has been shown to be an effective method of treatment. There is no question, however, of either form of therapy preventing recurrences. Of the antivirals available, adenine arabinoside (25,26), trifluorothymidine (26,27), and idoxuridine (15,26) all have some toxic effect on the corneal epithelium, as they are incorporated into normal cellular DNA. Because acyclovir is not taken up by normal cellular DNA, it would appear to be the best treatment available. There is a school of thought, however, that suggests that acyclovir should be kept in reserve for progressive severe disease, in order to reduce the possibility of resistance (28). There is, though, very little evidence that acyclovir produces any significant degree of resistance (28), and a strong case can be made for its use as a primary therapeutic agent. In healing time it is at least as good as idoxuridine or adenine arabinoside (7,17,29), and because of its low level of toxicity, it is a more acceptable method of treatment to clinicians and to patients. The therapeutic dose regime is a five times daily application of 3% ointment into the inferior fornix. The pattern of healing starts with a decrease in pain within 24 h. The ulcer then stops extending and begins to break up. Subsequently a small area of punctate keratopathy, or ghosting, will be present at the site of the lesion, and these changes clear subsequently. This localized keratopathy should not be confused with a toxic effect, as it is frequently a stage in the natural healing process of the ulcer.

Oral treatment may be used as a substitute for locally applied acyclovir. There is a group of patients that are best treated in such a manner. These include those that will not comply with instructions, mentally defective patients, those who are incapacitated physically and who are unable to instill medication into the eye and those with dry eye states. It has been shown that therapeutic levels are reached in both the tears and serum and that the effect of oral medication, given 400 mg, five times daily, is the same as locally applied acyclovir (9). In many instances systemic administration is more acceptable to the average patient than local application of ointment (9).

A number of these patients will have some extension of the disease into the superficial stroma, giving a light superficial reaction. In the typical case, this will clear fairly completely, without gross reduction in vision. However, ulcers in the center of the pupil, even though they heal quickly, will frequently leave a mild scar, and even the least corneal disruption in this position will produce a disproportionate visual disturbance.

Many of these patients will have some degree of ciliary spasm with some cells in the anterior chamber. The use of a cycloplegic, therefore, such as cyclopentolate, is frequently desirable. Because of the pain and watering, many patients are more comfortable if the eye is padded. There is little merit in combining antivirals with antibiotics in uncomplicated cases.

The problem of recurrence remains. If a patient has had one attack, then he has a 22% chance of getting a second, and those who have had two or more attacks have a 45% chance of getting a further episode (21). The longer the interval between attacks, the less likely is the patient to have a further outbreak.

Patients who have frequent recurrences should be considered for prophylactic treatment. Because no drug can identify and destroy the latent virus, there is a case to be made for using continuous antiviral therapy, and acyclovir is the treatment of choice. The suggested regimen is to give systemic acyclovir in low doses (400 mg per day), until it is felt that the pattern has been broken. The only contraindication is renal malfunction.

Geographic (Amoeboid) Ulceration

Geographic ulceration of the cornea is frequently associated with the previous use of corticosteroids. Steroids are absolutely contraindicated in herpetic epithelial disease, and if they are inadvertently given to a patient with a dendritic ulcer, the sequence of events frequently results in the formation of a geographic ulcer. This ulcer is a large area of epithelial loss (Fig. 3, after page 46). In its simple form it is superficial, although it may become complicated by secondary infection and extend deeper into the cornea. Because of its size it is slower to heal than dendritic ulcers and is not suitable for mechanical debridement. Acyclovir is the treatment of choice. Prolonged treatment with idoxuridine or other antivirals may produce epithelial complications, and therefore these are best avoided. It has been shown that the healing time in geographic ulceration, while being a little longer than in dendritic ulceration when treated with acyclovir, is still reasonable and that acyclovir is a good method of treatment of this lesion (17).

Stromal Keratitis

Stromal keratitis is a particularly difficult manifestation of herpetic disease. It is due to the virus, but the main response seems to be an immune reaction. The cornea becomes hazy, very frequently in a disc pattern, which leads to the use of the term disciform keratitis (Fig. 4, after page 46). In addition to corneal thickening, there are epithelial and stromal edema, prominence of the endothelial cells, and folds in Descemet's membrane. There are nearly always keratitic precipitates (KPs) on the posterior surface of the affected part of the cornea, and they are accompanied by the presence of flare and cells in the anterior chamber. The distribution of the KPs is not typical of that of iritis, which may suggest a specific active response to altered endothelial cells (30). A significant uveitis may be present in severe cases, with posterior synechiae and the complications associated therewith. The patient has extreme blurring of vision, and the eye is painful, red, photophobic, and watery. No age group is exempt, and once the patient has had the primary disease, stromal keratitis can occur in all, including children.

The management of the condition is prolonged (8). The inexperienced practitioner may make the mistake of treating stromal keratitis as a short-term disease, and this will result in a recurrence of the inflammation. When the attack seems to be completely healed, there is still a significant chance of a flareup. Because the virus is primarily involved, an antiviral is necessary, but because there is a large immune background, an immunosuppressive agent is usually desirable. The immunosuppressive agent most useful is a local corticosteroid, but because these can, in the presence of the virus, precipitate dendritic and geographic ulcers, it is essential that they be covered by an antiviral.

These patients frequently need medication for months and perhaps even years. For this reason acyclovir is, without any doubt, the treatment of choice (8,31). There is no question of using the other currently available antivirals, because their toxic effect is such that prolonged use will produce damage to the cornea, conjunctiva, and lacrimal system in many cases.

The regimen of treatment is to start on maximum therapy, which consists of acyclovir ointment five times daily together with corticosteroid drops five times daily. Careful monitoring of the patient should be carried out, and this dosage regimen can be reduced gradually, so that it may be possible to maintain the patient on a maintenance dose of a drop of corticosteroid and an application of acyclovir ointment, even as little as every second day.

It is our experience that premature withdrawal of the treatment will result in flareups. It is also our experience that the subsequent flareups are more difficult to control than the initial attack. An adjunct to therapy is the use of systemic acyclovir (32,33). This has the attraction that patients don't have the problems associated with applying ointment every day to the eye, leading to interference with work and social activities. A low maintenance dose of 200-400 mg of acyclovir, given orally, is usually sufficient to control the attack combined with a very low-dose local corticosteroid preparation. It has to be stressed that the treatment must not be withdrawn suddenly, or prematurely, as this will result in early recurrence.

The criteria for healing are the return of the cornea to normal thickness, disappearance of epithelial and stromal edema, disappearance of the folds in Descemet's membrane, absence of fresh KPs, and inactivity in the anterior chamber. When these criteria are observed, the treatment can be reduced, but treatment should not be withdrawn for a considerable period of time, and this can only be determined by an experienced observer. Long-term complications have been reduced significantly with the administration of acyclovir, but there is no doubt that permanent corneal scarring can result from a severe attack and will certainly result from recurrences. For this reason, every attempt to continue adequate treatment for a sufficient length of time must be made.

It is possible that some patients may respond to acyclovir alone, particularly those having a first attack or those who previously have never had corticosteroid treatment (32).

Endotheliitis

The endothelial cells are seen to be swollen in herpetic stromal keratitis. It is suggested that the primary problem in the development of stromal keratitis is at the endothelial level (34) and that it is there that the virus produces its effect. It is certainly true that endothelial cell changes can be seen, and the management of endotheliitis is the same as the management of the stromal disease—namely, acyclovir given topically or systemically, coupled with corticosteroid drops. In addition, in cases where there is severe anterior chamber activity, cycloplegics should be used.

Complicated Corneal Ulceration

Some herpetic corneal ulcers will become complicated by secondary infection. The ulceration may also be complicated by excess production of collagenase, which in turn will produce disturbances of the architecture of the cornea. Careful observation and laboratory investigations will be helpful in this situation. When the ulcer is complicated by bacterial superinfection, the appropriate antibiotic must be combined with the antiviral, and where there is excess collagenase production, anticollagenase agents, such as acetylcysteine, are beneficial. It is the case that many ulcers, labeled metaherpetic, no longer have an active viral component, and the antiviral should be discontinued in these patients. Debridement is useful to get rid of necrotic tissues, which in turn promotes healing.

An added problem in chronic herpetic keratitis is the destruction of corneal sensory nerves. An anesthetic cornea is unhealthy with atrophy of the microvilli of the epithelium and subsequently poor adherence and spread of tears, leading to the development of dry spots with later ulceration. This adds to the problems associated with the herpes infection, and in many instances where there are recurrences of keratitis, it is likely that they are not primarily herpetic but rather associated with some of the physiological upsets mentioned. Tarsorraphy may be indicated in these patients.

Uveitis

Uveitis often accompanies stromal disease. There is anterior chamber activity with cells and flare visible, but in severe cases all the problems of severe anterior uveitis, including dilatation of the iris blood vessels with spontaneous hyphaema and glaucoma, may occur (35). The diagnosis of herpetic anterior uveitis is difficult and can only be made with certainty by an anterior chamber tap. If there is a clinical suspicion of herpes simplex, and when all other causes are ruled out, it is reasonable to treat these patients with systemic acyclovir, and, as a therapeutic trial, it may give the correct diagnosis. A response will be obtained to the appropriate dose of systemic acyclovir—namely, 400 mg five times daily.

Herpetic uveitis may occur without an associated keratopathy. Presumably in these cases latency has been established in the superior cervical sympathetic ganglion from where the virus may get to the uveal tract by axoplasmic flow (35).

DIAGNOSIS OF OCULAR HERPES SIMPLEX

Dendritic ulceration of the cornea is almost pathognomonic of the herpes simplex virus. The only condition that mimics it is the transient dendrites associated with zoster. Geographic ulcers have a typical appearance and, in the uncomplicated state, do not present a diagnostic problem. Nonspecific ulcers and punctate keratopathy, however, are difficult. From the point of view of treatment, it is important to establish a correct diagnosis, since inappropriate therapy may so confuse the clinical picture as to make a positive diagnosis impossible at a later stage. There are, therefore, times when resort must be made to the laboratory. Traditionally, tests such as virus antibodies, virus cultures, cell cytology, and electron microscopic studies have been carried out (36-42).

Cell cytology may give a pointer toward the diagnosis, but it is certainly not diagnostic. Virus antibodies will simply suggest that there was a virus infection in the past, and only a significantly rising titer, during an attack, will be diagnostic. This is not usually found in localized infection in the eye. Virus cultures are helpful, but they take 3 or 4 days and are therefore not practical in ocular conditions, and unless treatment is instigated at an early stage, irrevocable damage can be done. Electron microscopy is accurate but not usually available in the average clinical situation. A simple quick, inexpensive test, easy to carry out and specific for simplex, is desirable, such as an immunocytochemical reaction for the detection of herpes simplex virus antigen. The technique is relatively simple

in that all that is necessary is to remove some cells and to use a prepre-
pared kit for the establishment of the presence of the antigen. This test is
specific and is enormously useful in the diagnosis of doubtful lesions (19,
20,43). It should be available in most ophthalmic centers and, if used
properly, will avoid the problems associated with inappropriate therapy.

PREVENTION

The major portion of this chapter has been devoted to the classification
and treatment of herpes simplex disease. It has been suggested that the
major problem is recurrence. A simple attack will not usually result in significant permanent damage. Each recurrence, however, takes its toll, and
frequent recurrences will produce a significant effect on visual function.

Acyclovir has a role to play in prophylaxis (29). Where patients are
having frequent attacks of corneal ulceration or stromal disease, it may
be given locally or systemically, either on its own or combined with corticosteroids. Oral acyclovir is the treatment of choice if renal function is
normal, as local medication is a nuisance for the patient. What is not
clear is the optimum dose for prophylaxis. The dosage suggested is 400-
800 mg daily. The problem is to decide when this treatment should be
discontinued. Experience shows that withdrawal of the medication too
soon will result in recurrence of the disease, and there is no clinical sign
or other indication as to when it is safe to do so.

Withdrawal of the treatment is therefore arbitrary. A rule of thumb
is that if the patient has been having frequent attacks and has been incapacitated socially, or from the point of view of occupation, 12 months of
therapy, at least, is indicated. There is no doubt that this type of preventive treatment has helped an enormous number of patients that, hereto-
fore, would have suffered considerably from recurrences of the attacks.

SUMMARY

Acyclovir has made a definite impact on the management of most forms
of herpetic eye disease, and, in addition, its role in prophylaxis is making
a significant contribution. That it is nontoxic makes it stand apart from
other antivirals and makes its long-term use acceptable. It is a major advantage that it can be given orally, as this is more acceptable to many patients, especially if long-term treatment is necessary. The problem with
acyclovir, however, is that, like all antivirals, it does not prevent recurrences, and this is still the major challenge in herpetic ocular disease.

PLATE I

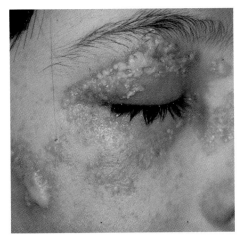

FIGURE 3.1 Primary herpes simplex infection.

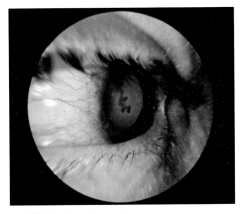

FIGURE 3.2 Corneal dendritic ulceration.

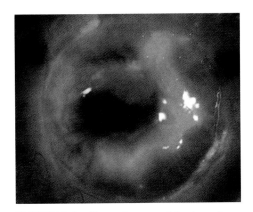

FIGURE 3.3 Corneal geographic ulceration.

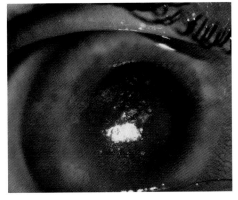

FIGURE 3.4 Corneal disciform keratitis.

PLATE II

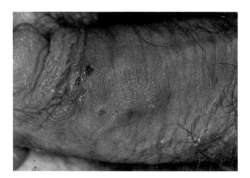

FIGURE 6.1 Primary genital herpes in a man (day 8): Development of new penile vesicles is apparent. The original lesions are crusted. The new vesicles are not contiguous with the original lesions.

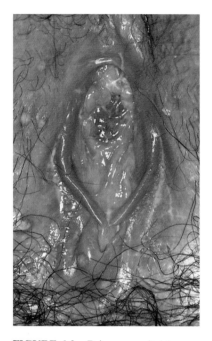

FIGURE 6.2 Primary genital herpes in a woman (day 2): (a) Painful bilateral vesicular and ulcerative lesions are present on the labiae minora and majora.

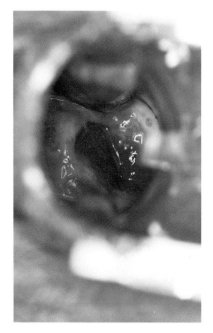

FIGURE 6.2 (continued) (b) Ulcerative lesions are seen on a friable cervix with a small amount of mucopurulent discharge.

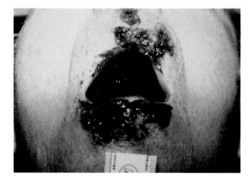

FIGURE 16.1 Orolabial herpes simplex virus infection in an immunocompromised host.

REFERENCES

1. Sorsby, A. (1972). *Reports on Public Health and Medical Subjects*, No. 128. London: HMSO.
2. Norn, M. S. (1970). Dendritic (herpetic) keratitis. 2. Follow up examination of corneal opacity. *Acta Ophthalmol.* 48:214.
3. Wilhelmus, K. R., Coster, D. J., Falcon, M. G., and Jones, M. C. (1981). Longitudinal analysis of ulcerative herpetic keratitis. In Sundmacher, R. (ed.): *Herpes Eye Diseases.* Munich, J. F. Bergmann Verlag, p. 375.
4. Wilhelmus, K. R., Falcon, M. G., and Jones, B. R. (1981). Bilateral herpetic keratitis. *Br. J. Ophthalmol.* 65:385-387.
5. Jones, B. R., Coster, D. J., Falcon, M. F., and Cantell, K. (1976). Clinical trials of topical interferon therapy of ulcerative viral keratitis. *J. Infect. Dis.* 133 (Suppl. A):93-95.
6. Sundmacher, R., Neumann-Haefelin, D., and Cantell, K. (1981). Therapy and prophylaxis of dendritic keratitis with topical human interferon. In Sundmacher, R. (ed.): *Herpetic Eye Diseases.* Munich, J. F. Bergmann Verlag, pp. 401-407.
7. Collum, L. M. T., Benedict-Smith, A., and Hillary, I. B. (1980). Randomised double blind trial of acyclovir and idoxuridine in dendritic corneal ulceration. *Br. J. Ophthalmol.* 64:766-769.
8. Collum, L. M. T., Logan, P., and Ravenscroft, T. (1983). Acyclovir (Zovirax) in herpetic disciform keratitis. *Br. J. Ophthalmol.* 67:115-118.
9. Collum, L. M. T., McGettrick, P., Akhtar, J., Lavin, J., and Rees, P. J. (1986). Oral acyclovir (Zovirax) in herpes simplex dendritic corneal ulceration. *Br. J. Ophthalmol.* 70:435-438.
10. Field, H. J., and Phillips, I. (eds.). (1983). Proceedings of the second international acyclovir symposium, London, 15-18 May 1983. *J. Antimicrob. Chemother.* 12B.
11. Hung, S. O., Patterson, A., Clarke, D. I., and Rees, P. J. (1984). Oral acyclovir in the management of dendritic herpetic corneal ulceration. *Br. J. Ophthalmol.* 68:398-400.
12. Collum, L. M. T., and Benedict-Smith, A. (1981). Acyclovir (Zovirax) in herpes simplex keratitis. In Sundmacher, R. (ed.): *Herpetic Eye Diseases.* Munich, J. F. Bergmann Verlag, p. 323-327.
13. Elion, G. B., Furman, P. A., Fyfe, J. A., De Miranda, P., Beauchamp, L., and Schaeffer, H. J. (1977). Selectivity of action of an antiherpetic agent, 9-(2-hydroxyethoxymethyl)-guanine. *Proc. Natl. Acad. Sci. USA* 74:5716-5720.
14. Schaeffer, H. J., Beauchamp, L., De Miranda, P., and Elion, G. B. (1978). 9-(2-Hydroxyethoxymethyl)guanine activity against virus of the herpes group. *Nature* 272:583-585.
15. Patterson, A., and Jones, B. R. (1967). The management of ocular herpes. *Trans. Ophthalmol. Soc. U.K.* 87:59-84.

16. Collum, L. M. T. (in preparation).
17. Collum, L. M. T., Logan, P., McAuliffe-Curtin, Hung, S. O., Patterson, A., and Rees, P. J. (1985). Randomised double-blind trial of acyclovir (Zovirax) and adenine arabinoside in herpes simplex amoeboid corneal ulceration. *Br. J. Ophthalmol.* 69:847-850.
18. Field, H. J., Bell, S., Elion, G. B., Nash, A. A., and Wildy, P. (1979). Effect of acycloguanosine treatment of acute and latent herpes simplex infections in mice. *Antimicrob. Agents Chemother.* 15:544-561.
19. Collum, L. M. T., Mullaney, J., and Hillery, M. (1985). A suggested rapid test for corneal herpes simplex (letter). *N. Engl. J. Med.* 314:245.
20. Collum, L. M. T., Mullaney, J., Hillery, M., Mullaney, P., and Lester, R. (1987). Two laboratory methods for diagnosis of herpes simplex keratitis. *Br. J. Ophthalmol.* 71:742-745.
21. Wellings, P. C., Awdry, P. N., Bors, F. H., Jones, B. R., Brown, D. C., and Kaufman, H. E. (1972). Clinical evaluation of trifluorothymidine in the treatment of herpes simplex corneal ulcers. *Am. J. Ophthalmol.* 73:932-942.
22. Whitcher, J. P., Dawson, C. R., Hoshiwara, I., Daghfous, T., Messadi, M., Triki, F., and Oh, J. O. (1976). Herpes simplex keratitis in a developing country. *Arch. Ophthalmol.* 94:587-592.
23. Coster, D. L., Jones, B. R., and Falcon, M. C. (1977). Role of debridement in the treatment of herpetic keratitis. *Trans. Ophthalmol. Soc. U.K.* 97:314-317.
24. Jones, B. R., Coster, D. J., Fison, P. N., Thompson, G. M., Cobo, L. M., and Falcon, M. G. (1979). Efficacy of acycloguanosine (Wellcome 248U) against herpes simplex corneal ulcers. *Lancet* 1:243-244.
25. Pavan-Langston, D., and Dohlman, C. H. (1972). A double-blind clinical study of adenine arabinoside therapy of viral keratoconjunctivitis. *Am. J. Ophthalmol.* 74:81-88.
26. Falcon, M. G., Jones, B. R., Williams, H. P., and Coster, D. J. (1981). Adverse reactions in the eye from topical therapy with idoxuridine adenine, arabinoside and trifluorothymidine. In Sundmacher, R. (ed.): *Herpetic Eye Diseases.* Munich, J. F. Bergmann Verlag, pp. 263-266.
27. Wellings, P. C., Awdry, P. N., Bors, F. H., Jones, B. R., Brown, D. C., and Kaufman, H. E. (1972). Clinical evaluation of trifluorothymidine in the treatment of herpes simplex corneal ulcers. *Am. J. Ophthalmol.* 73:932-942.
28. Falcon, M. G. (1987). Rational acyclovir therapy in herpetic eye disease. *Br. J. Ophthalmol.* 71:102-106.
29. McGill, M. G., and Tormey, P. (1981). The clinical use of acyclovir in the treatment of herpes simplex corneal ulceration. In Sundmacher, R. (ed.): *Herpetic Eye Diseases.* Munich, J. F. Bergmann Verlag, p. 319.
30. Sundmacher, R. (1987). Clinical aspects of herpetic eye diseases. In *Proceedings of the International Conference on Herpetic Eye Disease* 6:183-188.
31. Colin, J., Mazet, D., and Chastel, C. (1985). Treatment of herpetic keratouveitis: Comparative action of vidarabine, trifluorothymidine and acyclovir

in combination with corticoids. In Maudgal, L., and Missotten, L. (eds.): *Herpetic Eye Diseases.* W. Junk, pp. 227-232.

32. McGill, J. (1987). The enigma of herpes stromal disease. *Br. J. Ophthalmol.* 71:118-125.
33. Wilhelmus, K. R., Falcon, M. G., and Jones, B. L. (1982). Herpetic irido-cyclitis. *Int. Ophthalmol.* 4:143-150.
34. Sundmacher, R. (1981). A clinico-virologic classification of herpetic anterior segment diseases with special reference to intraocular herpes. In Sundmacher, R. (ed.): *Herpetic Eye diseases.* Munich, J. F. Bergmann Verlag, pp. 202-210.
35. Easty, D. L. (1985). *Virus Diseases of the Eye.* London, Lloyd Luke, pp. 152-153.
36. Grist, N. R., Bell, E. J., Follitt, E. A. C., and Urquhart, G. E. D. (1979). *Diagnostic Methods in Clinical Virology*, 3d Ed. Oxford, Blackwell.
37. Moore, D. F. (1984). Comparison of human fibroblast cells and primary rabbit kidney cells for isolation of HSV. *J. Clin. Microbiol.* 19:548-549.
38. McSwiggan, D. A., Darougar, S., Rahman, A. F. N. S., and Gibson, J. A. (1975). Comparison of the sensitivity of human embryo kidney cells, HeLa cells and WI38 cells for primary isolation of viruses from the eye. *J. Clin. Pathol.* 28:410-413.
39. Walpita, P., Darougar, S., and Thaker, U. (1985). A rapid and sensitive culture test for detecting herpes simplex virus from the eye. *Br. J. Ophthalmol.* 69:637-639.
40. Smith, I. W., Peutherer, J. F., and MacCallum, F. O. (1967). The incidence of herpes virus hominis antibodies in the population. *J. Hyg. (Lond.)* 65: 395-408.
41. Gardner, P. S., McQuillan, J., Black, M. M., and Richardson, J. (1968). Rapid diagnosis of HSV hominis in superficial lesions by immunofluorescent staining techniques. *Br. Med. J.* iv:89-92.
42. Kobayashi, S., Shogi, K., and Ishizu, M. (1972). Electron microscopic demonstration of viral particles in keratitis. *Jpn. J. Ophthalmol.* 16:247-253.
43. Corey, L. (1987). Laboratory diagnosis of HSV. Antiviral update. Reporting the Wellcome International Antiviral Symposium, 2-4 Dec., Monte Carlo, p. 8.

4

Treatment of Nongenital Herpesvirus Infections

G. Wayne Raborn *University of Alberta Hospitals, Edmonton, Alberta, Canada*

INTRODUCTION

Herpes simplex virus (HSV) infections account for a number of nongenital infections in immunocompetent patients. Primary gingivostomatitis can afflict children or young adults. Recurrent herpetic labialis or other more localized HSV infections can range from minor to debilitating in severity. In addition, HSV has been implicated in eczema herpeticum (Kaposi's varicelliform eruption) and recently in erythema multiforme (1).

The keys to successful management of most diseases are early diagnosis and rapid initiation of therapy with an appropriate drug at a concentration that will affect the infectious organism. This chapter contains a brief description of several nongenital herpetic diseases that can be treated with acyclovir (ACV) followed by suggested treatment regimens. The use of appropriate virological tests is described elsewhere. All treatment regimens are predicated on the positive clinical and/or laboratory diagnosis of herpes simplex infection.

Oral or paraoral infections caused by herpes simplex type 1 virus are quite common occurrences. In contrast, herpes simplex type 2 virus accounts for only 1-2% of the oral or paraoral infections (2,3). The actual incidence of herpetic labialis infections is unknown. However, Overall (2) placed the number of cases of primary oral herpes at 500,000 per year in the United States. The recurrent form of the disease is said to occur in approximately one third of the population of the United States in a single year (2). The recurrences are quite variable, with some being more severe and others mild. Patients are often unable to predict the severity of a recurrence in advance. This provides a problem for any type of therapy attempted, since mild episodes are often mistaken for treatment efficacy.

There are probably as many proposed therapies for recurrent oral herpes as there are for the common cold. However, until the advent of antiviral drugs, therapy was limited to palliative treatment that sometimes bordered on witchcraft or alchemy. The literature reveals that such diverse compounds as vitamin E (4), smallpox vaccinations (5), levamisole (6), and liquid nitrogen (7) were tested for their effect on "cold sores." Subsequently, antiviral compounds like cytosine arabinaside (8), adenine arabinaside (9), interferon (10), lithium carbonate (11), and idoxuridine (12) have been tested against oral herpes without marked success.

More recently, ACV has been shown by a number of researchers to be of value in treating genital herpes (13-15). With this success in mind, other researchers (16-18) tested various forms of ACV against herpes labialis. In comparison to the HSV-2 results, these tests have sometimes been disappointing and are dependent on the route of administration and the timing of treatment in early prodrome.

PRIMARY GINGIVOSTOMATITIS

The clinical manifestation of a primary oral herpes infection usually begins as a painful redness of the gingiva. In addition, involvement may occur on the buccal mucosa, palate, tonsils, and pharynx as well as the lips or face (Fig. 1). Several days after the onset of the gingival inflammation, yellowish fluid-filled vesicles develop which quickly rupture, leaving a painful ulcer covered by a gray membrane and surrounded by an erythematous halo. Constitutional symptoms of fever, malaise, headache, sore throat, and regional lymphadenopathy precede the onset of the oral inflammation (19). These lesions usually resolve without the formation of a scar in 7-14 days. The course of healing is variable, with reports that healing can occur over periods ranging from 3 to 21 days (20).

Primary oral infections with HSV-1 are rare in infants before the age of 6 months, as protection is provided by antibodies acquired from their mothers. The ages most frequently affected are 3-5 years and in adolescence. On occasion, cases of primary infection are also reported in young adults (18).

Latency, recurrence, and variability of episode severity pose problems for those persons who contract paraoral herpes. After the primary

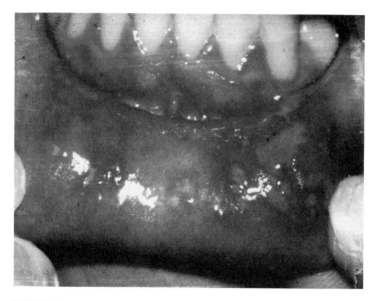

FIGURE 1 Intraoral manifestations of a primary herpetic attack in a 19-year-old female.

herpetic attack has subsided, the virus often lies dormant in the trigeminal nerve ganglion (19). Later, upon receipt of a proper stimulus known as a "trigger," the virus begins to replicate itself rapidly. The virus then migrates back along the axon of the nerve from the ganglion to the mucous membranes of the oral cavity or lips, replicates, and thus causes the formation of the familiar recurrent vesicles. According to Young et al. (21), the triggering factors for paraoral lesions are, in order of importance, emotions, illnesses, sun exposure, trauma, fatigue, menses, chapped lips, and seasonal changes. It is interesting to note that this process occurs despite the fact that the patients have a high antibody level (22).

Recently, some evidence has suggested that the virus may be active constantly but at a very low level in the host cell (23). For those patients who have already suffered through the primary episode of the disease, management therapy for recurrent episodes must concentrate on either ameliorating symptoms, preventing the formation of vesicles, or improving the time it takes for lesions to heal. Approximately 70% of herpes labialis patients experience a prodrome warning of the onset of recurrent herpetic disease (22). Prodromal symptoms may include pain, tingling, itching, and burning that occurs just prior to or concurrent with the macular stage of the disease. It has been demonstrated that viral replication is at its peak during the early stages of the disease (20,22). Since ACV is a virostatic drug, therapy must begin in early prodrome (23). One research group (24) has suggested that therapy that begins at prodrome may be late and intervention should start at the trigger or in a prophylactic manner as suggested by Gibson et al. (25). This prophylactic therapy with ACV has been shown to be quite effective in suppressing recurrent genital herpes attacks (26).

While herpes labialis is not usually life threatening for immunocompetent patients, the pain, tenderness, disfigurement, and recently the social stigma attached to recurrent episodes of this disease are at worst debilitating and at best uncomfortable and annoying. A typical outbreak of a recurrent infection with herpes type 1 virus is illustrated in Figure 2. The vesicles, like those of the primary infection, soon rupture and become secondarily infected (Fig. 3). This compounds the management of the

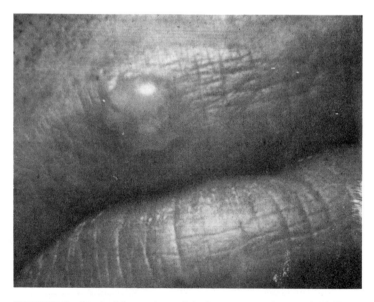

FIGURE 2 Typical herpetic vesicle in recurrent herpes labialis. Courtesy of American Dental Association, Council on Therapeutics.

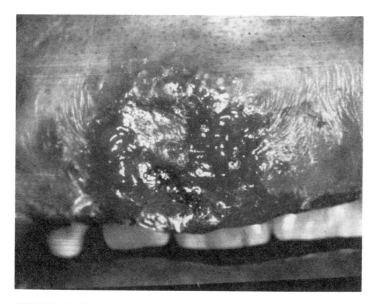

FIGURE 3 Secondary infection of a recurrent herpes labialis lesion. Courtesy of Dr. W. T. McGaw, Edmonton, Alberta (University of Toronto collection).

problem. Recurrent lesions appear on either the vermillion border of the lips or, intraorally, on the mucosa, which is firmly bound down to the underlying periosteum. Even though patients experience symptoms varying from moderate discomfort to severe pain, the disease is fortunately self-limiting in the majority of cases. Nevertheless, for immunocompromised patients, the disease can be life threatening. Whitley et al. (27,28) and other researchers (29) have shown ACV in its IV, oral capsule, and ointment forms to be of value in the management of HSV infections in immunocompromised patients.

TREATMENT REGIMENS

A special caveat is necessary at the beginning of this section, since exact drug regimens are not officially approved by the regulatory agencies of either Canada or the United States for the use of ACV in some of the disease entities discussed. The regimens are those suggested by the author in conjunction with the particular literature cited in each situation and should not constitute a recommendation for use in any unlicensed indication.

Primary Gingivostomatitis

Unfortunately, there are no published studies that relate the effectiveness of ACV in any form to the outbreak of primary disease in normal individuals. However, IV or oral capsule formulations should be the best route of drug administration for primary disease attacks. A suggested dosage would be 800 mg three times per day for 3-5 days. Careful monitoring of the patients is required if long-term IV therapy is contemplated because of the possibility of crystallization of the drug in the renal tubules. Short-term therapy with the oral drug should not present this complication.

Recurrent Herpes Labialis

Topical formulations are to be favored here if the patient's recurrences are mild. Unfortunately, the clinical trials conducted with ACV 5% ointment have failed to show efficacy (16,17,30). The modified aqueous cream with 5% ACV has shown some promise in a recent trial (24) but no definite efficacy. Gibson et al. (25) previously demonstrated efficacy in a small prophylactic cream trial, and Fiddian et al. (31) had originally shown efficacy in an earlier trial in the United Kingdom. The modified aqueous cream is not currently available in the United States or Canada.

However, if the patient has more severe and debilitating episodes, the oral formulation should be the drug of choice. In a recently published trial (32), 200 mg of oral ACV taken at early prodrome and five times per day for 5 days showed some promise, but the results were not as favorable as those with the same drug concentration and herpes genitalia (26). A trial utilizing the oral formulation in a concentration of 800 mg administered at early prodrome (within 1 h of onset of symptoms) and repeated four times per day for 4 days is now planned. Meanwhile, the clinician who wishes to treat his or her patients suffering with recurrent herpes labialis must choose an appropriate concentration without supporting clinical data. However, given the general safety record of ACV, a dose of 800 mg at early prodrome and repeated four times per day for at least 3 days is not an unreasonable approach.

Herpetic Whitlow

Another herpetic infection that can present special problems for those in the health care professions (33-35) is an infection of the finger caused by HSV-1 or HSV-2 (Fig. 4). The usual route of infection is from a patient's lesion to the ungloved finger through any small cut or abrasion. It was originally thought that health care workers had a much higher incidence

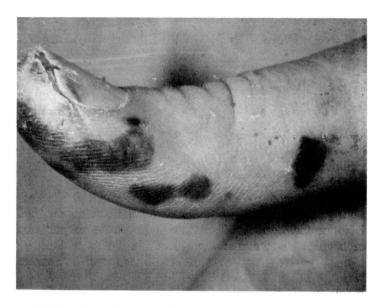

FIGURE 4   Herpetic Whitlow infection in a 28-year-old female physician. Courtesy of Dr. James Plecash, Edmonton, Alberta, Canada.

of this infection. However, a recent report by Gill et al. (36) suggests that other members of the community may also have a high incidence of this disease.

Self-inoculation is possible. Patients with oral lesions should be warned not to touch their herpetic lesions with unprotected fingers and should be warned against touching the lesions and then rubbing their eyes or genitals. Gill et al. (36) reported adult females who had recurrent genital herpes (HSV-2) associated with hand infections of the same strain. Likewise, children with a HSV-1 infection of the hand "commonly" had an associated herpetic gingivostomatitis.

As with herpes labialis, recurrences are possible (37). There is a prodrome associated with the recurrences just as with labialis. However, in the case of Whitlow's, the prodrome seems to be of a more prolonged duration and consists of tingling, pain, or aching in the arm or hand for sometimes as much as 24 h prior to lesion formation.

The onset of primary herpetic Whitlow is invariably painful with vesicular lesions usually forming in the site of inoculation (often adjacent to the nail bed). It is important to establish the diagnosis and rule out bacterial involvement, because it is possible for the lesions to become secondarily infected. Lesions should be carefully drained and dressed, and cultures should be taken at the earliest opportunity.

Given the safety record of ACV, it might be prudent to begin treatment even before an exact diagnosis is established because of the virostatic nature of the drug. Then, if bacteria are implicated via culture and sensitivity testing, an appropriate antibiotic can be prescribed. If the lesions are responding clinically to ACV, there would be no need to add antibiotics. The most effective means of administration of ACV is the intravenous route. However, in very high doses for prolonged periods of time, crystallization of the drug in the kidney tubules is possible. With the oral route of administration, that problem has not been apparent. In the event of a recurrent attack with its long prodrome, oral drug 800 mg repeated twice per day for 7 days was a successful approach reported by Gill et al. in an unblinded series of eight patients (36). For an initial, painful attack when the patient was hospitalized, the IV route was chosen with therapeutic benefit in one case report (38). From 800 to 1000 mg was administered IV every 6 h for 5-7 days with no further need for drug after that time.

Since there is no accepted regimen, clinicians will have to consider the severity of the presentation in the individual case for the selection of IV versus oral administration.

Eczema Herpeticum (Kaposi's Varicelliform Eruption)

This potentially fatal disease is a form of disseminated cutaneous herpes simplex infection which was first described in the early 1940s (39). Clinically, this disease is seen in patients with preexisting cutaneous disease such as atopic eczema or neurodermatitis who become infected with HSV-1 or HSV-2 (40). The diagnosis may be delayed if the new eruption is thought to be an exacerbation of the original disorder.

Clinical signs and symptoms may involve the appearance of tiny umbilicated vesicles often in the same areas of original disease that gradually enlarge and coalesce followed by crusting. Fissuring and erosion accompanied by edema and purulent hemorrhagic exudate are common. The patient's temperature can be elevated for weeks, and the patient will exhibit general lymphadenopathy and have a toxic appearance.

The symptoms can vary in intensity from mild transient disease to a fulminating disease that is life threatening (41). Viremia of the patient's internal organs, bone marrow suppression, and secondary bacterial infection can account for the fatal course of this disease. Previous to treatment with ACV, mortality rates were reported as high as 50%. With proper management and the use of systemic ACV therapy, this rate has declined to something less than 10%.

Swart et al. (43) reported using IV ACV (20 mg/kg three times per day) with success in 1983. Niimura et al. (44) reported that a dosage of 200 mg of oral ACV administered five times per day for 5 days was significantly more effective than placebo in a double-blind, placebo-controlled trial involving approximately 60 patients. As a result, ACV appears to be the treatment of choice in the treatment of eczema herpeticum (1).

Erythema Multiforme

Erythema multiforme (EM) is characterized as an acute inflammatory syndrome with involvement of the skin and mucous membranes (45). The disease can be precipitated by an allergic reaction or by a preceding herpes infection (46). As the name implies, the lesions of this disease can take many forms and may include erosions, bullae, macules, or the characteristic iris or target lesion, which consists of a erythematous circle surrounded by a halo.

The oral manifestations usually include vesiculobullous lesions with an affinity for the vermillion border of the lips, although the lesions may occur throughout the oral cavity. Sometimes the oral lesions appear without the dermatological lesions. When the bullae develop and then burst, they leave raw erosions and desquamatous areas (45).

Traditional treatment included supportive measures and the use of antipyretics, antihistamines, and prednisone. Soft, bland diets are recommended, and the patient must be encouraged to remain hydrated (45,46).

Leigh (1) reported that 70% of a cohort of 80 patients diagnosed as EM had oralabial HSV infections prior to their EM outbreaks. She reported successful treatment with topical (5% modified aqueous cream) or oral ACV when it was used at the early prodrome. Oral ACV actually suppressed the outbreaks of HSV and EM in 22 of 32 patients who were treated prophylactically. Interestingly, six of these 22 patients had no previous history of HSV, which she suggests means that occult HSV infections may cause further cases of EM.

Because of the lack of any accepted treatment regimen, the clinician will be required to choose an appropriate ACV dosage regimen based on the severity of the disease presentation and the age and general condition

60 RABORN

of the patient. However, based on the results reported by Leigh (1) and the drug's general safety record, a course of oral ACV (400-800 mg three times per day for 5 days) might be indicated prior to instituting the traditionally recommended steroid therapy.

REFERENCES

1. Leigh, I. (1987). Management of non-genital HSV infections in immunocompetent patients. Abstract. Wellcome International Antiviral Symposium, 2 Dec.
2. Overall, J. C. Jr. (1981). Antiviral chemotherapy of oral and genital herpes simplex virus infections. In Nahmias, A. J., Dowdle, W. R., and Schinazi, R. I. (eds.): *The Human Herpesviruses: An Interdisciplinary Perspective.* (Proc. Int. Conf. Human Herpesviruses, Atlanta, March 17-20, 1980.) New York, Elsevier, p. 447.
3. Nahmias, A. J., and Starr, E. (1977). Infections caused by herpes simplex viruses. In Hoeprich, P. D. (ed.): *Infectious Diseases.* New York, Harper and Row, pp. 726-735.
4. Fink, M., and Fink, J. (1980). Treatment of herpes simplex by alphatocopherol (vitamin E). *Br. Dent. J.* 148:246.
5. Funk, E. A., and Strausbaugh, L. J. (1981). Vaccina necrosum after smallpox vaccination for herpes labialis. *S. Med. J.* 74(3):383-384.
6. Russell, A. S., Brisson, E., and Grace, M. (1978). A double blind, controlled trial of levamisole in the treatment of recurrent herpes labialis. *J. Infect. Dis.* 137(5):597-600.
7. Adam, J. (1982). Recurrent herpes simplex. Letter to Editor. *Can. Med. J.* 126:894-895.
8. Marks, R., and Koutts, J. (1975). Topical treatment of recurrent herpes simplex with cytosine arabinoside. *J. Med. J. Aust.* 1:479-480.
9. Chein, L., Cannon, N. J., Charamella, L. J., Dismukes, W. E., Whitley, R. J., Buchanan, R. A., and Alford, J. R. (1973). *Can. J. Infect. Dis.* 128:658-663.
10. Cheeseman, S. H., Rubin, R. H., Stewart, J. A., Tolkoff-Rubin, N. E., Cosimi, A. B., Cantell, K., Gilbert, J., Winkle, S., Herrin, J. T., Black, P. H., Russell, P. S., and Hirsh, M. (1979). *N. Engl. J. Med.* 300:1345-1349.
11. Lieb, J. (1979). Remission of recurrent herpes infection during therapy with lithium. *N. Engl. J. Med.* 301:942.
12. Sklar, S. H., and Buiovici-Klein, E. (1979). Adenosine in the treatment of recurrent herpes labialis. *Oral Surg.* 48:416-417.
13. Thin, R. N., Nabarro, J. M., Parker, J. D., and Fiddian, A. P. (1983). Topical acyclovir in the treatment of initial genital herpes. *Br. J. Vener. Dis.* 59: 116-119.

14. Bryson, Y. J., Dillion, M., Lovett, M., Acuna, G., Taylor, S., Cherry, J. D., Johnson, B. L., Wiesmeir, E., Growdon, W., Creagh-Kirk, T., and Keeney, R. (1983). Treatment of first episodes of genital herpes simplex virus infections with oral acyclovir. *N. Engl. J. Med.* 308(16):916-921.
15. Corey, L., Nahmias, A. J., Guinan, M. E., Benedetti, J. K., Critchlow, C. W., and Holmes, K. K. (1983). A trial of topical acyclovir in genital herpes simplex virus infections. *N. Engl. J. Med.* 306(22):1313-1319.
16. Spruance, S. L., Schnipper, L. E., Overall, J. C. Jr., Kern, E. R., Wester, B., Modlin, J., Wenerstrom, G., Burton, C., Arndt, A., Chiu, G. L., and Crumpacker, C. S. (1982). Treatment of herpes simplex labialis with topical acyclovir in polyethelene glycol. *J. Infect. Dis.* 146(1):85-90.
17. Spruance, S. L., Crumpacker, C. S., Schnipper, L. E., Kern, E. R., Marlowe, S., Arndt, K. A., and Overall, J. C. (1984). Early patient-initiated treatment of herpes labialis with topical 10% acyclovir. *Antimicrob. Agents Chemother.* 25(5):553-555.
18. Shaw, M., King, M., Best, J. M., Banatvala, J. E., and Gibson, J. R. (1985). Failure of acyclovir cream in the treatment of recurrent herpes labialis. *Br. Med. J.* 291:7-9.
19. Shafer, G. S., Hine, N. K., and Levy, B. M. (1984). *Textbook of Oral Pathology*, 4th Ed. Philadelphia, Saunders.
20. Spruance, S. L., Overall, J. C. Jr., Kern, E. R., Krueger, G. G., Pliam, V., and Miller, W. (1977). The natural history of recurrent herpes simplex labialis. Implications for antiviral therapy. *N. Engl. J. Med.* 297:69-75.
21. Young, S. K., Rowe, N. H., and Buckanan, R. A. (1976). A clinical study for the control of facial mucocutaneous herpes virus infections. *Oral Surg.* April:498-507.
22. Bader, C., Crumpacker, D. S., Schnipper, L. E., Ransil, B., Clark, J. E., Arnot, K., and Fredburg, I. M. (1978). The natural history of recurrent facial-oral infections with herpes simplex virus. *J. Infect. Dis.* 138(6):897-905.
23. Spruance, S. L., and Wenerstrom, G. (1984). Pathogenesis of recurrent herpes simplex labialis: Implications for antiviral treatment. *Oral Surg. Oral Med. Oral Pathol.* 58(6):667-671.
24. Raborn, G. W., McGaw, W. T., Grace, M., Percy, J., and Samuels, S. (1988). Herpes labialis treatment with acyclovir 5% modified aqueous cream: A double-blind, randomized trial. *Oral Surg. Oral Med. Oral Pathol.* (in press).
25. Gibson, J. R., Klaber, M. R., Harvey, S. G., Tosti, A., Jones, D., and Yeo, J. M. (1986). Prophylaxis against herpes labialis with acyclovir cream: A placebo controlled study. *Dermatologica* 172:104-107.
26. Reichman, R. C., Badger, J., Mertz, G., Corey, L., Richman, D. D., Conner, J. D., Oxman, M. N., Bryson, Y., Tyrrell, D. L., Portni, J., Creagh-Kirk, T., Kenney, R. E., Ashikaga, T., and Dolin, R. (1984). Orally administered acyclovir in the treatment of recurrent herpes simplex genitalis: A controlled trial. *JAMA* 251:2103-2107.

27. Whitley, R., Barton, N., Collins, E., et al. (1982). Mucocutaneous herpes simplex virus infections in immunocompromised patients: A model for evaluation of topical antiviral agents. Proceedings of a symposium on acyclovir sponsored by Burroughs Wellcome Co. and the National Institute of Allergy and Infectious Diseases. *Am. J. Med.* 289:781-789.
28. Whitley, R. J., Levin, M., Barton, N., Hershey, B. J., Davis, G., Kenney, R. E., Wheichel, J., Diethelm, A. G., Kartus, P., and Soong, S. (1984). Infections caused by herpes simplex virus in the immunocompromised host: Natural history and topical acyclovir therapy. *J. Infect. Dis.* 150(3):323-329.
29. Meyers, J. D., Wade, J. C., Mitchell, C. D., Saral, R., Leitman, P. S., Durack, D. T., Levin, M. J., Segreti, A. C., and Balfour, H. H. (1982). Multicenter collaborative trial of intravenous acyclovir for treatment of mucocutaneous herpes simplex virus infection in the immunocompromised host. *Am. J. Med.* 73A:229-235.
30. Raborn, G. W., McGaw, W. T., Grace, M., Samuels, S., and Tyrrell, L. D. (1987). Oral acyclovir and herpes labialis: A double-blind, placebo-controlled clinical trial. *J. Am. Dent. Assoc.* 115:38-42.
31. Fiddian, A. P., Yeo, J. M., Stubbings, R., and Dean, D. (1983). Successful treatment of herpes labialis with topical acyclovir. *Br. Med. J.* 286:1699-1701.
32. Raborn, G. W., McGaw, W. T., Grace, M., and Houle, L. (1989). Herpes labialis treatment with 5% acyclovir ointment: A double-blind, randomized, placebo-controlled trial. *J. Can. Dent. Assoc.* 55:2 135-137.
33. Jones, J. G. (1985). Herpetic Whitlow: An infectious occupational hazard. *J. Occup. Med.* 10:725-728.
34. Rowe, N. H., Heine, C. S., and Kowalski, C. J. (1982). Herpetic whitlow: An occupational disease of practicing dentists. *J. Am. Dent. Assoc.* 105: 471-473.
35. Orkin, F. K. (1970). Herpetic whitlow: Occupational hazard to the anesthesiologist. *Anesthesiology* 33:671-673.
36. Gill, J., Arlette, J., and Tyrrell, D. J. L. (1987). Herpes simplex of the hand: Manifestation and management. Abstract. Wellcome International Antiviral Symposium, Monte Carlo, 2-4 Dec.
37. Merchant, V. A., Molinari, J. A., and Sabes, W. R. (1983). Herpetic whitlow: Report of a case with multiple occurances. *Oral Surg. Oral Med. Oral Pathol.* 55:568-571.
38. Schwandt, N. W., Mjos, D. P., and Lubow, R. M. (1987). Acyclovir and the treatment of herpetic whitlow. *Oral Surg. Oral Med. Oral Pathol.* 64:255-258.
39. Kaposi, M. (1887). Impetigo herpetiformis. Vieriel jahresschrift Dermatol Syphilis 14:273-296.
40. Wheeler, C., et al. (1966). Eczema herpeticum: Primary and recurrent. *Arch. Dermatol.* 93:162-173.
41. Hazen, P., and Eppes, R. (1977). Eczema herpeticum caused by herpesvirus type two. *Arch. Dermatol.* 113:1085-1086.

42. Sanderson, T., et al. (1987). Eczema herpeticum: A potentially fatal disease. *Br. Med. J.* 294:693-694.
43. Swart, R., et al. (1983). Treatment of eczema herpeticum with acyclovir. *Arch. Dermatol.* 119:13-16.
44. Niimura, M., and Nishikawa, T. (1987). Treatment of eczema herpeticum with oral acyclovir. Abstract. Wellcome International Antiviral Symposium, Monte Carlo, 2-4 Dec.
45. Eversole, L. (1984). *Clinical Outline of Oral Pathology: Diagnosis and Treatment*, Second Edition. Philadelphia, Lea and Febiger, p. 92.
46. Rose, L. F., and Kaye, D. (1983). *Internal Medicine for Dentistry.* Toronto, C. V. Mosby, pp. 922-924.

5
Herpes Simplex Virus Infections of the Hand

M. John Gill   *University of Calgary, Calgary, Alberta, Canada*

INTRODUCTION

Herpes simplex viruses (HSV) are capable of infecting almost any cutaneous site (1). Genital and labial HSV infections are common, and their clinical features and management are well described (2,3). However, HSV may also infect other cutaneous sites, including the scalp, toes, knees, elbow, and hand (4-7). The clinical manifestations of infections at these sites may be distinct and have unique characteristics. Unfortunately, their epidemiology, clinical features, and treatment are, by comparison, poorly described.

HSV infection of the hand is one such site. Since the original description of the infection by Adamson in 1909, comparatively little attention has been paid either to the clinical features or to the management of this condition (7). However, this infection would appear to have certain characteristics that are different from those of either labial or genital herpes and could be considered characteristic of HSV infections of the extremities (8,9). The preliminary treatment studies, which are described later, suggest that control of this infection using antiviral therapy may now be possible.

HISTORICAL PERSPECTIVE

For the 50 years following the original description of four children with HSV infection of the fingers, the condition was only rarely reported (7).

65

In 1940, Findlay and MacCallum discussed one new pediatric case, and they also reviewed four other adult cases in which recurrent HSV infection of the hand appeared to be precipitated by traumatic events (10). Over the next decade, in addition to several more pediatric cases, three cases of infection with an associated lymphangitis were reported in young adults (11,12).

Then in 1959 a series of 54 cases of HSV infection of the hand was reported in nurses attending a septic hand clinic at a large hospital (13). The term herpetic whitlow was used, as the infection was purulent and affected the digits. HSV was isolated from the hand in 13 of these patients, and in the remaining cases a presumptive diagnosis was based on history and clinical examination. All of the lesions affected the digits, with the thumb or index finger being most often involved. In five of the 54 cases, more than one digit was infected. The natural history of the infection was described as lasting 2½-3 weeks with an average of 3 weeks' loss of work per case. All of the infections described were the first episode of infection. Recurrence of infection was unusual and far milder by comparison. It occurred at the original site of infection in all seven cases.

Following that report, numerous case reports and small series have documented and discussed HSV infections of the hand occurring in health care workers (HCWs) (14-31). These papers have shown that all HCWs who come in contact with patients' oral secretions appear to be at some risk. Despite an initial concern about cost, the practice of gloving when dealing with patients' oral secretions has now become routine (32,33), and it may have significantly reduced this mode of infection.

Other groups apart from HCWs also appear to be at risk for acquiring HSV infection of the hand. Two papers have reported an association with genital herpes (33,34), and the association of herpes labialis or herpetic stomatitis with HSV infection of the hand (probably secondary to autoinoculation) also appears strong. This has usually been described in children secondary to thumb or finger sucking (35,36), but one paper suggests that it may also follow the practice of nail biting in adults (37).

A variety of different terms have been used to describe HSV infection of the hand. Following the initial term of herpes febrilis of the fingers, recurrent traumatic herpes, herpetic whitlow, aseptic felon, and herpetic paronychia have all been used to describe the infection (7,10,13,37). However, as many papers show that infection may involve any site on the hand and not just the nail bed and that it is seldom associated with obvious trauma; HSV infection of the hand, or herpes manus, would appear to be the most appropriate term to describe the homogeneous nature of HSV infections at this site.

EPIDEMIOLOGY

The literature mentioned above suggests that HSV infection of the hand is predominantly a problem affecting HCWs (1). However, as our clinical experience suggested that this was no longer the case, we undertook a survey vey to ascertain the current epidemiologic profile of this problem in southern Alberta, Canada (38).

The Public Health Laboratory of Southern Alberta provides the only viral diagnostic services to a population base of approximately 1.1×10^6. In order to determine the current epidemiologic pattern the clinical history was reviewed on all of the 79 isolates received between January 1983 and April 1986 in which a specimen taken from the hand was positive for HSV (38). Any additional details not on the original requisition were usually obtained by a discussion with the referring physician. Immunosuppressed patients were excluded from the survey.

Of 74 cases in whom the age was documented there existed a marked bimodal age distribution with 32 cases occurring in adults aged 21-30 years and 16 occurring in children less than 10 years (Fig. 1). The sex distribution differed markedly between adult and pediatric cases. The number of females approximated the males in the pediatric cases but outnumbered the males 2.3:1 in cases over 20 years.

In 67 cases clear evidence was available on the occupation of the patient. This is listed in Table 1. Twenty-five patients were either infants or schoolchildren. Thirty-five patients had non-health care occupations, and seven patients were HCWs. In the remaining 12 patients in the series, the occupation could not be ascertained.

In 43 cases the virus was saved, and the type of HSV was determined. The breakdown by patient age and type of HSV is shown in Figure 2. All patients under 20 years of age had HSV-1 isolated, whereas in the majority of patients above 20 HSV-2 was isolated. In 15 of the 20 patients with HSV-2 infection of the hand, a history of genital herpes was obtained, while in the remaining five cases no history of genital HSV infection or any sexually transmitted diseases could be elicited.

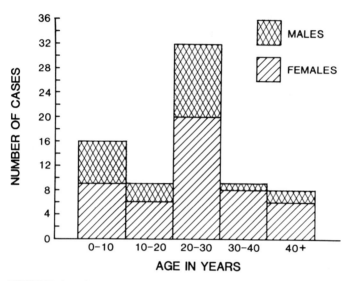

FIGURE 1 Distribution by age and sex of patients with culture-proven HSV infection of the hand.

In 35 cases (nine children, 26 adults), clear information was available as to whether this was a recurrent or the first episode of infection. Eight infections were the first episode, and 27 infections were described as being recurrent. Fifteen of the 16 recurrent infections were caused by HSV-2. One child in the study did have recurrent HSV-1 infection, and we have subsequently seen a second child with recurrent HSV-1 infection of the hand. Only one first-episode isolate was HSV-2, and that occurred

TABLE 1 Occupations of Patients with Herpetic Infection of the Hand

Occupation	Number of patients
Health care workers	7 (8%)
Nurses	3
Respiratory technologists	2
Physicians/dentists	2
Children/students	25 (31%)
Other non-health care occupations	35 (45%)
Not stated	12 (15%)

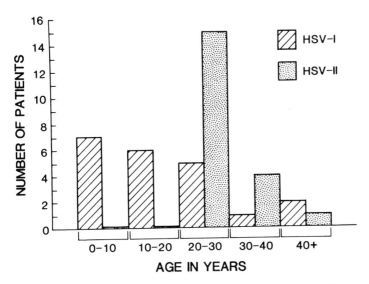

FIGURE 2   Distribution by age and viral type of patients with culture-proven HSV infection of the hand.

in a 24-year-old woman with a simultaneous recurrence of her genital herpes.

In this study known immunocompromised patients with disseminated HSV infection were excluded. No attempt was made to increase physician awareness of the problem or to achieve retrospective laboratory diagnoses of recurrent cases. A minimum incidence of 2.4/100,000 population per year was found. This is most likely an underestimate of the true incidence of this problem in our community. Misdiagnoses, diagnoses based on clinical grounds alone, and diagnoses using nonculture techniques (e.g., Tzanck preparation) undoubtedly account for many other "missed" cases. The observation that the majority of specimens were sent by a very small number of physicians practicing within the city of Calgary (population 600,000) also suggests that the true overall incidence may be higher than stated.

The population in southern Alberta is relatively young, with a higher proportion of individuals aged 20-30 years than many other areas of the continent. However, we are unaware of any other features of the population studied that would give a profile markedly different from many other such communities.

Although interpretation of such a study must be cautious, it does suggest that the traditional idea that HSV infection of the hand predominantly occurs in HCWs is no longer correct and that young adults with recurrent HSV-2 infection of the hand now account for many of the cases being seen in practice. This change in epidemiology most likely reflects both the increasing adherence of good infection control guidelines protecting HCW and the increasing incidence of genital HSV in a young population. Infection secondary to autoinoculation from labial herpes accounted for the majority of pediatric cases, as would be expected. A small number of unusual cases were found in whom no obvious association or route of infection was apparent, and these cases cannot be categorized readily.

CLINICAL FEATURES

First-Episode Infection

The first episode of infection, particularly in HCWs, can be severe, painful, and persistent. Soreness for a few hours localized to a small area precedes the infection, which usually starts as a swelling, then develops into vesicles often around the nail, and progresses quickly to a bullous pustular lesion. The skin may even become hemorrhagic and necrotic. HSV can usually be isolated for about 2 weeks. In 15-20% of patients described with this infection, lymphangitis occurs, and ipsilateral axillary lymphadenopathy is even more common (13). The site involved is usually the fingers, most often on the dominant hand, and it may involve several digits. The infection may be very painful. In many patients it may be their first contact with HSV and the attack may take 3-4 weeks to resolve if untreated. About 10-20% of HCWs are reported to suffer from recurrences.

In children HSV hand infection is usually acquired secondary to autoinoculation from a herpetic stomatitis or herpes labialis, and the clinical course can be overshadowed by the oral infection. Tenderness at the site of infection usually precedes the appearance of vesicles and pustules. One or more fingers may be involved. Ipsilateral lymphadenopathy can be present. The infection usually resolves in about 10-14 days without serious complications. Recurrences after the first episode of infection are reported but appear to be unusual.

The third group of patients with the first episode of HSV infection of the hand are those adults who have autoinoculated their hand from another site. Individuals who bite their nails are at particular risk (37). These infections are usually paronychial and painful. However, they appear significantly less severe than the first episode in HCW and resolve within 1-2 weeks.

Recurrent Infections

Recurrent infections account for the majority of cases seen in clinical practice. Of the 25 cases of recurrent HSV infections of the hand seen by myself and colleagues in Calgary, 23 were caused by HSV-2 and two by HSV-1. The predominance of HSV-2 recurrent infections could reflect an increased predisposition for HSV-2 to cause recurrences at this site, but it could also be explained if the majority of primary infections currently being acquired were HSV-2. An influence of both factors may also be occurring. No obvious differences in clinical features were seen between the HSV-1 and HSV-2 recurrences.

Most recurrent episodes appear to be preceded by a prodrome of pain, itchiness, aching, or burning, often affecting the area of eventual infection or even the whole arm. Prodromes often vary in the same individual from several hours even up to several days. In most patients the prodrome is a good predictor of a clinical attack.

The frequency of recurrences in the patients we followed varied considerably from one or two to over 12 episodes per year. A few patients with a very long history of infection felt that their attacks became less frequent with time. A variety of different factors triggering recurrences were described including physical and emotional stress, menstruation in females, and also local trauma. One right-handed patient regularly developed recurrences on the right thumb after playing racketball.

The fingers were the site of infection in about 60% of cases, with the thumb accounting for most of the remaining cases (Table 2). The pulp space of the finger was most commonly infected, and the nail fold was seldom involved. However, the palm and wrist were also involved in some recurrent episodes. In some patients the infection recurred at different

TABLE 2 Sites Involved by the Herpetic Infection of the Hand in 67 Patients

Site of infection	Number of cases
Fingers	45 (67%)
Thumb	15 (22%)
Palm/wrist	7 (11%)
Dorsum of hand	0 (0%)

sites within the same dermatome. Such patterns of infection, particularly if associated with lymphangitis, appeared to cause diagnostic difficulties.

Recurrences averaged 7-10 days in duration, although longer or shorter episodes were occasionally seen. The infection progressed from a prodromal pain to swelling of the predicted area of infection. Within 24 h vesicles appeared. However, probably because of the keratinization of the skin, they rarely became ulcerated but became enlarged and pustular.

In about 15% of recurrences, ipsilateral lymphangitis occurred. Some patients regularly had lymphangitis with recurrences, while in others it occurred only occasionally. This lymphangitis varied in severity from being mild and localized to a severe form spreading up to the axilla. The condition usually resolved spontaneously without therapy within 36 h. Mild lymphedema and lymphadenopathy were also occasionally seen during a recurrence.

The pain during a recurrence was usually localized to the area infected and only mild in severity. However, this pain and tenderness, particularly if involving the pulp space of the distal phalanx, occasionally caused problems necessitating time off work for some patients—e.g., secretarial work.

COMPLICATIONS

The complications noted with HSV infection of the hand support the need for correct diagnosis and good treatment. One paper has reported the case of a dental hygienist who did not wear gloves routinely. She developed a "worsening dermatitis" of the hand over several days which was initially treated with steroids and antibiotics before the correct diagnosis of HSV infection was eventually made (39). Twenty of 46 patients seen by this hygienist over a 4-day period developed an illness strongly suggestive of HSV oral infection. Restriction endonuclease mapping confirmed identity between the HSV-1 isolated from the hygienist's hands and the HSV-1 isolated from the pharyngeal swabs of nine of her patients. One further study has reported an outbreak of HSV-1 infection of the hand in a pediatric intensive care unit (40). Both patients and staff infected by nosocomial transmission of HSV-1 were documented, stressing the importance of good infection control techniques to prevent transmission.

The risks from HSV infection of the hand are not limited to infecting others. Eiferman and colleagues have reported identical strains of HSV-1 isolated from the hand and the conjunctival sac in two HCWs (41).

This suggests that autoincoulation of another site such as the eyes from an HSV hand infection may occur, and appropriate advice regarding precautions should be given patients, particularly if they use contect lenses.

We have seen one patient who developed chronic mild to moderate lymphedema of the hand following 10 years of recurrent HSV infection of the hand. Her case suggests that chronic multiple untreated infections may eventually cause some lymphatic scarring and result in chronic lymphedema. In addition to local tissue damage and the risks of autoinoculation to other sites, it should be appreciated that this infection, particularly the first episode of infection in HCWs, can be particularly painful and necessitate time off work. Stern et al. found that such patients on average require 3 weeks off work, and this has also been our experience (8,13). Even recurrent episodes can be problematic, particularly if they involve an area of the hand used during work.

Usually in healthy individuals HSV hand infection is self-limiting. However, in immunocompromised patients the clinical features, complications, and outcome may be different. Rapid diagnosis and appropriate therapy must be immediately instituted to prevent a chronic painful infection developing.

MANAGEMENT

A variety of different forms of management have been used in HSV hand infection. Surgical intervention is generally not advised, as it is believed that it may cause either local or systemic dissemination of the virus (14,42). One study, however, has reported that in nine patients with their first episode of infection (eight HCWs, one child) and one patient with recurrent infection involving the nail bed, decompression of the nail bed and segmental nail removal caused a major reduction in pain. No complications of this procedure were reported (43).

Two antiviral drugs have been used for therapy of HSV hand infections. Idoxuridine was the first agent used. Juel-Jensen successively evaluated, in an open study, 0.1%, 5%, and 40% idoxuridine dissolved in dimethyl sulfoxide (DMSO) applied to soaking lint and finger splinting as treatment for HCWs with first-episode infection (44,45). His results suggested that the highest concentration of idoxuridine (40%) was the most successful reducing the duration of viral shedding and pain. No recurrences of infection occurred after this treatment over a limited period of follow-up.

Acyclovir has been evaluated in several preliminary studies. In one HCW with multiple recurrent HSV infection (type not stated), recurrences could be suppressed with a 600-mg daily dose of acyclovir (46). We have also found that in three patients recurrent HSV-2 infections of the hand could be suppressed by daily acyclovir therapy. A second report has discussed the case of a dentist with the first episode of HSV hand infection who was treated with acyclovir and made an excellent clinical response (47). We have also seen a similar favorable response to acyclovir (200 mg PO × 5 daily × 7 days) in an HCW with a first episode of HSV-1 infection. However no blinded or placebo controlled trials have been conducted to confirm this data.

Little research has been described on the treatment of recurrent infections. In one open study 800 mg PO bid of acyclovir administered during the prodromal phase of a recurrent HSV-2 infection of the hand was evaluated (48). This study was based on the rationale that the prodromal phase of a recurrent HSV hand infection is often particularly long when compared to the prodrome of labial or genital infections, and it offers a large "window of opportunity" for therapeutic intervention.

In eight patients treated with acyclovir during the prodromal phase no recurrences were documented. These promising results have encouraged the initiation of a double-blind, placebo-controlled crossover study evaluating acyclovir administered during the prodromal phase of a recurrence. In eight of nine patients so far treated on both arms of the study, a distinct difference between episodes was apparent, suggesting that successful therapeutic intervention during one episode. In the ninth patient, during neither episode studied did any signs of a full recurrence develop, suggesting that an aborted prodrome may have occurred during at least the placebo arm of the study.

One case of a progressive HSV hand infection caused by an acyclovir-resistant virus in a patient with AIDS has been reported (49). However, the pressures to select for resistance were unusual in the case described, and the virus remained sensitive to a second systemic antiviral drug Vidarabine.

We have found the following management approach to be of value. For the first episode of HSV infection of the hand occurring in adults we use a 7 to 10-day course of 200 mg PO × 5 daily acyclovir. The drug can also be administered intravenously if necessary. If pain is very prominent and the infection involves the nail bed, a fine-needle aspiration on at least one occasion relieves the pain until the antiviral therapy has achieved an effect. In children, owing to limited toxicity data, we have not attempted routine antiviral therapy and rely on supportive management provided that the infection is relatively mild.

For recurrent infections in adults, suppression using a daily dose of acyclovir appears promising and should be evaluated prospectively. Early intervention during the lengthy prodromal phase of a recurrent hand infection also appears promising, and at least one formal study is under way to confirm this.

SUMMARY

HSV infection of the hand has some of the characteristics of genital and labial herpes. However, as outlined above, many features are relatively unique. The association with lymphangitis, the bullous/pustular nature of some lesions, the length of the prodrome, and the difficulty in isolation of virus without puncturing the skin are all unusual in genital or labial HSV infections but common in hand infections.

Because of its relative rarity and its changing epidemiology, the management of this HSV infection is poorly investigated. However, the preliminary studies described above suggest that acyclovir is a promising agent that will play an important role for both first-episode and recurrent infections.

REFERENCES

1. Corey, L., and Spear, P. G. (1986). Infections with herpes simplex viruses. *N. Engl. J. Med.* 314:686-691, 749-757.
2. Bader, C., Crumpacker, C. S., Schnipper, L. E., Ransil, B., Clark, J. E., Arndt, K., and Freedberg, I. M. (1978). The natural history of recurrent facial-oral infection with herpes simplex virus. *J. Infect. Dis.* 138:897-905.
3. Corey, L., Adams, H. G., Brown, Z. A., and Holmes, K. K. (1983). Genital herpes simplex virus infections: Clinical manifestations, course and complications. *Ann. Intern. Med.* 98:958-972.
4. Feder, H. M., and White, W. B. (1987). Herpes simplex virus infections. *N. Engl. J. Med.* 316:754-755.
5. Selling, B., Kibrick, S. (1964). An outbreak of herpes simplex among wrestlers (herpes gladatorum). *N. Engl. J. Med.* 270:979-982.
6. White, W. B., and Grant-Kels, J. M. (1984). Transmission of herpes simplex virus type I infection in rugby players. *JAMA* 252:533-535.
7. Adamson, H. G. (1909). Herpes febrilis attacking the fingers. *Br. J. Dermatol.* 21:323-324.
8. Gill, M. J., Arlette, J., and Buchan, K. A. (1989). Clinical manifestations of herpes simplex virus infection of the hand. *J. Am. Acad. Dermatol.* (in press).

9. Gill, M. J., Arlette, J., Buchan, K. A., and Tyrrell, D. L. J. (1988). Herpes simplex infection of the hand. Clinical features and management. *Am. J. Med.* 85(Suppl 2A):53-56.
10. Findlay, G. M., and MacCallum, F. O. (1940). Recurrent traumatic herpes. *Lancet* 1:259-261.
11. Trice, E., and Shafer, J. C. (1953). Recurrent herpes simplex infections of upper extremities with lymphangitis. *Arch. Dermatol. Syph.* 67:37-41.
12. NcNair Scott, T. F., Coriell, L., Blank, H., and Burgoon, C. F. (1952). Some comments on herpetic infection in children with special emphasis on unusual clinical manifestations. *J. Pediatr.* 41:835-843.
13. Stern, H., Elek, S. D., Millar, D. M., and Anderson, H. F. (1959). Herpetic whitlow: A form of cross-infection in hospitals. *Lancet* 2:871-874.
14. Louis, D. S., and Silva, J. (1979). Herpetic whitlow: Herpetic infections of the digits. *Am. J. Hand Surg.* 4:90-93.
15. LaRossa, D., and Hamilton, R. (1971). Herpes simplex infections of the digits. *Arch. Surg.* 102:600-603.
16. Rosato, F. E., Rosato, E. F., and Plotkin, S. A. (1970). Herpetic paronychia—an occupational hazard of medical personnel. *N. Engl. J. Med.* 283:804-805.
17. Hamory, B. H., Osterman, C. A., and Wenzel, R. P. (1975). Herpetic whitlow. (Letter.) *N. Engl. J. Med.* 292:268.
18. Gavelin, G. E., and Knight, C. R. (1965). Herpes simplex infection of the finger. *Can. Med. Assoc. J.* 93:366-367.
19. Hambrick, G. W., Cox, R. P., and Senior, J. R. (1962). Primary herpes simplex infection of fingers of medical personnel. *Arch. Dermatol.* 85:583-589.
20. Merchant, V. A., Molinari, J. A., and Sabes, W. R. (1983). Herpetic whitlow: A report of a case with multiple recurrences. *Oral Surg. Oral Med. Oral Pathol.* 55:568-571.
21. Sehayik, R. I., and Bassett, F. H. (1982). Herpes simplex infection involving the hand. *Clin. Orthop.* 166:138-140.
22. Chang, T. W., and Gorbach, S. L. (1977). Primary and recurrent herpetic whitlow. *Int. J. Dermatol.* 16:752-754.
23. Kanaar, P. (1967). Primary herpes simplex infection of fingers in nurses. *Dermatologica* 134:346-350.
24. Byth, P. L. (1984). Herpetic whitlow. *Intensive Care Med.* 10:321-322.
25. Orkin, F. K. (1970). Herpetic whitlow—occupational hazard to the anesthesiologist. *Anesthesiology* 33:671-673.
26. Giacobetti, R. (1979). Herpetic whitlow. *Int. J. Dermatol.* 18:55-58.
27. Brightman, V. J., and Guggenheimer, J. G. (1970). Herpetic paronychia—primary herpes simplex infection of the finger. *J. Am. Dent. Assoc.* 80:112-115.
28. Rowe, N. H., Heine, C. S., and Kowalski, C. J. (1982). Herpetic whitlow: An occupational disease of practicing dentists. *J. Am. Dent. Assoc.* 105:471-473.
29. Greaves, W. L., Kaiser, A. B., Alford, R. H., and Schaffner, W. (1980). The problem of herpetic whitlow among hospital personnel. *Infect. Cont.* 1:381-385.

30. Ward, J. R., and Clark, L. (1961). Primary herpes simplex virus infection of the fingers. *JAMA* 176:226-228.
31. Lucey, J., and Baroni, M. (1984). Herpetic whitlow. *Am. J. Nurs.* 84:60-61.
32. Orkin, F. K. (1975). Herpetic whitlow. *N. Engl. J. Med.* 292:648.
33. Glogau, R., Hanna, L., and Jawetz, E. (1977). Herpetic whitlow as part of genital virus infection. *J. Infect. Dis.* 136:689-692.
34. Crane, L. R., and Lerner, A. M. (1978). Herpetic whitlow: A manifestation of primary infection with herpes simplex virus type 1 or type 2. *J. Infect. Dis.* 137:855-856.
35. Novick, N. L. (1985). Autoinoculation herpes of the hand in a child with recurrent herpes labialis. *Am. J. Med.* 79:139-142.
36. Feder, H. M., and Long, S. S. (1983). Herpetic whitlow: Epidemiology, clinical characteristics, diagnosis and treatment. *Am. J. Dis. Child.* 137:861-863.
37. Muller, S. A., and Herrmann, E. C. (1970). Association of stomatitits and paronychias due to herpes simplex. *Arch. Dermatol.* 101:396-402.
38. Gill, M. J., Arlette, J., and Buchan, K. (1988). Herpes simplex virus infection of the hand. A profile of 79 cases. *Am. J. Med.* 84:89-92.
39. Manzella, J. P., McConville, J. H., Valenti, W., Menegus, M. A., Swierkosz, E. M., and Arens, M. (1984). An outbreak of herpes simplex virus type 1 gingivostomatitis in a dental hygiene practice. *JAMA* 252:2019-2022.
40. Adams, G., Stover, B. H., Keenlyside, R. A., Hooton, T. M., Buchman, T. G., Roizman, B., and Stewart, J. A. (1981). Nosocomial herpetic infections in a pediatric intensive care unit. *Am. J. Epidemiol.* 113:126-132.
41. Eiferman, R. A., Adams, G., Stover, B., and Wilkins, T. (1979). Herpetic whitlow and keratitis. *Arch. Ophthalmol.* 97:1079-1081.
42. Flatt, A. E. (1972). *Infections in the Care of Minor Hand Injuries*, 4d Ed. St. Louis, Mosby.
43. Polayes, I. M., and Arons, M. S. (1980). The treatment of herpetic whitlow—a new surgical concept. *Plast. Recon. Surg.* 65:811-817.
44. Juel-Jensen, B. E. (1970). Herpetic whitlow: Results of treatment with idoxuridine. *J. Am. Coll. Health Assoc.* 18:227-230.
45. Juel-Jensen, B. E. (1971). Herpetic whitlow: A medical risk. *Br. Med. J.* 4:681.
46. Laskin, O. L. (1985). Acyclovir and suppression of frequently recurring herpetic whitlow. *Ann. Intern. Med.* 102:494-495.
47. Schwandt, N. W., Mjos, D. P., and Lubow, R. M. (1987). Acyclovir and the treatment of herpetic whitlow. *Oral Surg. Oral Med. Oral Pathol.* 64:255-258.
48. Gill, M. J., Buchan, K., Arlette, J., and Tyrrell, D. L. J. (1986). Acyclovir therapy for herpetic whitlow. *Ann. Intern. Med.* 105:631.
49. Norris, S. A., Kessler, H. A., Fife, K. H. (1988). Severe progresive herpetic whitlow caused by an acyclovir resistant virus in a patient with AIDS. *J. Infect. Dis.* 157:209-210.

6
Treatment of First-Episode Genital Herpes

Cynthia L. Fowler* and Gregory J. Mertz *University of New Mexico School of Medicine, Albuquerque, New Mexico*

INTRODUCTION

Herpetic diseases have been noted for at least 25 centuries. The Greek word herpes means "to creep." Many different species from invertebrates to mammals are susceptible to infection with herpesviruses. Of the human herpesviruses, herpes simplex virus (HSV) is one of the most commonly encountered and extensively studied. Genital herpes was first described in 1736 by John Astruc, a French physician. By the early 1900s it was known to be a transmissible disease of viral etiology, and a tissue culture system was available. In the 1960s it was shown that there were two antigenic types, and the association between antigenic type and the site of infection was demonstrated. In the 1980s a new antiviral agent, acyclovir, became available for treatment of HSV infections. This chapter will deal with the diagnosis and treatment of first-episode genital herpes infection.

DESCRIPTION OF THE VIRUS

The human herpesvirus group includes herpes simplex virus (HSV), varicella zoster virus (VZV), Epstein-Barr virus (EBV), cytomegalovirus (CMV), and the recently recognized human herpesvirus-6 (HHV-6). This group of viruses is characterized by icosahedral shape, linear double-stranded DNA, and the presence of a lipid envelope (1,2). With the possible

---

**Present affiliation*: National Institutes of Health, Bethesda, Maryland

exception of HHV-6, for which information is incomplete, these viruses are all capable of establishing latency after initial infection. Herpes simplex virus can be divided into two types (HSV-1 and HSV-2) based on glycoprotein antigens located on the viral envelope and on the membranes of infected cells. There is approximately 50% base-sequence homology between the two types. There are type-common antigens (those shared by both types) and type-specific antigens (those found on only one type). Utilizing restriction endonuclease analysis of the viral DNA, each type can be further divided into strains, which are of epidemiologic interest but otherwise of no known clinical significance.

EPIDEMIOLOGY: INCIDENCE AND PREVALENCE

Herpes simplex virus infections are found in most populations throughout the world. Infection may occur at any time during the year.

Utilizing serological testing it has been demonstrated that HSV-1 infection usually occurs early in childhood (3). The prevalence of HSV-1 antibody is higher in persons from lower socioeconomic groups than in those from middle or upper socioeconomic groups. In the Western industrialized countries, the incidence of HSV-1 infection appears to be declining.

Antibody to HSV-2 first appears in the population at puberty, and the incidence increases with age and sexual experience (3,4). HSV-2 infection is more prevalent in persons from lower socioeconomic groups. However, because the incidence of HSV-1 infection is lower in persons from the middle and upper socioeconomic classes, true primary genital herpes infections (those that occur in persons without preexisting antibody to HSV-1 or HSV-2) are more common in this group.

Approximately 60-90% of first-episode genital herpes infections are caused by HSV-2, and 10-40% by HSV-1 (5,6). The two types cause clinically indistinguishable first episodes of genital herpes. However, patients with HSV-2 genital infections are much more likely to experience recurrences than those with HSV-1 genital infections, and the recurrences of genital HSV-2 infections occur more frequently than the recurrences of genital HSV-1 infections (7-9).

Patients are rarely infected at one anatomic site with both HSV-1 and HSV-2 or with more than one strain of the same type (10). However, most patients are infected with only one strain of HSV at a given site, and serial cultures of subsequent recurrences show the same virus type and strain (11).

In the United States, accurate figures on the incidence of genital herpes are lacking for a variety of reasons. Unlike some other sexually trans-

mitted diseases, physicians are not required to report genital HSV infections. There is a high rate of asymptomatic cases, and symptomatic patients
do not always seek medical care. Therefore most studies probably underestimate the incidence. To confuse the matter more, not all reported studies
have distinguished between the first and recurrent episodes. However,
data from a variety of sources indicate that the incidence of patients with
genital herpes seen by physicians is increasing (12,13). This most likely
represents both an increasing awareness of the disease and willingness to
seek care (especially with the advent of effective treatment), as well as a
true increase in incidence of infection.

MODE OF TRANSMISSION

Genital herpes is acquired by contact with virus-infected secretions. HSV
can penetrate mucosa but not intact skin. Entry is aided by mechanical
rubbing, resulting in abrasion of the skin. The incubation period ranges
from 1 to 26 days but averages 6-8. Persons with active lesions due to a
primary infection are the most contagious, because virus is present in
larger amounts than in persons who are experiencing a nonprimary infection or a recurrent episode. Although small amounts of herpesvirus may
be shed in the absence of symptoms (14), persons with active lesions shed
higher numbers of virus. Thus contact with a symptomatic partner is more
likely to lead to infection than contact with an asymptomatic partner who
is shedding virus. However, because the asymptomatic partner may be
unaware of the potential for transmission, he or she may be more likely
to engage in sexual activity. In one recent study it was shown that 60% of
the source contacts of new cases of genital herpes claimed to be asymptomatic at the time the disease was transmitted (15).

HSV can be transmitted by oral-genital contact. During oral sex a
person with oral herpes may transmit the infection to the partner, resulting
in genital herpes. Oral herpes infection can occur by contact with a partner's HSV-infected genitals.

Although HSV has been cultured from the surfaces of inanimate ob-
jects, the virus is susceptible to desiccation and to extremes of temperature, so that transmission via aerosolation or fomites is unlikely (16).

PATHOGENESIS

After the virus is inoculated onto susceptible mucosa or abraded skin,
productive replication occurs in the epidermal and dermal cells. The process
of viral replication is complex (2). Initially the virus attaches to receptors

on the cell membrane and enters the cytoplasm. The DNA is released and migrates to the nucleus. Inside the nucleus, viral DNA is synthesized and viral messenger RNA is transcribed. The messenger RNA migrates to the cytoplasm, where it is translated into the various viral-specific proteins. These proteins are the transported back to the nucleus, where viral DNA maturation and encapsidation occur. Next the nucleocapsids bud through the nuclear membrane, acquiring the viral envelope in the process. Traveling through the cytoplasm in vacuoles, the virus leaves the cell. Productive infection is fatal to the host cell.

Histologically, there is a ballooning of the cells and degeneration of cell nuclei. A vesicle forms from within the epithelium containing multinucleated giant cells and cells with the virus-induced eosinophilic nuclear inclusions (Cowdry type A bodies). Infection spreads to contiguous cells, progressing toward sensory and autonomic nerve endings. Once the peripheral nerve cells are infected, the viral nucleocapsids are transported inside the axons to the nerve cell bodies in the spinal cord ganglia. It is probably at this point that latent infection is established, often before the clinical appearance of lesions. Viral replication continues in the ganglia and contiguous neural tissue. Infectious virions then migrate distally along sensory nerves, resulting in spread of the infection to additional skin surfaces. This explains the large affected surface area and the high frequency of new lesions distant from the initial crop of vesicles that characterizes the initial infection (Fig. 1, before page 47).

Host immune responses influence the acquisition of infection, the severity of disease, the development of latency, the maintenance of latency, and the frequency of recurrences. Both antibody-mediated and cell-mediated immune reactions are involved (17,18). Patients with defective cell-mediated immunity have more severe and more extensive herpetic infections than patients with defective humoral immunity. It is not known whether immune response to any one particular viral glycoprotein is important in the course of disease, although suppression of the antibody response to one glycoprotein (gD) and one structural protein with acyclovir treatment in primary disease is associated with prolongation of symptoms during the first recurrence (19,20).

CLINICAL COURSE

The first clinically apparent episode of genital herpes may be a true first episode due to acute infection or the first symptomatic (i.e., first recognized) recurrence in a previously infected patient. A true first episode of genital herpes may be classified as either a primary infection or a nonprimary infection. Primary infection is that which occurs in a patient without previous exposure to either type of HSV. Nonprimary infection occurs in a patient who has had previous infection with the heterologous type. Patients with primary infection lack antibody to HSV in acute sera, whereas antibody to the heterologous type of HSV can be demonstrated in acute sera from patients with nonprimary infection. Primary infection is likely to produce a larger number of lesions that are more painful and that persist for a longer period of time than nonprimary infection. In addition, patients with primary infection are more likely to experience systemic symptoms (1,4,5).

Both men and women with symptomatic first episode of genital herpes most frequently present with multiple, widely spaced, bilateral, vesicular, or ulcerative lesions on the external genitalia (4,5) (Figs. 1, 2, before page 47). There may have been preceding erythema and edema of the area. Lesions typically start as multiple small vesicles or papules that rapidly spread over the external genitalia, coalescing into larger lesions. In men the glans and the penile shaft are most commonly involved. In women the lesions are typically found on the mons pubis and the labia. As the lesions age, the vesicules become pustular and then ulcerate. If located on dry skin, they will crust. When located on moist or intertriginous areas such as the labia minora, vaginal introitus, or anus, the vesicles quickly lose their epithelial covering, and moist ulcers are the most predominant lesion.

Herpetic lesions are usually described as painful or irritating. They are often associated with paresthesia that may precede the appearance of the vesicles. Discomfort is greatest early in the episode and tends to lessen as the lesions crust.

The lesions usually persist for 2-3 weeks, gradually healing without scar formation. During primary infection, formation of new lesions may occur in waves so that lesions in different stages of development will be present simultaneously (Fig. 1, before page 47). The entire course from first symptoms to healing of the last wave of lesions lasts for an average of 3 weeks (Fig. 3, before page 47).

Viral shedding correlates with the appearance of the genital lesions. The highest concentration of virus occurs as the vesicle forms and diminishes as it crusts or ulcerates. For example, in one study (21), cultures were positive from 94% of vesicular lesions, 87% of pustular lesions, 70% of ulcerated lesions, and 27% of crusted lesions. However, cultures may also be positive from sites without obvious lesions such as urethra, cervix, or rectum. During the first episode of illness, virus shedding occurs

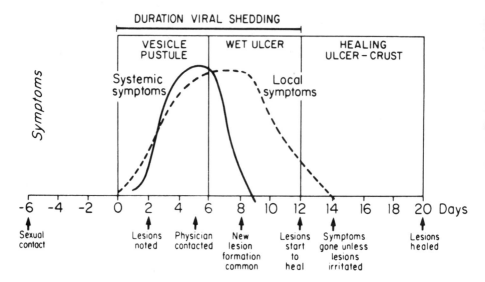

FIGURE 3   The clinical course of primary genital herpes simplex virus infection. (From Corey et al. (5), with permission.)

in higher numbers and for a longer period of time than in subsequent re-current episodes. On the average, patients with untreated primary infection excrete the virus for 11 days, those with untreated nonprimary infection for 7 days, and those with recurrent lesions for 4 days (5).

Tender inguinal lymphadenopathy frequently appears by the second to third week of illness and often persists until after the lesions have healed.

Symptoms tend to be more severe in women than in men (Table 1). Women often complain of pain, dysuria, itching, and vaginal discharge. In a recent study dysuria was noted by 83% of women with primary genital HSV infection. The virus was cultured from the urethra of 82% of those with dysuria (5). In addition to the dysuria due to urethritis, discomfort can be due to urine contacting sensitive and painful ulcers of the external genitalia during urination. Uncommonly HSV can cause urethritis without associated external lesions. In one study the virus was cultured from the urethra of 5% of women with acute urethral syndrome who had no visible lesions (22).

Symptoms of dysuria are less common in men. In one study, dysuria was noted in only 44% of male patients with first-episode genital herpes, and only 28% of these men had positive urethral cultures. However, of

FIRST-EPISODE GENITAL HERPES 85

TABLE 1   Clinical Symptoms and Manifestations of Primary Genital HSV-2 Infections in Men and Women

	Men (n = 63)	Women (n = 126)
Patients with systemic symptoms, %*	39	68
Patients with meningitis symptoms, %*	11	36
Patients with local pain, %	95	99
Mean duration of local pain (range), days	10.9 (1-40)	12.2 (1-37)
Patients with dysuria, %*	44	83
Mean duration of dysuria (range), days**	7.2 (2-20)	11.9 (1-26)
Patients with urethral or abnormal vaginal discharge, %*	27	85
Mean duration of discharge, days**	5.6	12.9
Patients with tender adenopathy, %	80	81
Mean duration of adenopathy, days**	8.6	14.2
Mean number of lesions (range)	15.7 (3-50)	15.4 (1-60)
Patients with bilateral lesions, %	77	82
Mean area of lesions (range), mm^2	427 (6-1671)	550 (8-3908)
Patients forming new lesions during infection, %	76	74
Mean number of days of new lesion formation (range)	7.2 (1-18)	8.1 (1-20)
Mean duration viral shedding from genital lesions, days	10.5	11.8
Patients with herpes simplex virus isolated from urethra, %*	28	82
Patients with herpes simplex virus isolated from cervix, %	NA	88
Mean duration viral shedding from cervix, days	NA	11.4
Mean duration of lesions, days**	16.5	19.7

*p < .05 (chi-square test).
**p < .05 (Student's t-test).
Source: Corey et al. (5), with permission.

those who noted a urethral discharge as well as dysuria, 90% were culture positive from the urethra (5). The discharge is usually clear and mucoid and less in quantity than would be expected from the severity of the symptoms. Gram stain of the discharge commonly shows 5-15 WBCs per 1000× field.

During the first episode of infection, HSV can be cultured from the cervix in 80-88% of the primary and 65% of the nonprimary cases. Cervical findings range from mild erythema to severe necrotic cervicitis, and typical ulcerative lesions may be seen on the ectocervix (Fig. 2b, before page 47). Cervicitis can be the only manifestation ot HSV infection and may be as asymptomatic (23).

Rectal and perianal HSV lesions are seen in homosexual men and heterosexual women who engage in receptive anal intercourse. Perianal ulcers without involvement of the rectum can occur by local spread from genital infection.

HSV is a common cause of proctitis in homosexual men. Symptoms and signs may include severe anorectal pain, tenesmus, constipation, sacral paresthesias, difficulty in urinating, fever, inguinal lymphadenopathy, rectal discharge, rectal bleeding, and ulceration of the perianal skin and the rectal mucosa (24).

Herpetic infection of the adult pharynx may be acquired by oral-genital contact. The patient complains of a severe sore throat. Findings in the pharynx range from a mild erythema to severe exudative pharyngitis. Ulcerative lesions are often present. Most patients will also have tender anterior cervical lymphadenopathy. Commonly, the patient with herpes pharyngitis has acquired genital infection as well. Because oral exposure and genital exposure usually occur simultaneously, sexually acquired herpes pharyngitis is usually seen in association with the signs and symptoms of genital herpes (5).

During the first episode, systemic symptoms are common, occurring more often in primary than in nonprimary infections and more often in women than in men (5). Patients often experience headache, malaise, myalgias (especially backache), and fever. The systemic manifestations usually coincide with the onset of the genital lesions, peak within 3-4 days, and then gradually subside.

COMPLICATIONS

Aseptic meningitis has been reported in approximately one third of women with primary HSV-2 genital infections. The percentage of men is lower. Symptoms include headache, stiff neck, and photophobia. In one study, from Seattle (5), 16% of patients with these symptoms required hospitalization. These patients all had fever, nuchal rigidity, positive Kernig's or Brudzinski's signs, lymphocytic pleocytosis of the CSF, and normal CSF glucose. Patients usually recover without neurological sequelae. Recurrence of the meningitis is rare with recurrent episodes of the genital lesions.

Herpes encephalitis in adults is almost always due to HSV-1. However, HSV-2 has been isolated from temporal lobe biopsies in two patients with AIDS and clinical findings of herpes encephalitis. Neither patient had genital lesions by history or exam.

Urinary retention is a frequent complaint of infected women. Usually this is due to voluntary inhibition of micturition because of pain, and the difficulty resolves as the painful genital lesions resolve.

Inability to urinate due to pain must be distinguished from urinary retention due to autonomic nerve dysfunction. The latter is suggested when urine retention develops when local pain is absent or is clearly improving. This is occasionally seen in patients with genital herpes (more common in women than in men, 25) and can be accompanied by sacral dysesthesia and constipation. In men, autonomic dysfunction is more commonly associated with herpes proctitis than with genital infection. In addition to the above symptoms, men may also experience impotence and decreased rectal sphincter tone. In many patients the dysfunction persists after the external lesions have resolved, then gradually improves over several months.

Transverse myelitis associated with herpes infection has been reported. This is characterized by a rapidly progressing bilateral lower-extremity weakness, decreased tendon reflexes, and autonomic dysfunction. Neurologic sequelae may occur (26).

Rarely some patients experience recurrent episodes of erythema multiforme triggered by herpes infections (27).

In immunocompetent hosts, extragenital lesions sometimes occur and are usually the result of autoinoculation. These extragenital lesions most often appear after the development of the genital lesions. They are most commonly located on the buttocks, thighs, groin, and fingers. Occasionally spread to the eye occurs with resultant HSV keratoconjunctivitis.

Immunocompromised patients, especially those with defects of cell-mediated immunity, are at risk for developing disseminated disease. Typical vesicles may appear at any location on the skin. Visceral involvement may include the lung, liver, kidney, joints, and adrenal glands. Mortality in these patients is high.

A recent study (28) showed that pregnant women who develop a primary HSV infection have a high risk (40%) of perinatal morbidity. The highest risk appears to be in those women who acquire primary genital herpes infection in the third trimester. Women with a primary first episode are more likely to have cervical involvement than women with non-primary or recurrent infections. Involvement of the cervix is thought to increase the chance for fetal infection. These women are likely to have premature labor or early fetal demise. Their babies are more likely to have intrauterine growth retardation or HSV infection in utero. Women with primary genital herpes shed higher concentrations of the virus and have a higher incidence of asymptomatic viral shedding from the cervix that persists for a longer period of time than women who have a nonprimary first episode or a recurrent episode. Thus, they are more likely to be shedding the virus at the onset of labor, and their babies are more likely to be exposed to HSV at birth.

Although uncommon, herpetic lesions may become infected with bacteria. Secondary infection occurs late in the course of the episode and is associated with increasing erythema, induration, and pain. Purulent drainage or abscess formation may occur. Causative organisms are most commonly derived from the skin or gut flora.

Presence of genital lesions, including those caused by HSV, has been associated with an increased incidence of AIDS. It is postulated that the lesions serve as ports of entry for the virus, facilitating infection upon exposure to HIV-containing secretions (29).

DIAGNOSIS

To treat and counsel a patient with genital herpes, it is important to make an accurate diagnosis. In the United States HSV is the most common cause of sexually acquired genital ulcers but still must be distinguished from other causes such as syphilis, chancroid, lymphogranuloma venereum, genital warts, molluscum contagiosum, and trauma. Most symptomatic patients can be diagnosed clinically on the basis of the previously described signs and symptoms. However, in patients with atypical findings or with asymptomatic infections, the diagnosis may be more difficult, and laboratory confirmation may be helpful. Genital infection with HSV-1 versus HSV-2 cannot be differentiated clinically. Since the prognoses for recurrence differ, determination of the type of virus is recommended whenever possible during the first clinical episode of infection.

Useful laboratory methods include viral culture, detection of viral antigens in clinical specimens, cytology, and serology (30,31). The sensitivity of all laboratory methods for detecting HSV depends on the number of virus particles present as well as accuracy in the collection and transportation of the specimen.

The gold-standard laboratory method for confirmation of HSV infection is culture. The virus grows well in a variety of tissue culture systems, producing a typical cytopathic effect in 24-72 h (40-50% within 24 h, 80% within 48 h, and 90% within 72 h) (32). Once the cytopathic effect is evident, typing of the isolate can be performed by staining of the HSV-infected cells with HSV type-specific monoclonal antibodies that are conjugated to a variety of agents (e.g., fluorescein, immunoperoxidase, or biotin-avidin with fluorescein) (33). A modified technique combines growth in tissue culture with early immunochemical staining for HSV antigens before cytopathic effect is evident (34).

Recently developed methods (35,36) that involve staining smears taken directly from suspicious lesions with conjugated type-specific monoclonal antibody are able to differentiate the two types of HSV as well as varicella zoster virus (VZV). Taking only 1-4 h, these direct staining techniques are quicker and less expensive than viral culture. They appear to have acceptable sensitivity and specificity compared to viral culture when large numbers of virus are present (such as specimens from early vesicular lesions) but are less sensitive when smaller numbers of virus are present (such as specimens from late ulcerative lesions or swabs from the rectum, urethra, or cervix).

Tzanck preps showing multinucleated giant cells are suggestive of HSV or VZV infection (37). To make a Tzanck prep, a suspicious lesion is unroofed and scraped. The scrapings are placed on a slide and then stained with Wright's stain. Although easy and quick to do, Tzanck preps are much less sensitive than either culture or fluorescent antibody staining. Also this technique cannot distinguish HSV from VZV or HSV-1 from HSV-2.

On PAP smears, HSV infection is suggested by the presence of cells with intranuclear inclusions or multinucleated giant cells. As with the Tzanck prep, the sensitivity and specificity are low.

Proper collection and handling of the specimen will ensure the highest possible recovery of virus. To obtain a specimen for culture or smear (32), preferably choose a vesicular or pustular lesion rather than an ulcerative or crusted one. Unroof the lesion with a sterile needle, and firmly swab the base of the lesion. Dacron-tipped swabs are preferred. Swabs containing calcium alginate should not be used, as the calcium alginate binds the herpesvirus, rendering the virus noninfectious (38). Place the swab in viral transport media for culture or fluorescent antibody staining. Gently roll the swab on a glass slide if a smear for Tzanck prep is desired. Prior to use, viral transport media should be frozen or stored at 4 °C. After inoculation the media should be kept at 4 °C but not frozen (39). HSV will remain viable in the transport media at this temperature for up to 72 h, allowing adequate time to transport the specimen to a virology laboratory.

As previously mentioned, there are type-specific and type-common antigens present on the virus. When patients who are infected with one type of HSV acquire infection with the heterologous type, the predominant antibody response is to the type-common antigens. In this case there is little induction of the type-specific antibody to the new type of virus (40). With conventional assays, detection of the type-specific antibodies in serum is very difficult owing to the overwhelming amount of the type-common antibodies. Thus, it has been difficult to diagnose newly acquired HSV-2 infections by serology in patients previously infected with HSV-1. Recently developed assays such as Western blot have a higher sensitivity and specificity for the type-specific antibodies (41,42).

Careful analysis of serologic data indicates that patients who present with their first clinical episode of genital herpes fall into several categories. The first group is patients who are experiencing their first infection with HSV. They will have no detectable antibody to either type of HSV initially but will develop antibodies within 4 weeks after the onset of symptoms. These patients have a primary first episode of genital herpes. The next group of patients is those who have been previously infected with one type of HSV (usually oral HSV-1) and have a newly acquired genital infection with the other type of HSV (usually HSV-2). These patients will have antibody to HSV that is detectable at the onset of their genital symptoms. Using the conventional assays, the presence of the old infection could be determined, but the new often could not be distinguished. Utilizing the newly developed and more specific assays, antibody to the previously acquired viral type can be found initially, and antibody to the newly acquired type will appear after a few weeks. These patients have a nonprimary first episode of genital herpes. The third group of patients can be shown to have antibody to both HSV-1 and HSV-2 at the time of initial presentation. Although it is the first clinically evident episode, these patients have had asymptomatic or unrecognized infection in the past and are actually experiencing a recurrent episode (43). A small number of patients have antibody to one type of HSV at presentation but do not develop antibody to the heterologous type following genital infection. Presumably these patients were previously infected at another anatomical site (e.g., the lips) with HSV-1 or HSV-2 and then acquired genital infection with the same type of HSV.

Although serologic testing is of great use to the researcher, it is not routinely obtained by the clinician. Documenting a primary versus nonprimary infection by serology adds to expense and does not alter therapy.

TREATMENT

Acyclovir is a nucleoside analog that has demonstrated specific activity against herpes simplex virus. Acyclovir is available as a 5% topical cream (in Europe) or ointment (in the United States), a 200-mg oral capsule, and an IV solution. Studies comparing the three formulations to placebo (44-49) in treatment of first episodes of genital herpes have demonstrated significant virologic and clinical benefit. Acyclovir has been shown to decrease the duration of local symptoms and viral shedding and to hasten resolution of existing lesions (Table 2). Effects of treatment were more dramatic in primary than in nonprimary episodes. Although there has not been a study that directly compares the three formulations of acyclovir, analysis of the data (50) from the sequential studies in the same clinic at the University of Washington suggested that the efficacies of IV and

TABLE 2 Signs and Symptoms of First-Episode Primary Genital Herpes in Acyclovir-Treated (ACV) Versus Placebo-Treated Patients

Median No. days after start of treatment	Treated patients					
	Topical ACV $n = 28$	Placebo ointment $n = 23$	Intravenous ACV $n = 14$	Placebo $n = 13$	Oral ACV $n = 33$	Placebo $n = 27$
Local itching	4*	8	2**	8	4*	6
Local pain	5*	7	3*	7	5**	9
Dysuria	4	5	4*	7	3*	6
Vaginal discharge	6	7	4**	11	6	8
Percentages with systemic symptoms at 7 days of treatment	18%	30%	0**	46%	9%	18%
Complete crusting of lesions	8*	13	6**	13	7**	13
Complete healing of lesions	11*	15	9**	21	13**	20
Percent forming new lesions after 48 h of therapy	69%	74%	20%**	69%	13%**	74%

*$p < .05$ Mantel-Cox test.
**$p < .01$ Mantel-Cox test.
All comparisons are between patients who had described symptoms at time of enrollment into the study.
Source: Corey et al. (50), with permission.

TABLE 3   Treatment of Primary Genital Herpes with Acyclovir: Comparison of Intravenous, Oral, and Topical Preparation (percent reduction as compared to control group)

Study size	Intravenous acyclovir $n = 27$	Oral acyclovir $n = 59$	Topical acyclovir $n = 51$
Duration of viral shedding: genital lesions	85%	80%	55%
Duration of viral shedding: cervix	89%	92%	65%
Reduction in new lesion formation	Yes	Yes	No
Time to complete crusting of lesions	54%	46%	34%
Time to complete healing of lesions	57%	35%	29%
Local itching	75%	33%	55%
Local pain	57%	44%	26%
Dysuria	43%	50%	12%
Vaginal discharge	64%	25%	16%
Systemic symptoms	Yes	± *	No

*Not statistically significant from placebo-treated control group.
Source: Corey et al. (50).

oral acyclovir are similar and that both are superior to topical treatment (Table 3). The systemic forms appeared to decrease local pain and itching quicker than topical acyclovir. Duration of viral shedding and time to crusting of lesions were shorter with the IV and oral preparations than with the ointment (Fig. 4). In addition, the systemic forms of acyclovir significantly shortened the duration of dysuria and suppressed the formation of new lesions during the course of therapy, but topical acyclovir did not. Combined treatment with topical and systemic therapy appears to offer no advantage over systemic therapy alone (51).

As a result of these comparisons, use of the systemic forms of acyclovir is recommended for treatment of first episode genital herpes. Oral acyclovir is preferred, because it is almost equal in efficacy to the intravenous form but is less expensive and more convenient to administer. The dosage for first episodes is 200 mg orally five times daily (every 4 h while awake) for a total of 10 days (Table 4). When started within 7 days

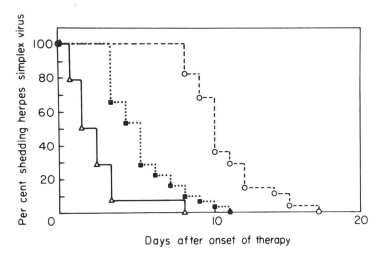

FIGURE 4 Duration of viral shedding from genital lesions in patients with primary genital herpes after stratification for differences in viral shedding and healing times in placebo-treated patients. Comparison of virological effects of intravenous, oral, and topical acyclovir ($p < .001$ for comparison between intravenous and oral with topical acyclovir; Mantel-Cox test). o --- o , Topical acyclovir, $n = 25$; △ --- △, intravenous acyclovir, $n = 15$; ■ --- ■ , oral acyclovir, $n = 26$. (From Corey et al. (50), with permission.)

TABLE 4 Recommendations for Acyclovir Treatment of Adults with First-Episode Genital Herpes

Dose	Route	Interval	Duration	Treatment of choice
Immunocompetent host				
200 mg	PO	q4h (5 × /day)	10 days	
5 mg/kg	IV	q8h	3-5 days	Complete 10-day course with PO
Immunocompromised host				
200-400 mg	PO	q4h (5 × /day)	10 days	
5 mg/kg	IV	q8h	3-7 days	Complete 10-day course with PO

of the onset of lesions, oral acyclovir shortens the clinical course of primary genital herpes by about 1 week (47-50). With treatment, the median duration of viral shedding is decreased from 9-15 days to 2-5 days, and the time to healing of lesions is decreased from 16-21 days to 10-12 days. The likelihood of forming new lesions decreases from 74% to 13% after 48 h on oral acyclovir. Treated patients experience a median decrease in itching of 2 days, in pain of 2-4 days, and in dysuria of 1-3 days compared to nontreated patients. Patients with nonprimary first episodes also benefit from treatment. However, because the symptoms are usually less severe and of a shorter duration in these patients, the advantage of treatment is less marked (47).

Although treatment of first-episode genital herpes with acyclovir is clearly of clinical benefit, it does not appear to affect the time to first recurrence, the frequency of recurrences, or the number of patients who experience recurrences in the first year after receiving treatment (8,9). One study (52) reported a significant reduction in the frequency of recurrences during the second year after treatment of primary genital herpes with oral acyclovir, but this was not seen in another similar group (53).

Acyclovir has been shown to have a very low incidence of side effects (54). The drug is cleared by the kidney via glomerular filtration and tubular secretion. Thus dosages must be adjusted in patients with abnormal renal function (Table 5) (55,56).

TABLE 5   Modification of Acyclovir Dosage in Patients with Renal Impairment

Creatine clearance (ml/min/1.73 M^2)	Dose (mg/kg)	Dosing interval (h)
Intravenous acyclovir		
>50	5	8
25-50	5	12
10-25	5	24
0-10	2.5	24
Oral acyclovir		
>10	200	4 (5× a day)
<10	200	12 (2× a day)

Note: There is a 60% decrease in plasma concentration following a 6-h hemodialysis. Therefore, patients on hemodialysis should receive their acyclovir dose after dialysis.

Oral acyclovir is the drug of choice for treatment of first-episode genital herpes. Clinicians should initiate therapy as early as possible in the course of the first episode. Because of the significant clinical benefit from oral acyclovir and the low toxicity of the drug, treatment of all first episodes is recommended. Any patient who has a clinical picture consistent with genital herpes and no past history of a similar episode should be treated as if he is having a first episode. Exceptions might be those patients who present late in the course of the episode in whom symptoms are definitely improving and lesions are crusted or healed. Some have argued that nonprimary first episodes need not be treated. However, clinical differentiation of primary and nonprimary first episodes is often difficult at the time of presentation. Even though the clinical benefits are less dramatic than in a primary first episode, significant reduction in duration of clinical symptoms and viral shedding does occur with treatment of a nonprimary first episode.

In patients with severe disease and complications who require hospitalization, treatment can be initiated with intravenous acyclovir (5 mg/kg IV over 1 h every 8 h). Once the patient is stable enough to go home, the 10-day course can be completed with oral acyclovir.

In immunocompromised patients, either intravenous or oral acyclovir treatment may be utilized. Many clinicians routinely employ doses of 400 mg orally five times daily for patients who do not require hospitalization. This dose (400 mg orally five times daily for 10 days) was also employed in a recent study that demonstrated the safety and efficacy of oral acyclovir treatment of first-episode herpes proctitis in homosexual men (57).

Anecdotal data from pregnant patients who were treated with acyclovir have not demonstrated any harmful drug effects on the fetus. Because of the high morbidity and mortality associated with primary infection during the second and third trimesters, some clinicians have administered acyclovir treatment in this setting (58). However, at the present time, acyclovir in any form is not approved for use in pregnant patients, and there are no data on the efficacy of acyclovir in reducing fetal morbidity and mortality.

There has been interest in the addition of immune stimulators or other antiviral agents to acyclovir for treatment of HSV infections in hopes of preventing establishment of latency. A recent clinical study of isoprinosine combined with acyclovir in first-episode genital herpes did not demonstrate any increased benefit over acyclovir alone (59). Animal studies involving interferon (60), immunoglobulins (61), and vidarabine

(62) in combination with acyclovir have shown some synergistic antiviral effects, but data in humans are not yet available. Recently, a placebo-controlled trial in women with first-episode genital herpes demonstrated acceleration in healing and cessation of viral shedding in women treated with human leukocyte interferon alone, but there was no reduction in the duration of pain (63).

ADJUNCTIVE TREATMENT

In addition to acyclovir, there are measures that can decrease symptoms while awaiting healing. Usually mild analgesics such as aspirin or acetaminophen are adequate for control of discomfort, but narcotics may occasionally be necessary.

Both men and women can be treated with Domeboro soaks to accelerate drying and healing. Patients with bladder retention due to autonomic dysfunction may need to perform in-and-out self-catheterization. Women with severe dysuria or urinary retention secondary to pain can be told to sit in a tub of warm water and urinate to prevent the urine from touching the external genitalia. Since concentrated urine is more irritating, fluids should be encouraged. Sitz baths are also beneficial for women with genital herpes and men or women with anorectal herpes.

Patients with severe symptoms of genital HSV-associated aseptic meningitis should be hospitalized and treated with supportive care. However, most patients who develop meningitis will have milder symptoms and can be managed at home with close follow-up. Whether acyclovir affects the course of the meningitis is not known, because in placebo-controlled trials the number of patients with meningitis has been too small to evaluate the effect of treatment on the course of the meningitis.

Patients should be cautioned about the possibility of autoinoculation, especially to the eye. Good hygiene with frequent hand washing should be encouraged.

Secondary bacterial infection can be treated with local care and topical antibiotic ointments. Occasionally, oral antibiotics or drainage of an abscess may be necessary.

Emotional support is very important (64). Counseling the patient on how the disease is acquired and spread should be done at the first visit. Patients will usually be quite concerned about the source of infection, especially if they are in a monogamous relationship. It is important to emphasize that because the disease may be asymptomatically acquired and transmitted, it is often difficult to establish the exact time and source of the infection (except in the case of a true primary infection). In addition, patients need to know that the partner who transmitted the infection may have acquired the infection years earlier. Referral to a herpes support group (such as HELP) may be of benefit.

PREVENTION

Physicians should discuss means of preventing infected patients from spreading the disease to others. Since viral shedding is highest from active lesions, patients are most likely to infect their sexual partners during times when lesions are present. Patients with true primary infection are especially contagious. Therefore, patients should be advised to avoid sexual activity until all lesions are completely healed. The possibility of future recurrences and the need for similar sexual abstinence until the recurrent lesions are healed should also be discussed. However, because of asymptomatic viral shedding, transmission of the infection can occur even in the absence of lesions. Use of condoms should reduce the risk of acquiring or transmitting HSV during asymptomatic periods (65). Since the risk of asymptomatic shedding appears greatest during the first year following first-episode herpes, use of condoms should be especially encouraged during this period.

SUMMARY

Genital HSV infection is a commonly encountered sexually transmitted disease. Patients presenting with their first clinical episode may have a primary or nonprimary true first episode or a first recognized recurrent episode. Primary infection is associated with severe local symptoms, systemic involvement, and a higher incidence of complications. Diagnosis is usually made on the basis of clinical findings. Several rapid diagnostic tests are available for confirmation, but the most sensitive and reliable means of diagnosis is still tissue culture.

Although not necessary to initiate treatment, viral isolation and typing are recommended to aid in prediction of the risk and frequency of subsequent recurrences. Serology for differentiation of primary and nonprimary first-episode disease is not usually obtained.

Acyclovir is the only available antiviral compound that has demonstrated efficacy in controlled studies for the treatment of genital herpes infections. Oral and IV formulations appear to be more efficacious than topical. Because of lower cost and ease of administration, oral acyclovir is the preferred treatment for most patients with first-episode genital herpes. Therapy should be initiated as early as possible at 200 mg five times daily for 10 days (Tables 4, 5). Used correctly, acyclovir significantly decreases the duration of lesions, formation of new lesion, severity of clinical symptoms, and duration of viral shedding. Although it is known that acyclovir treatment of the first episode of genital herpes does not prevent establishment of latent infection, there is conflicting evidence as to whether treatment will lessen the frequency of subsequent recurrences. Thus, acyclovir is useful to reduce the duration of viral shedding and clinical symptoms, but it does not effect a cure.

REFERENCES

1. Nahmias, A. J. and Roizman, B. (1973). Infection with herpes-simplex viruses 1 and 2. *N. Engl. J. Med.* 289:667-674,719-725, 781-789.
2. Rapp, F. (1984). Herpes simplex viruses. In Holmes, K. K., et al. (eds.): *Sexually Transmitted Diseases.* New York, McGraw-Hill, pp. 438-449.
3. Straus, S. E., et al. (1985). Herpes simplex virus infection: Biology, treatment, and prevention. *Ann. Intern. Med.* 103:404-419.
4. Corey, L. (1984). Genital herpes. In Holmes, K. K., et al. (eds.): *Sexually Transmitted Diseases.* New York, McGraw-Hill, pp. 449-474.
5. Corey, L., Adams, H. G., Brown, Z. A., and Holmes, K. K. (1983). Genital herpes simplex virus infections: Clinical manifestations, course, and complications. *Ann. Intern. Med.* 98:958-972.
6. Kalinyak, J. E., Fleagle, G., and Docherty, J. J. (1977). Incidence and distribution of herpes simplex virus type 1 and 2 from genital lesions in college women. *J. Med. Virol.* 1:175-181.
7. Reeves, W. C., Corey, L., Adams, H. G., et al. (1981). Risk of recurrence after first episodes of genital herpes: Relation to HSV type and antibody response. *N. Engl. J. Med.* 305:315-319.
8. Mindel, A., Weller, I. V. D., et al. (1986). Acyclovir in first attacks of genital herpes and prevention of recurrences. *Genitourin. Med.* 62:28-32.
9. Corey, L., Mindel, A., et al. (1985). Risk of recurrence after treatment of first-episode genital herpes with intravenous acyclovir. *Sex. Transm. Dis.* 12:215-218.
10. Buchman, T. G., Roizman, B., and Nahmias, A. J. (1979). Demonstration of exogenous genital reinfection with herpes simplex virus type 2 by restriction endonuclease fingerprinting of viral DNA. *J. Infect. Dis.* 140:295-304.
11. Schmidt, O. W., Fife, K. H., and Corey, L. (1984). Reinfection is an uncommon occurrence in patients with symptomatic genital herpes. *J. Infect. Dis.* 149:645-646.
12. Schmidt, O. W., Fife, K. H., and Corey, L. (1986). Genital herpes infection—United States, 1966-1984. *MMWR* 35:402-404.

13. Becker, T. M., Blount, J. H., and Guinan, M. E. (1985). Genital herpes infections in private practice in the United States, 1966 to 1981. *JAMA* 253: 1601-1603.
14. Rooney, J., Felser, J. M., Ostrove, J. M., and Straus, S. E. (1986). Acquisition of genital herpes from an asymptomatic sexual partner. *N. Engl. J. Med.* 314:1561-1564.
15. Mertz, G. J., Schmidt, O., Jourden, J. L., et al. (1985). Frequency of acquisition of first-episode genital infection with herpes simplex virus from symptomatic and asymptomatic source contacts. *Sex. Transm. Dis.* 12:33-39.
16. Douglas, J. M. and Corey, L. (1983). Fomites and herpes simplex viruses: A case for nonvenereal transmission? *JAMA* 250:3093-3094.
17. Corey, L., Reeves, W. C., and Holmes, K. K. (1978). Cellular immune response in genital herpes simplex virus infection. *N. Engl. J. Med.* 299:986-991.
18. Zweerink, H. J. and Corey, L. (1982). Virus-specific antibodies in sera from patients with genital herpes simplex virus infection. *Infect. Immun.* 37:413-421.
19. Ashley, R. L. and Corey, L. (1984). Effect of acyclovir treatment of primary genital herpes on the antibody response to herpes simplex virus. *J. Clin. Invest.* 73:681-688.
20. Bernstein, D. I., Stanberry, L. R., et al. (1987). Antibody response to herpes simplex virus glycoprotein D: Effects of acyclovir and relation to recurrence. *J. Infect. Dis.* 156:423-429.
21. Moseley, R. C., Corey, L., Benjamin, D., et al. (1981). Comparison of viral isolation, direct immunofluorescence, and indirect immunoperoxidase techniques for detection of genital herpes simplex virus infection. *J. Clin. Microbiol.* 13:913-918.
22. Stamm, W. E., Wagner, K. F., Amsel, R., et al. (1980). Causes of the acute urethral syndrome in women. *N. Engl. J. Med.* 303:409-415.
23. Ferrer, R. M., Kraiselburd, E. N., and Kouri, Y. H. (1984). Inapparent genital herpes simplex infection in women attending a venereal disease clinic. *Sex. Transm. Dis.* 11:91-93.
24. Goodell, S. E., Quinn, T. C., et al. (1983). Herpes simplex virus proctitis in homosexual men: Clinical, sigmoidoscopic, and histopathological features. *N. Engl. J. Med.* 308:868-871.
25. Caplan, L. R., Kleeman, F. J., and Berg, S. (1977). Urinary retention probably secondary to herpes genitalis. *N. Engl. J. Med.* 297:920-921.
26. Klastersky, J., Cappel, R., et al. (1972). Ascending myelitis in association with herpes-simplex virus. *N. Engl. J. Med.* 287:182-184.
27. Britz, M. and Sibulkin, D. (1975). Recurrent erythema multiforme and herpes genitalis (type 2). *JAMA* 233:812-813.
28. Brown, Z. A., Vontver, L. A., et al. (1987). Effects on infants of a first episode of genital herpes during pregnancy. *N. Engl. J. Med.* 317:1246-1251.
29. Holmberg, S. D., Stewart, J. A., et al. (1988). Prior herpes simplex virus type 2 infection as a risk factor for HIV infection. *JAMA* 259:1048-1050.

30. Vestergaard, B. F. (1985). Laboratory diagnosis of herpesviruses. *Scand. J. Infect. Dis.* 47(Suppl):22-32.
31. Richman, D. D., Cleveland, P. H., et al. (1984). Rapid viral diagnosis. *J. Infect. Dis.* 149:298-310.
32. Mead, P. B. (1986). Proper methods of culturing herpes simplex virus. *J. Reprod. Med.* 31(5 Suppl):390-394.
33. Goldstein, L. C., Corey, L., McDougall, J. K., et al. (1983). Monoclonal antibodies to herpes simplex viruses: Use in antigenic typing and rapid diagnosis. *J. Infect. Dis.* 147:829-837.
34. Nerurkar, L. S., Namba, M., and Sever, J. L. (1984). Comparison of standard tissue culture, tissue culture plus staining, and direct staining for detection of genital herpes simplex virus infection. *J. Clin. Microbiol.* 19:631-633.
35. Hoffman, B. E., Jungkind, D. L., et al. (1985). Evaluation of two rapid methods for the detection of herpes simplex virus antigens in patient specimens. *Ann. Clin. Lab. Sci.* 15:418-427.
36. Pouletty, P., Chomel, J. J., et al. (1987). Detection of herpes simplex virus indirect specimens by immunofluorescence assay using monoclonal antibody. *J. Clin. Microbiol.* 25:958-959.
37. Solomon, A. R., Rasmussen, J. E., et al. (1984). The Tzanck smear in the diagnosis of cutaneous herpes simplex. *JAMA* 251:633-635.
38. Crane, L. R., Gutterman, P. A., et al. (1980). Incubation of swab materials with herpes simplex virus. *J. Infect. Dis.* 141:531.
39. Bettoli, E. J., Brewer, P. M., et al. (1982). The role of temperature and swab materials in the recovery of herpes simplex virus from lesions. *J. Infect. Dis.* 145:399.
40. McClung, H., Seth, P., and Rawls, W. E. (1976). Relative concentrations in human sera of antibodies to cross-reacting and specific antigens of herpes simplex virus types 1 and 2. *Am. J. Epidemiol.* 104:192-201.
41. Bernstein, D. I., Bryson, Y. J., and Lovett, M. A. (1985). Antibody response to type-common and type-unique epitopes of herpes simplex virus polypeptides. *J. Med. Virol.* 15:251-263.
42. Lee, F. K., Coleman, R. M., et al. (1985). Detection of herpes simplex virus type 2-specific antibody with glycoprotein G. *J. Clin. Microbiol.* 22:641-644.
43. Bernstein, D. I., Lovett, M. A., and Bryson, Y. J. (1984). Serologic analysis of first-episode nonprimary genital herpes simplex virus infection: Presence of type 2 antibody in acute serum samples. *Am. J. Med.* 77:1055-1060.
44. Mindel, A., Adler, M. W., Sutherland, S., and Fiddian, A. P. (1982). Intravenous acyclovir treatment for primary genital herpes. *Lancet* 1:697-700.
45. Corey, L., Fife, K. H., Benedetti, J. K., et al. (1983). Intravenous acyclovir for the treatment of primary genital herpes. *Ann. Intern. Med.* 98:914-921.
46. Corey, L., Nahmias, A. J., Guinan, M. E., et al. (1982). A trial of topical acyclovir in genital herpes simplex virus infections. *N. Engl. J. Med.* 306:1313-1319.

47. Mertz, G. J., Critchlow, C. W., Benedetti, J., et al. (1984). Double-blind placebo-controlled trial of oral acyclovir in first-episode genital herpes simplex virus infections. *JAMA* 252:1147-1151.
48. Nilsen, A. E., Aasen, T., Halsos, A. M., et al. (1982). Efficacy of oral acyclovir in the treatment of initial and recurrent genital herpes. *Lancet* 2:571-573.
49. Bryson, Y. J., Dillon, M., Lovett, M., et al. (1983). Treatment of first episodes of genital herpes simplex virus infection with oral acyclovir: A randomized double-blind controlled trial in normal subjects. *N. Engl. J. Med.* 308:916-921.
50. Corey, L., Benedetti, J., Critchlow, C., et al. (1983). Treatment of primary first-episode genital herpes simplex virus infections with acyclovir: Results of topical, intravenous, and oral therapy. *J. Antimicrob. Chemother.* 12(Suppl. 8):79-88.
51. Kinghorn, G. R., Abeywickreme, I., et al. (1986). Efficacy of combined treatment with oral and topical acyclovir in first episode genital herpes. *Genitourin. Med.* 62:186-188.
52. Bryson, Y., Dillon, M., Lovett, M., et al. (1985). Treatment of first episode genital HSV with oral acyclovir: Long-term follow-up of recurrences. *Scand. J. Infect. Dis.* 47(Suppl.):70-75.
53. Mertz, G. J., Benedetti, J., Critchlow, C., and Corey, L. (1985). Long-term recurrence rates of genital herpes infections after treatment of first episode genital herpes with oral acyclovir. In Kano, R. (ed.): *Herpes Viruses and Virus Chemotherapy.* Amsterdam, Elsevier, pp. 141-144.
54. Laerum, O. D. (1985). Toxicology of acyclovir. *Scand. J. Infect. Dis.* 47 (Suppl.):40-43.
55. Brigden, D. and Whiteman, P. (1985). The clinical pharmacology of acyclovir and its prodrugs. *Scand. J. Infect. Dis.* 47(Suppl.):33-39.
56. Laskin, O. L., Longstreth, J. A., et al. (1982). Effect of renal failure on the pharmacokinetics of acyclovir. *Am. J. Med.* 73(1A):197-201.
57. Rompalo, A. M., Mertz, G. J., Davis, L. G., et al. (1988). Oral acyclovir for the treatment of first episode herpes simplex virus proctitis. *JAMA* 259:2879-2881.
58. Lagrew, D. C., Furlow, T. G., et al. (1984). Disseminated herpes simplex virus infection in pregnancy: Successful treatment with acyclovir. *JAMA* 252:2058-2059.
59. Mindel, A., Allason-Jones, E., Barton, I., et al. (1987). Treatment of first-attack genital herpes—acyclovir versus inosine pranobex. *Lancet* 1:1171-1173.
60. Connell, E. V., Cerruti, R. L., and Trown, P. W. (1985). Synergistic activity of combinations of recombinant human alpha interferon and acyclovir, administered concomitantly and in sequence, against a lethal herpes simplex virus type 1 infection in mice. *Antimicrob. Agents Chemother.* 28:1-4.
61. Hilfenhaus, J., DeClereq, E., Kohler, R., et al. (1987). Combined antiviral effects of acyclovir or bromovinyldeoxyuridine and human immunoglobulin in herpes simplex virus infected mice. *Antiviral Res.* 4:227-235.

62. Karim, M. R., Marks, M. I., et al. (1985). Synergistic antiviral effects of acyclovir and vidarabine on herpes simplex infection in newborn mice. *Chemotherapy* 31:310-317.
63. Pazin, G. J., Harger, J. H., Armstrong, J. A., et al. (1987). Leukocyte interferon for treating first episodes of genital herpes in women. *J. Infect. Dis.* 156:891-898.
64. Derman, R. J. (1986). Counseling the herpes genitalis patient. *J. Reprod. Med.* 31(5 Suppl.):439-444.
65. Conant, M. A., Spicer, D. W., and Smith, C. D. (1984). Herpes simplex virus transmission: Condom studies. *Sex. Transm. Dis.* 11:94-95.

7
Acyclovir for Recurrent Genital Herpes

H. Reid Mattison and Richard C. Reichman   *University of Rochester School of Medicine and Dentistry, Rochester, New York*

INTRODUCTION: EPIDEMIOLOGY AND NATURAL HISTORY

Genital herpes infections represent a major public health problem causing significant morbidity, particularly in sexually active young adults and adolescents. In addition, genital herpes infections during pregnancy often result in serious infant morbidity and mortality. Indirect estimates of the incidence and prevalence of genital herpes have shown recent marked increases (1-4), with speculation that as many as 1.2 million new cases occur in the United States per year (5) and result in a cumulative prevalence of greater than 20 million (6). Epidemiologic investigation of the spread of genital herpes has been slowed, because the majority of these infections are felt to be asymptomatic, making the source and spread of infection difficult to identify (7-9). Seroepidemiologic investigation has shown that less than 25% of seropositive individuals have been knowingly infected (10). Long-term natural history studies are not available to reliably predict whether and/or when recurrences decrease or change over time.

Patients followed for 3 years after the initial episode of HSV type 2 genital herpes have not shown a significant change in the median recurrence rate of disease (11). The risk of recurrence after the first clinical episode has been estimated to vary between 55% and 88% in follow-up studies of 1-2 years after disease onset (12,13). The likelihood of recurrence of genital herpes differs between HSV types (14), with genital HSV type 2 disease recurring more than 15 times more commonly than genital HSV type 1 disease, when mean monthly frequencies of recurrences are compared (15). Studies of the natural history of genital herpes infections have shown that recurrent disease is not as severe as primary infection (6,12, 16,17). Commonly lacking in recurrent infection are the systemic manifestations of illness and distal site inoculations that characterize primary disease. In addition, in recurrent disease the duration of symptoms, viral shedding, and time to crusting and healing of lesions are approximately halved in comparison to primary infections.

Although individual episodes of recurrent genital herpes are relatively mild compared to first-episode infections, the cumulative morbidity associated with recurrent disease (pain, psychological trauma, and potential for transmission) has made the treatment and suppression of this entity an important area of investigation.

TOPICAL ACYCLOVIR THERAPY

Topical administration of acyclovir in the treatment of recurrent genital herpes was initially viewed with great interest because of the theoretical advantage of delivering high drug concentrations locally without incurring the risk of systemic toxicity. Investigations in the United States have employed the U.S. and Canadian approved formulation of 5% acyclovir in a polyethylene glycol base. A second preparation of the medication, 5% acyclovir in a propylene glycol base, has been studied in several European countries.

Corey et al. (18) reported their experience in treating 111 patients with frequently recurring genital herpes in a double-blind, placebo-controlled, multicenter treatment trial using 5% acyclovir ointment applied four times per day for 5 days. Patients were required to report to the study center within 48 h of prodrome or lesion onset to receive and begin using the study medication. The results revealed a modest antiviral effect but no clear-cut clinical benefit. Topical acyclovir therapy decreased the duration of viral shedding in men but not in women. Topical acyclovir use did not produce a significant reduction in the time to lesion crusting or healing, or in the duration of symptoms, in either men or women. It did appear to hasten the time to crusting and healing of lesions in men, and more so when lesions present at study entry were compared to all lesions appearing during the recurrence. A modest reduction was seen in new lesion formation during therapy when the entire population (men and women) was examined, but similar benefit was not demonstrated when men and women were examined separately.

A similar protocol was employed by Reichman et al. (19) in the treatment of 88 patients, except that study medication was applied six times per day. Results again demonstrated a significant reduction only in the duration of viral shedding in men, but no clinical effect was seen in men or women in the time to lesion crusting and healing, cessation of pain, or frequency of new lesion formation during therapy. Corey et al. subsequently presented an expanded report of their earlier study, following a similar protocol, with acyclovir applied topically either four or six times per day (20). A reduction in the duration of viral shedding was reported in men and women but again without clinical benefit demonstrable in either group. An increase in the number of acyclovir applications from four to six per day offered no advantage.

These studies demonstrated differences in the nature of recurrent genital herpes in men and women (18-20). Men showed a 1-log higher mean titer of virus isolated from lesions at the first clinic visit of each recurrence. Placebo-treated male patients shed virus significantly longer than female counterparts and required a significantly longer time to heal. Lesion characteristics of later stages were seen more often in women when they were first observed, and women tended to enroll in the study later after lesion onset than men. The decreased antiviral effect seen in women may have reflected either a shortened disease course or enrollment in the study at a point further along in the recurrence. Such factors would reduce the likelihood of detecting a drug effect and suggest that earlier treatment in the course of the recurrence might be more beneficial.

These considerations led to a patient-initiated treatment trial employing 5% acyclovir ointment applied six times per day for 5 days (21).

A total of 309 patients were enrolled in this study, which required patients to initiate treatment within 24 h of the prodrome or lesion onset. The mean time from symptom onset to treatment initiation was 5-8 h. The early initiation of treatment failed to result in significant antiviral or clinical benefits. The only significant difference compared to physician-initiated treatment trials was a reduction in the duration of viral shedding in women. This benefit was observed when the group of women initiating treatment at prodrome and the group initiating treatment after lesion onset were taken together, but no such benefit was seen when the group of women initiating treatment at prodrome was viewed separately. Disappointingly, the results showed that patient-initiated treatment with topical acyclovir had no clinical effect on the course of recurrent genital herpes.

Also of note was that the group of patients initiating treatment between the onset of prodrome and the appearance of lesions failed to gain either antiviral or clinical benefit.

Other investigations have been directed to improving drug penetration into the skin. An in vitro model of 5% acyclovir ointment penetration of guinea pig skin showed that acyclovir penetrated the stratum corneum very poorly (22). An accompanying in vivo guinea pig treatment trial demonstrated results similar to the human trials. A modest antiviral effect without clinical benefit was obtained. Acyclovir cream, which is licensed in some European countries, uses propylene glycol as a base. Propylene glycol may facilitate transdermal penetration of acyclovir by increasing the aqueous solubility of the drug in this vehicle, with resultant increased availability (23). Studies with animal models of cutaneous herpes have shown an improved treatment response when acyclovir cream was compared to ointment, including a reduction in the titer of virus shed (24). One human treatment trial evaluated the efficacy of 5% acyclovir cream, applied five times per day for 5 days in a patient-initiated treatment protocol, and reported a significant reduction in the time to healing, duration of symptoms, viral shedding, and new lesion formation during therapy (25). However, the number of patients enrolled was too small for statistically valid comparisons between men and women. Patients were enrolled if recurrences were greater than or equal to two per year, which is less severe recurrent disease than reported for comparison acyclivor ointment studies and may represent a patient population with a different natural history of disease. Data from the above studies are summarized in Table 1.

ORAL ACYCLOVIR THERAPY

In the treatment of recurrent genital herpes, oral acyclovir appears to be more effective than topical acyclovir, although a study has not been done that directly compares the two treatments. Reichman et al. (26) evaluated 212 patients with frequently recurring genital herpes in a double-blind, placebo-controlled, two-part treatment trial. In part A, patients reported to the study center within 48 h of symptom onset to receive a course of either placebo or acyclovir (200 mg taken five times per day for 5 days). During a subsequent recurrence, 165 of the same patients were enrolled in part B of the study. In part B, patients received the same treatment (either acyclovir or placebo) under a similar protocol as in part A, except that treatment was patient initiated at the onset of symptoms.

TABLE 1 Oral Acyclovir (ACV) Treatment of Recurrent Genital Herpes

	Enrolled	200 mg ACV tablets/day	Rx duration in days	Viral shedding	Time to crust	Time to healing all lesions	Lesions at study entry	Symptom reduction Pain	Symptom reduction Itching	Formation of lesions during treatment
Reichman et al. (26) Part A (physician-initiated treatment)	$n = 212$ 106 ACV 55 M 51 F 106 Placebo 58 M 48 F	5	5	↓*	↓	↓	—a	—	—	—
Part B (patient-initiated treatment)	$n = 165$ 82 ACV 45 M 37 F 83 Placebo 43 M 40 F	5	5	↓	↓	↓	↓	—	—	↓
Significant difference in results in part B vs. part A				+	+	+	+	—	—	+
Nielsen et al. (27)	$n = 85$ 42 ACV 31 M 11 F 43 Placebo 35 M 8 F	5	5	↓	—	↓	NA	—	—	↓

*Significant ($p \leq .05$) reduction in parameter measured for ACV compared to placebo treatment.
aLack of a significant reduction comparing ACV to placebo.

TABLE 2 Topical Acyclovir (ACV) Treatment of Recurrent Genital Herpes

	Enrolled	Rx applications per day	Rx duration in days	Virus shedding (M/F)	Time to crusting (M/F)	Time to healing (M/F)	Symptom (pain) reduction (M/F)	Formation of lesions during treatment (M/F)
5% ACV ointment Physician-initiated treatment								
Corey et al. (18)	$n = 111$ 53 ACV 31 M 22 F 58 Placebo 32 M 26 F	4	5	↓*/—[a]	—/—	—/—	—/—	—/—
Reichman et al. (19)	$n = 88$ 42 ACV 27 M 15 F 46 Placebo 27 M 19 F	6	5	↓/—	—/—	—/—	—/—	—/—
Corey et al. (20)	$n = 111$ 51 ACV 31 M 20 F	4 ($n = 27$) 6 ($n = 24$)	5	↓/↓	—/—	—/—	—/—	—/—

	60 Placebo 35 M 25 F			—/↓	—/—	—/—	—/—
Patient-initiated treatment Luby et al. (21)	$n = 309$ 147 ACV 85 M 62 F 162 Placebo 91 M 71 F	6	5	—/↓	—/—	—/—	—/—
5% ACV cream Patient-initiated treatment Fiddian et al. (25)	$n = 85$ 44 ACV 30 M 14 F 41 Placebo 22 M 19 F	5	5	↓/NA	—/NA	↓/NA	—/NA	↓/NA

*Significant ($p \leq .05$) reduction in parameter measured for ACV comapred to placebo treatment.
aLack of a significant reduction comparing ACV to placebo.

In both parts A and B of the study, acyclovir treatment was associated with a significant reduction in the duration of virus shedding and the time to healing of all lesions arising during the recurrence, but it did not affect the duration of symptoms. Acyclovir recipients in part B demonstrated a reduction in the time to healing of lesions present at study entry and all lesions arising during the recurrence. In part A, acyclovir treatment reduced the time to healing of all lesions arising during a recurrence but did not affect those lesions present at study entry. A significant reduction in the proportion of patients forming new lesions during the study medication period was seen when acyclovir and placebo groups were compared in part B; a similar effect was not apparent with acyclovir use in part A. When the effects of acyclovir in part A were directly compared with part B, a significantly reduced duration of virus shedding and time to crusting and healing of all lesions were seen in the patient-initiated treatment group. Treatment via patient- or physician-initiated schedule did not alter the natural history of genital herpes, as the time to next recurrence was similar for acyclovir and placebo recipients in both parts A and B. The study demonstrated a beneficial antiviral and clinical effect of orally administered acyclovir in the treatment of recurrent genital herpes, which was more pronounced when treatment was initiated earlier in the course of the recurrence.

Another study followed a double-blind, placebo-controlled, physician-initiated treatment design to report on 85 patients with recurrent genital herpes (27). Patients were begun on treatment within 48 h of symptom onset with either placebo or 200 mg acyclovir, taken five times per day for 5 days. When all patients (male and female) were evaluated, treatment with oral acyclovir produced a significant reduction in the duration of virus shedding, time to healing, and new lesions formed during treatment. Acyclovir and placebo treatment groups did not differ in the time to lesion crusting or symptom duration. Similar effects of acyclovir treatment were demonstrated when the male enrollees were viewed separately, but the female enrollment was too small for separate, statistically valid comparison.

A recent study (28) evaluated chronic suppressive and acute short-term oral acyclovir therapy of recurrent genital herpes and provided an additional opportunity to compare the outcome of oral acyclovir treatment with placebo over the 1-year period of patient observation. Therapy was begun within 24 h of symptom onset with either placebo or 200 mg of oral acyclovir, taken five times per day for 5 days. The acyclovir treatment group had a significant reduction in the duration of recurrent episodes. Oral acyclovir treatment initiated at symptom onset did not alter the pattern of disease recurrence, as no significant difference in either

recurrence rate or time to first recurrence, both during and after completion of the study, was noted when compared to placebo treatment. Data
from the above studies are summarized in Table 2.

SUMMARY

The effects of topical acyclovir in the treatment of recurrent genital herpes
have been well studied. Use of acyclovir ointment, a 5% acyclovir preparation using polyethylene glycol as a base, produces antiviral effects without associated clinical benefit when used in the treatment of recurrent
genital herpes. Its use results in a decrease in the duration of viral shedding but does not change the time to crusting or healing of lesions, the
duration of symptoms, or the development of new lesions during the treatment period. These measurements of clinical efficacy have not been affected by increased frequency of treatment application or by initiation of
treatment earlier in the course of the recurrence. Topical acyclovir cream,
a 5% acyclovir preparation using propylene glycol as a base, may be a
more effective form of therapy for recurrent genital herpes because of increased skin penetration and bioavailability. Its use in preliminary treatment trials has been associated with a reduction in the duration of virus
shedding, the duration of symptoms, the time to healing, and development
of new lesions during treatment. These findings need to be confirmed by
additional studies.

Oral acyclovir has shown both antiviral effects and clinical benefit
when used in the treatment of recurrent genital herpes. Its use is associated
with a reduction in the duration of virus shedding, the time to crusting
and healing of lesions, and the number of new lesions formed during therapy. Treatment is more effective when therapy is initiated by the patient
early in the course of a recurrence. Administration of oral acyclovir can,
therefore, shorten the course and reduce the severity of recurrent genital
herpes episodes. Use of oral acyclovir to treat episodes of recurrent genital herpes needs to be individualized and put in perspective with chronic
suppression of the disease. Chronic suppression is clearly superior to intermittent therapy among patients with frequently recurring disease (28). Patients who are good candidates for intermittent therapy with oral acyclovir
are probably those with infrequent but severe recurrent episodes (29).

REFERENCES
1. Centers for Disease Control (1982). Genital herpes infection—United States,
   1966-1979. *MMWR* 31:137-139.

112   MATTISON AND REICHMAN

2. Chuang, T. Y., Su, W. P. D., Ustrup, D. M., et al. (1983). Incidence and
   trend of herpes progenitalis. *Mayo Clin. Proc.* 58:436-441.
3. Publisher (1984). Sexually transmitted diseases. *Br. J. Vener. Dis.* 60:99-203.
4. Becker, T. M., Blount, J. H., and Guinan, M. E. (1985). Genital herpes infections in private practice in the United States, 1966-1981. *JAMA* 253:1601-
   1603.
5. Institute of Medicine. (1985). *New Vaccine Development: Establishing Priorities*,
   Vol. 1. *Diseases of Importance in the United States, Appendix I: Prospects
   for Immunizing Against Herpes Simplex Viruses.* Report by a committee at
   the Institute of Medicine, Washington, D.C., National Academy Press, 1985.
6. Guinan, M. E., Wolinsky, S. M., and Reichman, R. C. (1985). Epidemiology
   of genital herpes simplex virus infection. *Epidemiol. Rev.* 7:27-46.
7. McCaughtry, M. L., Fleager, G. S., and Docherty, J. J. (1982). Inapparent
   genital herpes simplex virus infection in college women. *J. Med. Virol.* 10:
   283-290.
8. Bernstein, D. I., Lovett, M. A., and Bryson, Y. J. (1984). Serologic analysis
   of first-episode nonprimary genital herpes simplex virus infection. *Am. J.
   Med.* 77:1055-1060.
9. Rooney, J. F., Felser, J. M., Ostrove, J. M., and Straus, S. E. (1986). Acquisition of genital herpes from an asymptomatic sexual partner. *N. Engl. J.
   Med.* 314:1561-1564.
10. Stavraky, K. M., Rawls, W. E., Chiavetta, J., Donner, A. P., and Wanklin,
    J. M. (1983). Sexual and socioeconomic factors affecting the risk of past in-
    fections with herpes simplex virus type 2. *Am. J. Epidemiol.* 118:109-121.
11. Corey, L., and Spear, P. G. (1986). Infections with herpes simplex viruses.
    N. Engl. J. Med. 314:686-691.
12. Corey, L., Adams, H. G., Brown, Z. A., and Holmes, K. K. (1983). Genital
    herpes simplex virus infections: Clinical manifestations, course, and compli-
    cations. *Ann. Intern. Med.* 98:958-972.
13. Mertz, G. J., Benedetti, J., Critchlow, C., and Corey, L. (1985). Long term
    recurrence rates of genital herpes infections after treatment of first episode
    genital herpes with oral acyclovir. In Kono, R., and Nakajima, A. (eds.):
    *Herpes Viruses and Virus Chemotherapy: Pharmacology and Clinical Ap-
    proaches.* New York, Excerpta Medica, pp. 141-144.
14. Reeves, W. C., Corey, L., Adams, H. G., Vontver, L. A., and Holmes, K.
    K. (1981). Risk of recurrence after firs episodes of genital herpes. *N. Engl. J.
    Med.* 305:315-319.
15. Lafferty, W. E., Coombs, R. W., Benedetti, J., Critchlow, C., and Corey,
    L. (1987). Recurrences after oral and genital herpes simplex virus infection.
    N. Engl. J. Med. 316:1444-1449.
16. Guinan, M. E., MacCalman, J., Kern, E. R., Overall, J. C., and Spruance,
    S. L. (1981). The course of untreated recurrent genital herpes simplex infec-
    tion in 27 women. *N. Engl. J. Med.* 304:759-763.

17. Mindel, A., Coker, D. M., Faherty, A., and Williams, P. (1988). Recurrent genital herpes: Clinical and virological features in men and women. *Genitourin. Med.* 64:103-106.

18. Corey, L., Nahmias, A. J., Guinan, M. E., et al. (1982). A trial of topical acyclovir in genital herpes simplex virus infections. *N. Engl. J. Med.* 22: 1313-1319.

19. Reichmen, R. C., Badger, G. J., Guinan, M. E., et al. (1983). Topically administered acyclovir in the treatment of recurrent herpes simplex genitalis: A controlled trial. *J. Infect. Dis.* 147:336-340.

20. Corey, L., Benedetti, J. K., Critchlow, C. W., et al. (1982). Double-blind, placebo-controlled trial of topical acyclovir in genital herpes simplex virus infections. *Am. J. Med.* 73:326-334.

21. Luby, J. P., Grann, J. W., Alexander, W. J., et al. (1984). A collaborative study of patient-initiated treatment of recurrent genital herpes with topical acyclovir or placebo. *J. Infect. Dis.* 150:1-6.

22. Spruance, S. L., McKeough, M. B., and Cardinal, J. R. (1984). Penetration of guinea pig skin by acyclovir in different vehicles and correlation with the efficacy of topical therapy of experimental cutaneous herpes simplex virus infection. *Antimicrob. Agents Chemother.* 25:10-15.

23. Kingsley, S. R., And Fiddian, A. P. (1985). Acyclovir cream—an effective therapy for cutaneous herpes simplex infections. In Kono, R., and Nakajama, A. (eds.): *Herpes Viruses and Virus Chemotherapy: Pharmacologic and Clinical Approaches.* New York, Excerpta Medica, pp. 133-137.

24. *Collins, P., and Oliver, N. M. (1982). Acyclovir treatment of cutaneous herpes in guinea pigs and herpes encephalitis in mice. Am. J. Med. 73:96-99.*

25. Fiddian, A. P., Kinghorn, G. R., Goldmeier, D., Rees, E., Rodin, P., Thin, R. N. T., and DeKonig, G. A. J. (1983). Topical acyclovir in the treatment of genital herpes: A comparison with systemic therapy. *J. Antimicrob. Chemother.* 12(Suppl. B):67-77.

26. Reichman, R. C., Badger, G. J., Mertz, G. J., et al. (1984). Treatment of recurrent genital herpes simplex infections with oral acyclovir. *JAMA* 2103-2107.

27. Nilsen, A. E., Aasen, T., Halsos, A. M., Kinge, B. R., Tjotta, E. A. L., Wikstrom, K., and Fiddian, A. P. (1982). Efficacy of oral acyclovir in the treatment of initial and recurrent genital herpes. *Lancet* 2:571-573.

28. Mattison, H. R., Reichman, R. C., Benedetti, J., et al. (1988). Double-blind, placebo-controlled trial comparing long-term suppressive with short-term oral acyclovir therapy for management of recurrent genital herpes. *Am. J. Med.* (in press).

29. Gold, D., and Corey, L. (1987). Acyclovir prophylaxis for herpes simplex virus infection. *Antimicrob. Agents Chemother.* 31:361-367.

8
Suppressive Acyclovir Treatment for Herpes Simplex Virus Infections

Gregory J. Mertz and Clifton C. Jones*   *University of New Mexico School of Medicine, Albuquerque, New Mexico*

INTRODUCTION

Although genital herpes infections may be asymptomatic or unrecognized (1-3), many normal adults experience frequent symptomatic episodes which may have substantial medical, social, and psychological impact (4,5). Herpes simplex infections can be severe and even life-threatening in immunosuppressed patients, and patients with long-term immunosuppression, such as patients with AIDS, may suffer from chronic, progressive mucocutaneous lesions that may persist indefinitely unless treated (6-16). This chapter will review the natural history and diagnosis of mucocutaneous herpes infections and the indications for suppressive acyclovir therapy.

NATURAL HISTORY OF GENITAL HERPES

In normal adults there is variation in the duration and severity of recurrent episodes of genital herpes and even more variability in their frequency (17,18). Approximately 50% of adults with recurrent genital herpes will experience a prodrome, often described as tingling, numbness, or pain, for a few hours to a few days prior to the appearance of lesions. As in first-episode genital herpes, lesions progress through typical stages of vesiculation, ulceration, crusting, and healing. In contrast to lesions in first episodes, those in recurrent herpes tend to be unilateral and localized

Present affiliation: Internal Medicine, Professional Association, Topeka, Kansas

and are less likely to form crops of new lesions (18). The mean duration of viral shedding is about 4 days, and the mean time to healing is about 10 days. Symptoms of local pain and itching are typically mild to moderate but may be absent. Systemic symptoms such as fever and malaise and complications such as aseptic meningitis, which are common with primary first-episode genital herpes, are exceedingly uncommon in recurrent episodes (18).

Influence of Virus Type and Site of Infection on Frequency of Recurrence

Although neither the severity nor the duration of first-episode or recurrent genital herpes is influenced by virus type, virus type is a major determinant of the frequency of recurrences. Reeves et al. first showed that the risk of recurrence of genital herpes was substantially reduced following primary first-episode HSV-1 as compared to HSV-2 infections (19). In a recent review of the natural history of genital herpes, Corey et al. noted that the risk of recurrence was 55% versus 88% within 6 months after primary first-episode HSV-1 and HSV-2 infections, respectively, and the median number of recurrences in the first year were one and four, respectively (18). More recently, Lafferty et al., in a study of patients with concurrent primary first-episode oropharyngeal and genital herpes, found that genital HSV-2 infections recurred most frequently at a mean of 0.33 recurrences per month, followed by oral-labial HSV-1 infections with 0.12 per month, genital HSV-1 with 0.02 per month, and oral-labial HSV-2 infections with 0.001 per month (20).

Although both virus type and the site of infection clearly influence the frequency of recurrences, it is not clear why there is so much variation in the frequency of recurrences in normal adults with the same virus type and site of infection. Studies of the seroprevalence of HSV-2 infection suggest that more than three fourths of persons with HSV-2 antibody have no history of genital herpes (3). Although the median number of recurrences in the first year after primary first-episode genital infection with HSV-2 is about four, many normal adults have extremely frequent recurrences. In a mail survey of members of a national organization of persons with genital herpes, Knox et al. found that 33% of 3069 members who completed questionnaires had 12 or more recurrences per year. including 26% of those who had genital herpes for 6 or more years (4).

Infections in Immunocompromised Patients

Although normal adults may experience frequent recurrences of genital herpes, the immunologic status of the host is an important factor in determining the severity, duration, and the frequency of recurrent herpes simplex virus infections. Animal experiments suggest that the cellular immune response is more important than the humoral immune response (22), and infections in patients with defective cell-mediated responses tend to be more severe than those in patients with defects in humoral immunity (17).

Approximately 80-90% of HSV-seropositive patients undergoing bone marrow transplantation experience mucocutaneous herpes episodes, which are typically severe and may be associated with persistence of viral shedding, pain, and lesions for periods of 3 or 4 weeks or more (8,11,15, 16,23,24). Severe recurrences have also been reported in patients receiving cardiac and renal transplants and in patients receiving chemotherapy for malignancies such as those with leukemia receiving induction chemotherapy (6,9,10,12,14,25,26). Finally, culture-proven HSV infection persisting for 4 or more weeks in a person with evidence of human immunodeficiency virus (HIV) infection and without evidence of underlying immunosuppression fulfills criteria for the diagnosis of AIDS. In the absence of effective treatment, these infections in patients with AIDS may persist indefinitely, causing severe, progressive, local or disseminated infection (7,13).

Complications of Recurrent Herpes Infections

Complications of recurrent herpes infections in the normal host are rare (17,18). Recurrent episodes of erythema multiforme may be triggered by recurrent mucocutaneous HSV episodes (27,28). Recent studies suggest that herpes infections may be the most common cause of recurrent erythema multiforme, even among those not clearly associated with herpes. Persons with eczema, especially when the eczema is under poor control, may develop eczema herpeticum, involving cutaneous or visceral dissemination of HSV infection.

In the immunocompromised host, visceral dissemination may occur. Sites of infection include the central nervous system, lung, esophagus, liver, pancreas, adrenyls, and other organs. With the exception of esophagitis, most infections complicated by visceral dissemination are fatal unless treated.

DIAGNOSIS

When a patient has a history of recurrent vesicles and ulcers and a typical episode is observed by the clinician, many clinicians are comfortable making a clinical diagnosis (29). However, many experts recommend virologic confirmation of the diagnosis, especially if suppressive therapy is contemplated. Acceptable confirmation would include either a viral culture or a direct test employing fluorescein-labeled monoclonal antibodies or enzyme immunoassay (29,30). In either case, a positive culture or direct test is most likely in the first 48-72 h of a recurrence when lesions are vesicular, pustular, or wet ulcers. In the immunocompromised host, lesions and viral shedding may persist for prolonged periods, and the yield of viral culture or direct tests remains high so long as lesions have not dried or crusted. Following isolation of HSV in cell culture, typing of HSV-1 and HSV-2 with commercially available monoclonal antibodies is quick, accurate, and inexpensive (31).

Serologic diagnosis is rarely employed outside the research setting. Currently available commercial serologic assays lack acceptable specificity in differentiating antibody responses to HSV-1 and HSV-2 and responses to dual infection with HSV-1 and HSV-2 (2,32,33). However, if conclusions about virus type are ignored, virtually any commercially available serologic assay should be able to detect past HSV infection. Thus, for example, a commercially available serologic test for herpes simplex virus could be used to determine whether suppressive therapy should be given following bone marrow transplantation in a person without a clear history of HSV infection.

As will be discussed in subsequent sections, there is little evidence in the normal adult that incomplete suppression of recurrent herpes episodes with oral acyclovir results from selection of virus less sensitive to in vitro inhibition by acyclovir (34-36). Thus, in normal adults treated with suppressive acyclovir therapy, there does not appear to be an indication for routine cultures or for sensitivity testing of HSV cultured during breakthrough episodes. In contrast, although uncommon, persistent acyclovir-resistant HSV infections have been clearly documented in the immunocompromised host (7,37).

If acyclovir-resistant HSV infection is suspected, in vitro sensitivity of HSV to acyclovir can be determined at a number of laboratories (34). In addition, if poor compliance or inadequate absorption after oral administration is suspected, plasma acyclovir levels can also be determined (34).

TREATMENT

Suppressive Therapy in the Normal Adult

A number of published reports have documented the safety and efficacy of chronic, suppressive acyclovir treatment in the normal adult with frequent

recurrences of genital herpes. Based on a series of reports from randomized, placebo-controlled studies documenting the safety and efficacy of
acyclovir 200 mg orally two, three, four, or five times daily for 3-6 months
(36,38-42), the U.S. Food and Drug Administration in 1985 approved the
use of oral acyclovir 200 mg tid for periods up to 6 months in normal adults
with frequently recurring genital herpes. Subsequently, single daily doses
of 800 mg, twice-daily doses of 400 mg, and other combinations with total
daily doses of from 200 to 1000 mg have been evaluated for periods of 1-4
years (34,43-46). To date, no serious adverse effects have been noted in
these studies.

Recently, Mertz et al. have reported the results of a study comparing
suppressive versus episodic treatment for periods of up to 2 years (34,43).
In the first year of this study, over 1100 patients at 24 study centers were
randomized to receive either acyclovir 400 mg orally tice daily or placebo.
Patients in either treatment group with genital herpes episodes confirmed

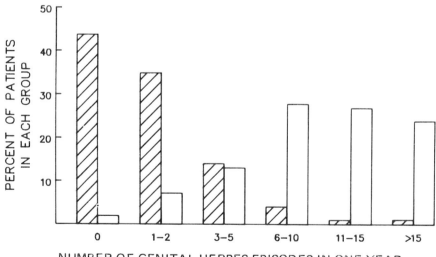

NUMBER OF GENITAL HERPES EPISODES IN ONE YEAR

FIGURE 1   Frequency of genital herpes episodes in 1 year among 519 patients
receiving continuous suppression (stippled bars) with acyclovir 400 mg orally twice
daily for 1 year and among 431 patients (open bars) receiving placebo (episodic
treatment) for 1 year. All patients received open-labeled acyclovir for 5 days during investigator-confirmed genital herpes episodes. From Mertz et al. (34).

by the investigator were treated episodically with acyclovir 200 mg five times daily for 5 days. In the year prior to entry, patients reported a mean of 12.8 recurrences. During the 1-year study, patients receiving episodic treatment continued to have a mean of 11.4 episodes, whereas those receiving suppressive treatment experienced a mean of only 1.8 episodes per year (34).

Only 2% of patients on episodic treatment were free of recurrences, whereas 44% of patients on suppressive treatment remained recurrence-free for 1 year (Fig. 1). The median time to the first recurrence was 18 days in patients on placebo treatment versus 246 days for patients on suppressive acyclovir therapy. In the second year of the study, subjects were allowed to choose between suppressive and episodic treatment, and 89% chose suppressive therapy (43). Among 289 patients who received continuous suppressive treatment for 2 years, 45-50% remained recurrence free each year, and 29% remained recurrence free for 2 years (Table 1).

Safety and Tolerance During Suppressive Treatment

In published studies in which suppressive therapy has been continued for up to 4 years, suppressive acyclovir therapy has been safe and remarkably well tolerated (34,43-46). Mertz et al. reported that nausea was reported more frequently by patients on suppressive therapy than by those

TABLE 1   Percent of Patients Having No Genital Herpes Recurrences in Year 1, Year 2, and Years 1 + 2 Among Patients Receiving Suppressive Acyclovir Treatment Continuously for 2 Years (suppressive-suppressive), Acute Treatment in Year 1 and Suppressive Treatment in Year 2 (acute-suppressive), Suppressive Followed by Acute Treatment (suppressive-acute), and Acute Treatment for 2 Years (acute-acute)

Treatment group	Number[a]	Year		
		1	2	1 + 2
Suppressive-suppressive	289	44.6%	49.5%	29.1%
Acute-acute	31	0%	0%	0%
Suppressive-acute	19	42.1%	5.3%	5.3%
Acute-suppressive	245	1.2%	38.8%	0.8%

[a]Prolonged continuous versus intermittent oral acyclovir treatment in normal adults with frequently recurring genital herpes simplex virus infection. [*Source*: Mertz et al. (43).]

on episodic treatment (34,43). However, this difference was present only in the first 3 months of the study, and only one patient discontinued treatment because of nausea. No other adverse effect was associated with suppressive treatment. No significant laboratory abnormalities have been associated with chronic suppressive therapy with oral acyclovir. Thus, routine monitoring for hematologic, renal, or hepatic toxicity does not appear warranted in the normal adult during chronic suppressive therapy with oral acyclovir. In addition, no effect was noted in sperm motility or morphology in men receiving total daily doses of 400 or 1000 mg acyclovir for 6 months (50). Some investigators have noted an increase in the frequency of prodromes not followed by episodes (false prodromes) during suppressive treatment (36,47), but others have failed to confirm this finding (34).

Breakthrough Recurrences During Suppressive Treatment

Genital herpes episodes in normal adults that occur during suppressive treatment are shorter, less severe, and less likely to be associated with viral shedding than are episodes in patients not receiving suppressive treatment (34,38). Thus, it is not clear whether there is any benefit in increasing the dose or frequency of oral acyclovir administration when episodes occur during suppressive treatment. Patients should be advised to abstain from sexual contact despite the decreased likelihood of viral shedding during these episodes, since both viral shedding and transmission to sexual partners have been clearly documented during breakthrough recurrences (34,36,38,48). There are no data available regarding the risk of asymptomatic shedding or the relative risk of transmitting genital herpes to a sexual partner during asymptomatic periods while on suppressive acyclovir treatment.

**Duration and Frequency of Episodes After Discontinuing
Suppressive Therapy**

Based on what is known about the mechanism of action of acyclovir and the natural history of recurrent genital herpes infections, it is unlikely that suppressive therapy would have a clinically significant or sustained effect on the duration or frequency of recurrent episodes following discontinuation of therapy. Douglas et al. (38) and Sacks et al. (47) found that recurrence rates returned to pretreatment frequencies once suppressive treatment was discontinued, and recurrence rates off therapy were similar among drug and placebo-treated patients. Mindel et al. noted a decrease in recurrence rates after discontinuing 1 year of suppressive treatment, but comparisons were made with historical pretreatment rates and did not include a placebo-control group (44).

Douglas et al. did find that the first recurrence following discontinuation of suppressive therapy occurred significantly sooner than in placebo-treated patients (38), and Mertz et al. found that the time to healing of lesions was prolonged by a mean of 2 days in the first episode following discontinuation of 1 year of suppressive versus episodic treatment (34).

In Vitro Sensitivity to Acyclovir

Although acyclovir-resistant HSV may be isolated from normal patients before, during, or after courses of suppressive acyclovir therapy, there is no evidence that suppressive therapy can induce permanent selection of resistant strains and little evidence that resistance is more likely in isolates cultured during suppressive therapy (34-36,49). Straus et al. did find acyclovir resistance in three isolates cultured from patients during suppressive therapy, but subsequent isolates in the same patients were sensitive to acyclovir (36). Subsequently Nusinoff Lehrman et al. (35) and Mertz et al. (34) have reported sensitivity to testing in HSV cultured before, during, and after suppressive therapy, and no association between acyclovir resistance and suppressive therapy has been found. Of note, in the latter two studies, none of the 13 isolates cultured during suppressive therapy demonstrated acyclovir resistance in vitro.

Short-Term Suppression

Short-term prophylaxis has been shown to decrease oral-labial HSV triggered by sun exposure in skiers (60). Short-term suppressive therapy could also be considered in situations such as facial dermabrasion or surrounding trigeminal ganglion surgery (51). Short-term prophylaxis late in the third trimester might decrease rates of cesarean section or decrease the risk of transmission of HSV at delivery, but no studies demonstrating either safety or efficacy have been performed in this setting. Finally, no studies have been performed evaluating the efficacy of short-term prophylaxis in HSV-uninfected persons following sexual or laboratory exposure to HSV. Although short-term empiric treatment in the latter situation might be considered, suppressive acyclovir treatment in pregnant women should be discouraged until more data are available.

Who Should Receive Suppressive Treatment?

Rather than adhere to strict guidelines for indications for suppressive therapy, many clinicians prefer to discuss the potential benefits as well as the cost and inconvenience associated with suppressive therapy so as to allow the patient to participate in the decision. In general, however, most patients with fewer than six to eight recurrences per year elect not to consider acyclovir suppression. Patients with very frequent recurrences have been shown to suffer the greatest psychological and social impact among patients with recurrent genital herpes (5), and these patients are likely to derive the greatest benefit from suppressive therapy. Unless deterred by financial considerations, most patients with frequent recurrences prefer suppressive rather than episodic therapy (34,43).

Suppressive therapy is occasionally indicated despite relatively infrequent recurrences. Some patients may have such great psychological distress with their outbreaks that a period of suppressive therapy may be considered in conjunction with counseling. Other individuals such as health care professionals with recurrent herpetic whitlow may find that suppressive therapy is indicated to prevent loss of work associated with even two or three outbreaks per year (52). In addition, patients with infrequent recurrences may benefit from suppressive therapy if recurrences are associated with serious complications. Examples include patients with erythema multiforme, recurrent aseptic meningitis, and eczema herpeticum (27,53).

Dose and Duration of Therapy

As indicated earlier, a variety of oral doses and dosing intervals including 200 mg two, three, four, or five times daily; 400 mg twice daily; and 800 mg once daily have been shown to be effective in reducing the frequency of recurrences in placebo-controlled studies in normal adults (34,36,38-46). Although the efficacy of these various regimens has appeared similar, only rarely have different regimens been directly compared in trials employing appropriate controls (38). Intermittent suppressive therapy administered for several days each week has been evaluated and found to be ineffective (54).

Recently Mindel et al. reported the results of a 1-year suppressive study in which various regimens were initiated at 3-month intervals and continued until the patient experienced a genital herpes recurrence (44). Although this study was not blinded or placebo controlled, analysis of the time to first recurrence with each regimen suggests that both dose and frequency of administration influence the degree of efficacy of suppressive acyclovir therapy (Fig. 2). In this study, the most effective regimens were 200 mg four times daily and 400 mg twice daily. Of interest, none of the once-daily regimens (800 mg, 400 mg, or 200 mg) appeared as effective as

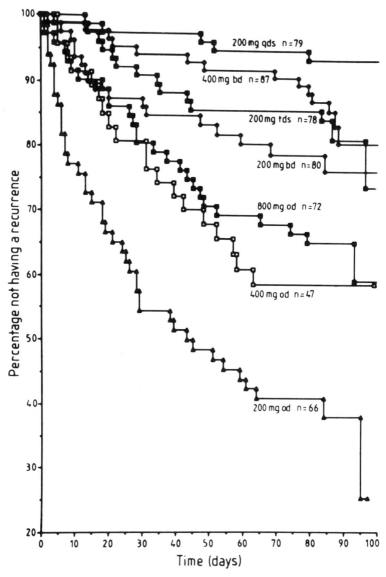

FIGURE 2   Time to first recurrence with different doses of oral acyclovir. Key: od, once daily; bd, twice a day; tds, three times daily; qds, four times daily. From Mindel et al. (44).

any regimen employing twice, three-times, or four-times daily dosing, including 200 mg twice daily. At the least effective regimen, 200 mg once daily, the median time to first recurrence was about 40 days. Mertz et al. found the median time to first recurrence in a similar population to be 246 days in patients receiving 400 mg twice daily and 18 days in placebo-treated patients (34). Thus, although 200 mg once daily is probably more effective than placebo, the same dose administered two to four times daily or 400 mg twice daily appears substantially more effective.

Although 200 mg four or five times daily appears highly effective in suppressing recurrences, we have found that many patients find such frequent dosing difficult to comply with. Because less frequent dosing intervals appear to have equivalent efficiency, we prefer to begin suppressive therapy with 200 mg three times dialy or 400 mg twice daily (Table 2). We often decrease the dose to 200 mg twice daily in patients who are concerned about the cost of treatment. We do not routinely recommend treatment

TABLE 2   Authors' Recommendations for Suppressive Therapy with Oral Acyclovir

Indication	Dose	Frequency	Duration	Comments
Normal host				
Frequent recurrences, complications, or herpetic whitlow interfering with profession	400 mg 200 mg	bid bid or tid	6 mo to 2 yr same	Consider longer treatment if complications are severe or for whitlow in health care workers
Sun-induced oral HSV, dermabrasion, or trigeminal ganglian surgery	400 mg	bid	1-2 weeks or more	Start several days before and continue for 1 week after procedure or sun exposure
Immunocompromised host				
Bone marrow transplant or induction chemotherapy if HSV seropositive	200 mg 400 mg	qid qid	see text	
Renal transplant if HSV seropositive	200 mg	bid or tid	1-2 mo	See text for dosing with renal impairment
AIDS with HSV episodes	400 mg	tid or qid	Indefinitely	

with 200 mg once daily, since both our anecdotal experience and results reported by Mindel et al. suggest that this regimen is substantially less effective.

At present, suppressive therapy is approved by the U.S. Food and Drug Administration for periods of up to 6 months, although a request for approval for treatment for longer periods has been submitted to the U.S. Food and Drug Administration. As indicated earlier, there are now published data documenting that treatment is safe for periods of 1 to 4 years (34,43-46). Although some evidence that treatment appears safe when continued for up to 4 years, it has also been shown that significant changes in recurrence patterns may occur in up to 25% of patients when comparing rates before and after a period of suppressive therapy (38). Therefore, we encourage our patients to interrupt treatment after 1 or 2 years and to stay off suppressive therapy long enough to reassess the frequency of recurrences. For patients with well-documented complications such as erythema multiforme or eczema herpeticum or health care workers with recurrences of herpetic whitlow that clearly interfere with their ability to work, longer periods of suppression may be indicated.

Suppression in Immunocompromised Patients

Both oral and intravenous acyclovir has been shown to be effective in preventing or modifying the course of recurrent HSV episodes in bone marrow and renal transplant patients and during induction chemotherapy for leukemia (6,10,11,14-16,23,25,26). In contrast to the normal host, the decision to initiate prophylactic treatment is based on a history of prior HSV infection or the presence of HSV antibody rather than a history of frequent or severe recurrences (6,9-12,23,25,26). As indicated earlier, 60-90% of placebo-treated or untreated patients develop severe, prolonged recurrences after bone marrow transplantation, whereas 10% or less of patients treated with prophylactic acyclovir develop culture-proven infections. Half of these are asymptomatic, and the majority of the symptomatic infections are mild and of short duration (11,12,16).

A variety of doses and dosing intervals have been evaluated, including intravenous acyclovir 250 mg/m² every 8-12 h and oral dosing with 200-400 mg four or five times daily (6,11,12,14,16,23,25). Once-daily dosing of intravenous acyclovir (250 mg/m²) has been evaluated in bone marrow transplant patients with normal renal function, but this dosing interval was found to be ineffective (24). Oral doses of 200 mg two or three times daily have been employed in renal transplant patients with impaired creatinine clearance (26). Oral regimens appear to have acceptable efficacy except in patients who cannot tolerate oral medication such as bone marrow transplant patients with severe oral mucositis.

Although there is little published experience regarding acyclovir prophylaxis in patients with AIDS, anecdotal experience suggests that suppressive treatment is usually effective (7).

Acyclovir-Resistant HSV in Immunocompromised Hosts

Although acyclovir resistance can develop through loss of viral thymidine kinase or alteration in substrate specifically of viral thymidine kinase or DNA polymerase, most acyclovir-resistant clinical isolates show thymidine kinase (TK) deficiency (7,15,21,37,49,55-59). Of interest, these TK-deficient viruses are usually less virulent in animal studies (55,59). Although TK-deficient strains have been isolated from immunocompromised patients during treatment with acyclovir, there has been some controversy over the role of TK deficiency in causing persistent infection (46). Until recently only a few well-documented cases had been reported, and in some cases the infections with TK-deficient viruses resolved during treatment with acyclovir as patients recovered from severe immunosuppression. Recently, however, cases of chronic TK-deficient HSV infection without clinical or virologic response to acyclovir therapy have been documented in patients with AIDS (7,29,61). Although rare, these cases leave little doubt that TK-deficient HSV can cause persistent infection in the immunocompromised host despite acyclovir therapy. In cases of TK-deficient HSV in patients with AIDS, patients have usually been treated with acyclovir in the past and present with large, chronic mucotaneous ulcers (61).

Treatment Guidelines in the Immunocompromised Host

In contrast to decisions for treatment in the normal adult, decisions about suppressive treatment in the immunocompromised patient are often based on the expected severity and duration of immunosuppression rather than on the frequency or severity of past recurrences. Although employing the lowest effective dose is widely practiced in the normal host, there are some theoretical concerns regarding use of very low doses in immunocompromised patients, especially when treating very large lesions or if immunosuppression is not expected to be transient. Acyclovir-resistant, TK-deficient mutants can be produced in vitro through exposure of HSV to subtherapeutic levels of acyclovir, and TK-deficient mutants also occur spontaneously in the absence of acyclovir treatment (57). The chances of having

TK-deficient HSV may therefore be greater in large lesions in immunocompromised patients. Thus, we do not try to determine the lowest effective dose and encourage early, aggressive treatment, especially for large lesions.

Routine serologic screening for HSV antibody is recommended for patients receiving bone marrow or other organ transplants, induction chemotherapy for leukemia, or equivalent high-dose chemotherapy, and prophylaxis is recommended for seropositive patients. Prophylaxis should begin at the time of induction therapy or transplantation, whichever occurs sooner. Treatment with intravenous acyclovir at doses of 5 mg/kg per dose or 250 mg/m^2 per dose every 8 h can be employed perioperatively or when patients have severe mucositis, but most suppressive therapy can be accomplished with oral acyclovir. Doses of 200 or 400 mg orally four or five times daily are effective and well tolerated in most patients (Table 2). Routine laboratory monitoring is probably not necessary during suppressive therapy with oral acyclovir, but renal function should be monitored during administration of intravenous acyclovir.

Renal transplant patients should have dose adjustments based on creatinine clearance. They can be treated intravenously with 5 mg/kg or 250 mg/m^2 q12h if the creatinine clearance is $\geq$ 50 ml/min, treated at the same dose every 24 h for a creatinine clearance of 20 to 50, and treatment with 2.5 mg/kg or 125 mg/m^2 q24h for a creatinine clearance of < 20 ml/min/1.73 m^2.

Oral acyclovir should be administered at a dose of 200 mg three times daily for a creatinine clearance of $\geq$ 30 and 200 mg twice daily for a creatinine clearance < 30 (Table 2).

The duration of prophylactic treatment is based on the likelihood of development of a severe recurrence. In general, prophylaxis can be discontinued once the granulocyte count is $\geq$ 500/mm^3 following induction chemotherapy. In contrast, prophylaxis is often continued for 6 weeks after bone marrow or organ transplant, and prophylaxis for longer periods may be appropriate if marrow engraftment is delayed or if high-dose immunosuppressive therapy is continued for treatment of graft rejection. Although not as severe as episodes occurring shortly after transplant or during granulocytopenia, the first episode following a course of prophylaxis may be more severe and prolonged than subsequent episodes, and episodic treatment may be appropriate.

Suppressive Therapy in Patients with HIV Infection

Many HIV-infected patients can be managed with episodic treatment. We treat episodes with oral acyclovir at a dose of 400 mg four or five times daily for at least 10 days or until all lesions are healed. When HIV-infected patients report frequent recurrences (e.g., once a month or every other month), we encourage suppressive therapy. In addition, we tend to consider suppressive therapy in patients with advanced AIDS-related complex or AIDS and those with less than 200 T4 cells/mm³, since recurrent infections tend to be more severe and prolonged in this setting. For suppressive therapy in HIV-infected patients, we routinely use doses of 400 mg three or four times daily (Table 2) and make no attempt to determine a minimal effective dose for reasons described earlier. Higher oral acyclovir doses are being employed in studies evaluating the safety and efficiency of combination therapy with acyclovir and zidovudine (Retrovir) for treatment of HIV infection, but no recommendations for treatment in this setting can be made until these studies are completed.

In view of the safety and efficacy demonstrated thus far in acyclovir suppression studies, the morbidity of HSV infections in patients with AIDS, and the limited life expectancy once AIDS is diagnosed, we generally recommend that suppressive treatment be continued indefinitely in patients with AIDS or with T4 counts < 200/mm³. For patients with earlier stages of HIV infection, recommendations for treatment duration in normal adults are probably more appropriate (Table 2).

CONCLUSION

Suppressive therapy with oral acyclovir is safe, well tolerated, and highly effective. In normal adults, the usual clinical indications for suppressive therapy include frequent recurrences, history of complications or interruption of work associated with recurrences, or predictable triggers. Continuous therapy for at least 4 years appears safe, but periodic interruption of therapy to evaluate the frequency of recurrences is recommended. Emergence of acyclovir resistance does not appear to be a problem in HSV infections in the normal host despite prolonged suppressive or episodic therapy.

Short-term suppressive therapy is recommended in patients with HSV antibody or with a history of HSV who undergo bone marrow transplant, organ transplant, or induction chemotherapy for leukemia. Suppressive therapy is also recommended in patients with AIDS who have HSV episodes. Although rare, in immunocompromised patients HSV isolates that demonstrate acyclovir resistance in vitro may cause severe, progressive disease, which is unresponsive to treatment with acyclovir.

REFERENCES

1. Mertz, G. J., Schmidt, O., Jourden, J. L., et al. (1985). Frequency of acquisition of first-episode genital infection with herpes simplex virus from symptomatic and asymptomatic source contacts. *Sex. Transm. Dis.* 12:33-39.

2. Mertz, G. J., Coombs, R. W., Ashley, R., et al. (1988). Transmission of genital herpes in couples with one symptomatic and one asymptomatic partner: A prospective study. *J. Infect. Dis.* 157:1169-1177.

3. Nahmias, A., Keyserling, H., Bain, R., et al. (1985). Prevalence of herpes simplex virus (HSV) type-specific antibodies in a U.S.A. prepaid group medical practice population. Programme of the 6th International Meeting, International Society for STD Research, Brighton, England, 31 July-2 Aug. 1985, p. 40 (abstract 43).

4. Knox, S. R., Corey, L., Blough, H. A., and Lerner, A. M. (1982). Historical findings in subjects from a high socioeconomic group who have genital infections with herpes simplex virus. *Sex. Transm. Dis.* 9:15-20.

5. Mertz, G. J., Skipper, B. J., Schaab, C., et al. (1987). Psychosocial responses to genital herpes infection and other sexually transmitted diseases. Presented at the VII Annual Meeting of the International Society for STD Research, Atlanta, Georgia, 2-5 Aug. 1987 (abstract 79).

6. Anderson, H., Scarffe, J. H., Sutton, R. N., et al. (1984). Oral acyclovir prophylaxis against herpes simplex virus in non-Hodgkin lymphoma and acute lymphoblastic leukemia patients receiving remission induction chemotherapy. A randomised double blind, placebo controlled trial. *Br. J. Cancer* 50:45-49.

7. Drew, W. L., Buhles, W., and Erlich, K. S. (1988). Herpesvirus infections (cytomegalovirus, herpes simplex virus, varicella-zoster virus): How to use ganciclovir (DHPG) and acyclovir. *Infect. Dis. Clin. North Am.* 2:495-509.

8. Meyers, J. D., Fluornoy, N., and Thomas, E. D. (1980). Infection with herpes simplex virus and cell-mediated immunity after marrow transplant. *J. Infect. Dis.* 142:338-346.

9. Pass, R. F., Whitely, R. J., Whelchel, J. D., et al. (1979). Identification of patients with increased risk of infection with herpes simplex virus after renal transplantation. *J. Infect. Dis.* 140:487-492.

10. Pettersson, E., Hovi, T., Ahonen, J., et al. (1985). Prophylactic oral acyclovir after renal transplantation. *Transplantation* 39:279-281.

11. Saral, R., Burns, W. H., Laskin, O. L., et al. (1981). Acyclovir prophylaxis of herpes simplexvirus infections. A randomized, double-blind, controlled trial in bone-marrow-transplant recipients. *N. Engl. J. Med.* 305:63-67.

12. Shepp, D. H., Newton, B. A., Dandliker, P. S., et al. (1985). Oral acyclovir therapy for mucocutaneous herpes simplex virus infections in immunocompromised marrow transplant recipients. *Ann. Intern. Med.* 102:783-785.

13. Siegal, F. P., Lopez, C., Hammer, G. S., et al. (1981). Severe acquired immunodeficiency in male homosexuals, manifested by chronic perianal ulcerative herpes simplex lesions. *N. Engl. J. Med.* 305:1439-1444.
14. Straus, S. E., Seidlin, M., Takiff, H., et al. (1984). Oral acyclovir to suppress recurring herpes simplex virus infections in immunodeficient patients. *Ann. Intern. Med.* 100:522-524.
15. Wade, J. C., McLaren, C., and Meyers, J. D. (1983). Frequency and significance of acyclovir-resistant herpes simplex virus isolated from marrow transplant patients receiving multiple courses of treatment with acyclovir. *J. Infect. Dis.* 148:1077-1082.
16. Wade, J. C., Newton, B., Flournoy, N., and Meyers, J. D. (1984). Oral acyclovir for prevention of herpes simplex virus reactivation after marrow transplantation. *Ann. Intern. Med.* 100:823-828.
17. Corey, L., and Spear, P. G. (1986). Infections with herpes simplex viruses (1 and 2). *N. Engl. J. Med.* 314:686-691, 749-757.
18. Corey, L., Adams, H. G., Brown, Z. A., and Holmes, K. K. (1983). Genital herpes simplex virus infection: Clinical manifestations, course and complications. *Ann. Intern. Med.* 98:958-972.
19. Reeves, W. C., Corey, L., Adams, H. G., et al. (1981). Risk of recurrence after first episodes of genital herpes: Relation to HSV type and antibody response. *N. Engl. J. Med.* 305:315-319.
20. Lafferty, W. E., Coombs, R. W., Benedetti, J., et al. (1987). Recurrences after oral and genital herpes simplex virus infection: Influence of site of infection and viral type. *N. Engl. J. Med.* 316:1444-1449.
21. Coen, D. M., and Schaffer, P. A. (1980). Two distinct loci confer resistance to acycloguanosine in herpes simplex virus type 1. *Proc. Natl. Acad. Sci. USA* 77:2265-2269.
22. Kapoor, A. K., Nash, A. A., Wildy, P., et al. (1982). Pathogenesis of herpes simplex virus in congenitally athymic mice: The relative roles of cell mediated and humoral immunity. *J. Gen. Virol.* 60:225-233.
23. Gluckman, E., Lotsberg, J., Devergie, A., et al. (1983). Oral acyclovir prophylactic treatment of herpes simplex infection after bone marrow transplantation. *J. Antimicrob. Chemother.* 12(Suppl. B):161-167.
24. Shepp, D. H., Dandliker, P. S., Flournoy, N., and Meyers, J. D. (1985). Once-daily intravenous acyclovir for prophylaxis of herpes simplex virus reactivation after marrow transplantation. *J. Antimicrob. Chemother.* 16:389-395.
25. Prentice, H. G. (1983). Use of acyclovir for prophylaxis of herpes infections in severely immunocompromised patients. *J. Antimicrob. Chemother.* 12 (Suppl. B):153-159.
26. Seale, L., Jones, C. J., Kathpalia, S., et al. (1985). Prevention of herpesvirus infections in renal allograft recipients by low-dose oral acyclovir. *JAMA* 254:3435-3438.

27. Bean, S. F., and Quezada, R. K. (1983). Recurrent oral erythema multiforme. Clinical experience with 11 patients. *JAMA* 249:2810-2812.
28. Green, J. A., Spruance, S. L., Wenerstrom, G., and Piepkorn, M. W. (1985). Post-herpetic erythema multiforme prevented with prophylactic oral acyclovir. *Ann. Intern. Med.* 102:632-633.
29. Mertz, G. J. (1987). Diagnosis and treatment of genital herpes infections. In Antiviral Chemotherapy, Infectious Disease Clinics of North America. Knight, V., and Gilbert, B. E. (eds.): *Antiviral Chemotherapy.* Philadelphia, Saunders, Vol. 1, pp. 341-366.
30. Goldstein, L. C., Corey, L., McDougall, J., et al. (1983). Monoclonal antibodies to herpes simplex viruses/ use in antigenic typing and rapid diagnosis. *J. Infect. Dis.* 147:829-837.
31. Peterson, E., Schmidt, O. W., Goldstein, L. C., et al. (1983). Typing of clinical herpes simplex virus isolates with mouse monoclonal antibodies to herpes simplex virus types 1 and 2: comparison with type-specific rabbit antisera and restriction endonuclease analysis of viral DNA. *J. Clin. Microbiol.* 17: 92-96.
32. Bernstein, D. I., Bryson, Y. J., and Lovett, M. A. (1985). Antibody response to type-common and type-unique epitopes of herpes simplex virus polypeptides. *J. Med. Virol.* 15:251-263.
33. Bernstein, D. I., Lovett, M. A., and Bryson, Y. J. (1984). Serologic analysis of first-episode nonprimary genital herpes simplex virus infection. Presence of type 2 antibody in acute serum samples. *Am. J. Med.* 77:1055-1060.
34. Mertz, G. J., Jones, C. C., Mills, J., et al. (1988). Long-term acyclovir suppression of frequently recurring genital herpes simplex virus infection: A multicenter double-blind trial. *JAMA* 260:201-206.
35. Nusinoff Lehrman, S., Douglas, J. M., Corey, L., and Barry, D. W. (1986). Recurrent genital herpes and suppressive oral acyclovir therapy: Relationship between clinical outcome and in vitro drug sensitivity. *Ann. Intern. Med.* 104:786-790.
36. Straus, S. E., Takiff, H. E., Seidlin, M., et al. (1984). Suppression of frequently recurring genital herpes, a placebo-controlled double-blind trial of oral acyclovir. *N. Engl. J. Med.* 310:1545-1550.
37. Crumpacker, C. S., Schnipper, L. E., Marlowe, S. I., et al. (1982). Resistance to antiviral drugs of herpes simplex virus isolated from a patient treated with acyclovir. *N. Engl. J. Med.* 306:343-346.
38. Douglas, J. M., Critchlow, C., Benedetti, J., et al. (1984). A double-blind study of oral acyclovir for suppression of recurrences of genital herpes simplex virus infection. *N. Engl. J. Med.* 310:1551-1556.
39. Halsos, A. M., Salo, O. P., Lassus, A., et al. (1985). Oral acyclovir suppression of recurrent genital herpes: Double-blind, placebo-controlled crossover study. *Acta Derm. Venereol.* 65:59-63.
40. Mindel, A., Weller, I. V. D., Faherty, A., et al. (1984). Prophylactic oral acyclovir in recurrent genital herpes. *Lancet* 2:57-59.

41. Portnoy, J., and Taussig, A. (1984). A double blind placebo controlled six month trial of prophylactic oral acyclovir in recurrent genital herpes. Read before the International Conjoint Sexually Transmitted Diseases Meeting, Montreal, 17-21 June 1984, p. 237 (abstract 185).

42. Thin, R. N., Jeffries, D. J., Taylor, P. K., et al. (1985). Recurrent genital herpes suppressed by oral acyclovir: A multicentre double blind trial. *J. Antimicrob. Chemother.* 16:219-226.

43. Mertz, G. J., Eron, L., Kaufman, R., et al. (1988). Prolonged continuous versus intermittent oral acyclovir treatment in normal adults with frequently recurring genital herpes simplex virus infection. *Am. J. Med.* 85(2A):14-19.

44. Mindel, A., Faherty, A., Carney, O., et al. (1988). Dosage and safety of long-term suppressive acyclovir therapy for recurrent genital herpes. *Lancet* 1:926-928.

45. Mostow, S. R., Mayfield, J. L., Marr, J. J., Drucker, J. L. (1988). Suppression of recurrent genital herpes by single daily dosages of acyclovir. *Am. J. Med.* 85(2A):30-33.

46. Straus, S. E., Croen, K. D., Sawyer, M. H., et al. (1988). Acyclovir suppression of frequently recurring genital herpes: Efficacy and diminishing need during successive years of treatment. *JAMA* 260:2227-2230.

47. Sacks, S. L., Fox, R., Levendusky, P., et al. (1988). Chronic suppression for six months compared with intermittent lesional therapy of recurrent genital herpes using oral acyclovir: Effects on lesions and nonlesional prodromes. *Sex. Transm. Dis.* 15:58-62.

48. Rooney, J. F., Felser, J. M., Ostrove, J. M., and Straus, S. E. (1986). Acquisition of genital herpes from an asymptomatic sexual partner. *N. Engl. J. Med.* 314:1561-1564.

49. Parris, D. S., and Harrington, J. E. (1982). Herpes simplex virus variants restraint to high concentrations of acyclovir exist in clinical isolates. *Antimicrob. Agents Chemother.* 22:71-77.

50. Douglas J. M., Davis, L. G., Remington, M. L., et al. (1988). A double-blind placebo-controlled trial of the effect of chronically administered oral acyclovir on sperm production in men with frequently recurrent genital herpes. *J. Infect. Dis.* 157:588-593.

51. Pazin, G. J., Ho, M., and Jannetta, P. J. (1978). Reactivation of herpes simplex virus after decompression of the trigeminal nerve root. *J. Infect. Dis.* 138:405-409.

52. Laskin, O. L. (1985). Acyclovir and suppression of frequently recurring herpetic whitlow. *Ann. Intern. Med.* 102:494-495.

53. Steel, J. G., Dix, R. D., and Baringer, J. R. (1982). Isolation of herpes simplex type 1 in recurrent (Mollaret) meningitis. *Ann. Neurol.* 11:17-21.

54. Straus, S. E., Seidlin, M., Takiff, H. E., et al. (1986). Double-blind comparison of weekend and daily regimens of oral acyclovir for suppression of recurrent genital herpes. *Antiviral Res.* 6:151-159.

55. Sibrack, C. D., Gutman, L. T., Wilfert, C. M., et al. (1982). Pathogenicity of acyclovir-resistant herpes simplex virus type 1 from an immunodeficient child. *J. Infect. Dis.* 146:673-682.

56. Burns, W. H., Saral, R., Santos, G. W., et al. (1982). Isolation and characterization of resistant herpes simplex virus after acyclovir therapy. *Lancet* 1: 421-423.

57. Crumpacker, C. S. (1986). Resistance of herpes viruses to nucleoside analogues—mechanisms and clinical importance. In Mills, J., and Corey, L. (eds.): *Antiviral Chemotherapy. New Directions for Clinical Application and Research.* New York, Elsevier, p. 226.

58. Schnipper, L. E., and Crumpacker, C. S. (1980). Resistance of herpes simplex virus to acycloguanosine: Role of viral thymidine kinase and DNA polymerase loci. *Proc. Natl. Acad. Sci. USA* 77:2270-2273.

59. Field, H. J., and Darby, G. (1980). Pathogenicity in mice of strains of herpes simplex virus which are resistant to acyclovir in vitro and in vivo. *Antimicrob. Agents Chemother.* 17:209-216.

60. Spruance, S. L., Hamill, M. L., Hoge, W. S., Davis, L. G., Mills, J. (1988). Acyclovir prevents reactivation of herpes simplex labialis in skiers. *JAMA* 260:1597-1599.

61. Erlich, K. S., Mills, J., Chatis, P., et al. (1989). Acyclovir-resistant herpes simplex virus infections in patients with the acquired immunodeficiency syndrome. *N. Engl. J. Med.* 320:293-296.

9
Acyclovir in Pregnancy

Zane A. Brown   *University of Washington, Seattle, Washington*

Acyclovir (ACV) is remarkably effective in treating primary, recrudescent, and life-threatening herpes simplex virus (HSV) and varicella zoster virus (VZV) infections of the normal adult, the immunocompromised adult, and the newborn infant (1-10). Other than case reports and preliminary pharmacokinetic data, there are no published clinical trials of ACV in pregnancy. Therefore, this review will address what is known of its pharmacokinetics and reported uses in pregnancy while emphasizing that at this writing, neither the safety nor the efficacy of this drug for any indication in pregnancy has been demonstrated.

PHARMACOKINETICS AND SAFETY OF ACYCLOVIR IN PREGNANCY

To evaluate the pharmacokinetics of orally administered ACV in late pregnancy, Brown et al. administered oral ACV 200 mg every 8 h to women with a history of recurrent genital herpes. Therapy was initiated prophylactically at approximately 38 weeks' gestation and continued until the onset of labor. The mean duration of ACV therapy was 9.8 days with a range of 6-15 days. Peak maternal plasma levels on the day of delivery ranged from 1.48 to 2.52 μM (0.225 μg/ml ACV = 1 μM ACV) at 1.5-3.0 h after last dose.

The highest plasma level observed in any newborn was 1.28 μM at 8.5 h of life. Acyclovir was significantly concentrated in amniotic fluid and gastric aspirate but not in fetal blood. At the time of delivery all newborn levels were less than those of the mother. The ratio of time-averaged plasma concentrations of ACV in mothers and newborns was 1.12. In the five mother/newborn pairs, there was no evidence of toxicity (11). The peak levels observed in these term pregnant patients were somewhat lower than those observed by Van Dyke et al. in nonpregnant patients where mean peak levels of 1.4-4.0 μM were observed 1.5-1.75 h after oral administration of a 200-mg dose of ACV (12). The differences are most likely secondary to the increased renal clearance and volume of distribution of ACV during pregnancy. Recently, the pregnancy pharmacokinetics were repeated with twice the dose of oral acyclovir (i.e., 400 mg every 8 h). The maternal blood levels that were attained seemed to be more comparable to those reported for nonpregnant patients (13).

In a patient 4 months postpartum, breast feeding, with a primary episode of orolabial herpes and receiving ACV 200 mg every 4 h, Lau et al. demonstrated a maximum plasma concentration of 4.23 μM at 1.5 h postdose, measured on the fourth day of therapy. The elimination half-life was approximately 3 h. The concentration of ACV in breast milk was 3.3 μM at the start of the study period and prior to a 200-mg dose of ACV. This fell to 1.9 μM one-half hour after the dose and rose to 5.8 μM at 3.2 h, indicating a lag before appearing in the milk. The concentrations in breast milk exceeded those in maternal plasma at all times except at the time of the peak plasma concentrations. They calculated a plasma-to-milk ratio of 0.15. As would be anticipated, ACV was measurable in the infant's urine (14). Meyer et al. also measured the concentration of acyclovir in the breast milk of a patient 1 year postpartum with herpes zoster for which she was receiving ACV 200 mg five times daily. The average concentration in milk was 1.06 μg/ml (4.71 μM) and 0.33 μg/ml (1.46 μM) in serum with a plasma-to-milk ratio of 0.31. The half-life of acyclovir in breast milk for this patient was 2.8 h. Based on an average breast milk concentration of 1.06 μg/ml (4.71 μM), they calculated that the infant received a daily dose of approximately 1 mg of acyclovir (15).

Very few data are available following intravenous use of acyclovir in late pregnancy. Lagrew et al. measured peak and trough levels of ACV following intravenous doses of 7.5 mg/kg every 8 h to a woman at 31-32 weeks' gestation. Trough maternal acyclovir levels drawn 5 min prior to doses 12, 13, and 18 were 2.7, 3.4, and 2.7 μg/ml. Peak levels drawn 20 min following the 1-hour administration period of the same doses were 13.2, 8.6, and 12.8 μg/ml (16).

In 1986, Kingsley reported on 116 pregnant patients from 15 countries that had received ACV. Fifty-eight patients received the drug in the first trimester. Eight terminated, and eight had reached term at the time of the report and were normal. At the time of the abstract, 36 of the 42 third-trimester exposures to ACV had reached term and showed no ill effects due to the drug. Acyclovir levels in cord blood from 18 neonates exposed to ACV in utero ranged from $<0.5\ \mu M$ to $1.23\ \mu M$. Fourteen amniotic fluid samples had ACV levels ranging from $<0.5\ \mu M$ to $5.58\ \mu M$. One patient receiving oral ACV had a breast milk level of $8.0\ \mu M$ (17).

No fetal toxicity or teratogenicity was observed in rabbits and rats given doses up to 25 mg/kg by subcutaneous injection. Mice given doses of 450 mg/kg/day by gavage (the usual oral adult human dose is approximately 15 mg/kg/day) showed no impairment of reproduction or development over two generations (18). Evaluations in mammalian cell systems demonstrated that ACV did not damage individual genes or components, even in huge doses. Chromosomal damage was observed in cultured human lymphocytes exposed to 250 μg/ml ACV (approximately 25 times the peak levels achieved with intravenous dosing in pregnancy (16) but not at $\leqslant 125$ μg/ml. No chromosomal damage was seen in Chinese hamsters given doses of 100 mg/kg (19).

Though these animal data would suggest that ACV is probably safe for use during pregnancy, it is difficult to apply animal data to humans, and data from large numbers of human pregnancies are not available.

To supplement published cases of ACV use during pregnancy, Burroughs Wellcome Co., the manufacturer of ACV, and the Centers for Disease Control have established an international case registry to evaluate the safety of ACV by epidemiological methods (20). As of June 30, 1987, a total of 274 pregnancies in which ACV was used have been reported. More than half have been from the United States. Unfortunately, these numbers are still far too small to draw conclusions regarding the use of the drug in any specific trimester of pregnancy (20). Practitioners are encouraged to report all known exposures to ACV during pregnancy to Dr. Elizabeth Andrews, Senior Epidemiologist, Division of Epidemiology, Burroughs Wellcome Co., 3030 Cornwallis Road, Research Triangle Park, NC 27709. Telephone reports should be made to (919)248-4017.

ACYCLOVIR IN PREGNANCIES COMPLICATED BY HSV INFECTIONS

Primary Genital Herpes

Primary genital herpes is the initial episode of genital herpes in individuals seronegative for HSV-1 and HSV-2 and demonstrating signs and symptoms such as headache, fever, malaise, myalgias, numerous bilateral genital lesions, and severe local pain for at least 10 days. The genital lesions usually persist for more than 16 days, with HSV lesions frequently appearing at distal sites such as the fingers, buttocks, and oropharynx. In contrast, nonprimary first episodes of genital herpes occur in patients who have had prior HSV-1 infections and are associated with less frequent and usually milder systemic signs and symptoms. Healing is faster than with primary genital herpes (21).

In a recent study comparing the pregnancy outcomes of 15 patients with primary genital herpes and 14 with nonprimary first-episode disease complicating pregnancy, 6 of the 15 (40%) patients with primary disease developed serious obstetrical and perinatal complications. These included spontaneous abortion (1 case), intrauterine growth retardation (3 cases), preterm labor (4 cases), neonatal HSV infection (2 cases), and neonatal death (1 case). The chance of adverse outcome increased with advancing gestation with one of five cases in the first trimester, one of five cases in the second trimester, and four of five cases in the third trimester demonstrating one or more of these complications.

Recurrences following healing of the primary episode during the pregnancy were more commonly asymptomatic and from the cervix in contrast to recurrences following a nonprimary first episode which were most commonly symptomatic and from the external genitalia. The pattern of symptomatic recurrences and asymptomatic shedding following nonprimary first episodes was similar to that reported for patients entering pregnancy with recurrent genital herpes (22). Other investigators have also reported an association between primary genital HSV infection and spontaneous abortion, preterm labor, and neonatal HSV infection (23-26).

The mechanisms for this perinatal morbidity are uncertain. Primary cervical HSV infection may progress to an ascending HSV chorioamnionitis and placentitis which either directly or in conjunction with a secondary bacterial infection activates the arachidonic prostaglandin pathway within the fetal membranes and decidua stimulating the local production of prostaglandins and initiating parturition (27-29). Using in vitro models, prostaglandin E_2 has been shown to significantly enhance viral replication and the cell to cell spread of HSV-2, possibly by modifying the local and systemic immune response (30,31).

The role of primary genital herpes in the pathogenesis of preterm labor is supported by the observations that approximately one third of the infants developing neonatal herpes are born prematurely, usually between 30 and 37 weeks of gestation (25,32). This is in contrast to infants delivered of mothers entering pregnancy with recurrent genital herpes where the prematurity rate is 3-4%—i.e., a rate comparable to that of a white middle-class population (33). It is possible that a viral placentitis damages the mechanisms for nutrient transport across the placenta. If the pregnancy remains undelivered because of either spontaneous waning of uterine activity or drug control of the preterm labor, then intrauterine growth retardation may result. Not only are women who acquire primary genital herpes during pregnancy at increased risk of direct adverse perinatal outcome such as intrauterine growth retardation and preterm labor, additionally because of the increased likelihood of asymptomatic cervical viral shedding rather than symptomatic recurrences subsequent to their primary episode, they are more likely to be permitted to labor and thereby transmit the infection to their newborns during vaginal delivery.

Utley et al. reported a case of primary genital herpes with onset at 23.5 weeks. Membranes ruptured at 25.5 weeks. Because of the extreme prematurity, acyclovir 500 mg every 8 h was administered. On the sixth day of therapy, the patient labored and delivered a 26.5-week gestation by cesarean section. Neonatal cultures were negative. The maternal and cord acyclovir levels at birth were 7.9 and 9.9 nmol/ml, respectively (34).

The unpublished experience of the author would suggest that the treatment of primary genital herpes infections during pregnancy with acyclovir 200 mg orally five times daily until resolution of symptoms is probably without immediate adverse effects for either mother or fetus. However, it is as yet not established that ACV therapy will modify the virologic course of the primary infection during pregnancy or its associated adverse obstetrical and perinatal outcomes. As in the nonpregnant patient, it is likely that ACV therapy will accelerate the healing of lesions and decrease the time of pain and viral shedding (1). Using type-specific neutralizing antibody titers, Bernstein et al. demonstrated that in nonpregnant adults, ACV therapy for primary genital HSV infections could delay the humoral response. This alteration in antibody response did not modify the rates of subsequent symptomatic recurrences, and at 6-12 months following their primary episode, all patients had achieved a normal antibody complement (35). An ACV-mediated delay in the humoral response following an episode of primary genital herpes in late pregnancy could result in delayed or diminished transfer of immunoglobulins to the fetus, making the fetus more vulnerable to HSV asymptomatically present in the genital tract during labor. Since transplacentally acquired antibody has been demonstrated to be protective for the neonate exposed to infectious HSV during vaginal delivery, any decrease or delay in the transfer of maternally acquired anti-HSV antibody to the fetus could increase the risk of neo-natal HSV infection (36). Ashley and Corey demonstrated a suppression of the cellular immune response following ACV therapy for primary genital HSV infection (37). Since pregnancy is already characterized by a progressive decline in the cellular immune response, this ACV-mediated effect could further increase the rate of asymptomatic shedding following the primary episode.

Transmembranous spread of the herpes simplex virus with congenital infection of the fetus has been well documented (38,39). Though accelerated resolution of the maternal primary infection might occur, ACV therapy may be ineffective in treating an established intrauterine infection of the fetoplacental unit (40). In the author's unpublished experience, ACV therapy has not uniformly prevented the intrauterine growth retardation subsequent to the primary episode. These issues of efficacy and safety can only be resolved by prospective (and probably collaborative) controlled studies.

Disseminated Maternal HSV Infection

The selective decline in the cellular immune response with advancing pregnancy is associated with an increased risk of acquisition and severity for certain infectious diseases in which cell-mediated immunity plays an important defense role (41-43). Included are mycobacterial, intracellular bacterial, systemic fungal, viral, protozoan, and helminthic infections (44,45). Disseminated HSV infection has been reported in immunocompromised patients, pregnancy, and, rarely, in normal immunocompetent adults. Presenting almost exclusively in the latter half of pregnancy with an encephalitis and/or hepatitis together with severe constitutional signs and symptoms, maternal and fetal mortalities in excess of 50% have been reported (40,46-50). A patient with a disseminated HSV infection was treated with ACV 7.5 mg/kg every 8 h for 7 days at 32 weeks. Though the mother rapidly improved with ACV, she developed an amnionitis, necessitating delivery of a normal 2320-g fetus on the seventh day of ACV therapy (48).

Another patient with a severe HSV encephalitis at 29 weeks' gestation was treated with 5 mg/kg ACV IV every 8 h and survived with only right focal motor seizures. She delivered a normal infant at term who remains normal at 3.5 years (49). A patient with a severe HSV-2 encephalitis at 32 weeks received three doses of intravenous ACV 10 mg/kg. Simultaneously, intravenous adenine arabinoside was started as a single

infusion of 30 mg/kg/day. On her 13th day of therapy, the adenine arabinoside was discontinued, and IV ACV was reinstituted at 10 mg/kg every
8 h. On her 18th day of therapy or 5 days after ACV was reinstituted, a
2850-g female infant was delivered. The mother died 2 days later. The infant had neonatal HSV at birth and was treated with ACV 5 mg/kg every
8 h for 10 days (39). Chazotte et al. reported a case of disseminated herpes
simplex infection in a patient with systemic lupus erythematosus. She was
treated with 400 mg IV every 6 h with rapid improvement and discharge
from the hospital after 10 days of ACV therapy (50).

Recurrent Genital Herpes

There is little doubt at present that the prevalence of genital herpes has
markedly increased in the last several decades with the greatest increase
in the more affluent segments of our reproductive age population. This
increase in the prevalence of genital herpes in the adult population has
been paralleled by a similar increase in the incidence of the neonatal infection. In King County, Washington, the incidence of the neonatal infection increased from 2.6/100,000 live births in 1966 to 28.5/100,000 (or
about 1/3,500 live births) in 1985 (51). This increase in the incidence of
neonatal herpes has occurred in spite of an aggressive national policy of
antepartum HSV cultures and cesarean section. Data derived from analysis of birth certificates in the State of Washington indicated a cesarean
section rate in excess of 50% for patients entering pregnancy with recurrent genital herpes (52). It is obvious that the extraordinary economic
and social costs of this excess cesarean section in addition to the associated
maternal morbidity and mortality has created a public health problem of
greater significance than the disease it was meant to prevent.

   Probably because of the decreased cellular immune response, the
frequency of symptomatic reactivation of genital herpes progressively increases with advancing gestation. This increases the likelihood of a recurrence appearing in proximity to the onset of labor. Since the prematurity
rate for patients entering pregnancy with recurrent genital herpes is very
low (reflecting their predominantly middle-class background, prophylactic
ACV therapy could be initiated at or close to 37 weeks' gestation, thereby
suppressing symptomatic recurrences of genital herpes, reducing patient
and physician anxiety, and obviating the need for cesarean section (33).
Ciraru-Vigneron et al. reported using prophylactic oral acyclovir at 800
mg/day in nine patients from 36 weeks' gestation to the onset of labor
(53). Though the concept is attractive, many issues remain to be resolved
before this therapy can be recommended.

Since therapy is initiated for a maternal indication without probable measurable benefit to the fetus, fetal safety, both short and long term, is of prime concern. With the increased renal clearance and volume of distribution of late pregnancy, the oral dosing of prophylactic ACV is likely to be substantially different from that for the nonpregnant patient. Since prophylactic oral ACV effectively suppresses symptomatic recurrences in immunosuppressed patients, it is likely that it will be equally effective in pregnancy. However, it has not been demonstrated in any group of patients that asymptomatic shedding is similarly suppressed. It is possible that symptomatic recurrences in late pregnancy could be incompletely suppressed and present as asymptomatic HSV shedding. Until these and other issues of efficacy and safety are resolved by appropriate prospective trials, the use of ACV for suppressing symptomatic recurrences in late pregnancy cannot be recommended.

ACYCLOVIR IN PREGNANCIES COMPLICATED BY VARICELLA ZOSTER VIRUS INFECTIONS

Varicella (chickenpox) is an acute, highly contagious, but benign disease of childhood due to a primary infection with the varicella zoster virus (VZV). It presents with a generalized maculovesicular eruption that appears in crops and rapidly passes through pustular, crust, and scab stages. Over 70% of young adults report a past history of varicella, and the incidence of seropositivity in temperate climates reaches 100% by age 60 (54, 55). When acquired by adults, it is usually a more severe disease with high fever, malaise, and frequent pulmonary symptoms. Although less than 2% of reported cases of varicella occur over the age of 20 years, 25% of fatalities occur in this age group (56). Like the HSV, the VZV persists in a latent form in the dorsal nerve root ganglia and reactives with waning immunity as zoster (shingles), which can be a severe, painful, and often debilitating disease, particularly among the immunocompromised and elderly. The available studies of VZV infections complicating pregnancy suggest that the infection occurs at a minimum frequency of 2.3 cases per 10,000 pregnancies (57).

Varicella Pneumonia Complicating Pregnancy

Harris et al., in a 1965 review of 17 cases of maternal VZV pneumonia, reported a maternal mortality of 41%. This was in contrast to an 11% mortality for the same condition in 236 nonpregnant adults (58). In the series of 43 cases of maternal varicella reported by Paryani and Arvin, four were complicated by VZV pneumonia, of which two required ventilatory support and one died (59). Because of significant reporting bias, it is difficult to assess from the literature whether varicella pneumonia imposes a graver risk to a pregnant woman. From this author's experience, however, both the frequency and severity of varicella pneumonia increase with advancing gestation. Because of its substantial morbidity and mortality, maternal varicella pneumonia should be treated with intravenous ACV. However, prospective data proving efficacy in modifying the natural history of the disease, safety for the fetus, and the optimum dosage and duration of therapy are lacking.

Glaser et al. reported a successful treatment with 400 mg every 8 h. The drug was discontinued after 12 doses when lesions began to heal (60). Hankins et al. reported a patient who was critically ill with VZV pneumonia, disseminated itnravascular coagulopathy, and renal shutdown. ACV was administered intravenously for 7 days, initially at 350 mg every 8 h for 2 days. Owing to an increasing serum creatinine, the dosage was decreased (61). Eder et al. used 500 mg every 8 h for two patients with VZV pneumonia. One patient acquired varicella pneumonia at 30 weeks' gestation and was treated with intravenous ACV for 7 days. She delivered a mildly growth retarded infant at 38 weeks. The placenta showed evidence of acute chorioamnionitis with foci of infarction, calcifications, and intervillous fibrinous material. The other patient acquired the varicella pneumonia at 27 weeks' gestation and received less than 2 days of acyclovir before precipitously delivering. The premature infant was treated with acyclovir and varicella zoster immune globulin (VZIG) and did not develop varicella (62).

Leen et al. reported six cases of varicella infections during pregnancy of which four had varicella pneumonia at gestational ages ranging from 16 to 33 weeks. They were treated successfully with 10 mg/kg every 8 h for 5 days, and all delivered at term (63). Boyd et al. reported four cases of varicella complicating pregnancy of which three had pneumonia. One patient who acquired her varicella pneumonia at 26 weeks' gestation received intravenous ACV 5 mg/kg every 8 h and was delivered by cesarean section. The infant died shortly after birth. The mother died 1 month later from intestinal obstruction.

Two other patients with varicella pneumonia were treated with 15 and 18 mg/kg every 8 h with rapid improvement of pulmonary status. Both were delivered at term. The fourth patient had uncomplicated varicella at 38 weeks' gestation and was treated with 10 mg/kg with rapid resolution of her rash (;64). Landsberger et al. reported three cases of varicella

pneumonia complicating pregnancy. One patient who acquired her varicella pneumonia at 31 weeks' gestation ruptured her membranes and delivered 36 h after initiation of intravenous ACV 10 mg/kg every 8 h. The
infant was treated with zoster immune globulin and did not develop a
varicella infection. The maternal serum concentration of ACV was 1.4
μg/ml with the cord serum level of 2.0 μg/ml and the amniotic fluid concentration of 5.5 μg/ml.

   Two other patients were treated with adenine arabinoside at 26 and
27 weeks' gestation, respectively. Both recovered and delivered healthy
infants at term (67). From meager data it seems that intravenous ACV
has a logical but unproven role in the therapy of critically ill gravid women
with varicella pneumonia. However, until careful pharmacokinetic studies
of the drug in pregnancy are performed, no recommendations can be made
about dosing schedules.

   Because of the morbidity associated with maternal varicella, some
experts recommend the use of VZIG for patients at high risk in whom
prior immunity cannot be established. However, since there is no evidence
that administering VZIG to a susceptible pregnant woman will prevent
viremia, fetal infection, or the congenital varicella syndrome, its use in
pregnancy should be to prevent maternal complications. In fact, it is theoretically possible that the use of maternal VZIG may render the maternal
infection subclinical without preventing fetal infection and disease (56).
In the only randomized, placebo-controlled study of uncomplicated varicella in normal, nonpregnant adults, intravenous acyclovir 10 mg/kg every
8 h for 5 days had little overall effect on the course of the disease (66).
Since there is no evidence that uncomplicated chickenpox in the absence
of pneumonia is a more serious illness during pregnancy, the definitive
statement about the use of acyclovir with or in place of VZIG for otherwise uncomplicated varicella during pregnancy cannot be made at this
time. In any case, neonates born to mothers who develop varicella within
the 5 days preceding or 48 h following delivery should receive VZIG regardless of whether the mother received VZIG (56).

The Neonatal Effects of Maternal Varicella Infections

It is now well established that VZV infection during the first 12-16 weeks
of pregnancy can result in a congenital varicella syndrome characterized
by an array of defects including microcephaly, encephalitis, intrauterine
growth retardation, chorioretinitis, cataracts, microphthalmia, skin scarring, and limb atrophy. Using data compiled from four studies, Preblud
et al. estimated the risk of delivering an infant with a congenital varicella

syndrome as 2.3% (3/131) of cases of first-trimester maternal VZV infection. The 95% confidence limits for this observed risk were 0.5-6.5%
(67). The role of treatment of first-trimester maternal VZV infections
with zoster immune globin and/or ACV, though possible, remains to be
clarified by prospective studies in addition to studies of the teratogenic
potential of ACV in human pregnancies (20).

Young and Gershon have calculated that approximately 5% of infants will die of congenital varicella infection when a varicella rash appears in the mother less than 5 days prior to delivery (57). This mortality
rate is apparently due to the lag in the production and transmission of
protective anti-VZV IgG antibody. No neonatal deaths were noted when
the rash appeared 5 or more days prior to delivery. To provide this protective antibody, it is recommended that VZIG be administered intramuscularly to the infant as soon as possible after birth from a mother with
active varicella. Though it appears to modify the course of neonatal varicella infection, mortalities have been reported in spite of neonatal ZIG
therapy (68). Because of its efficient placental transfer and amniotic fluid
concentration, ACV for the high risk mother and VZIG for the exposed
infant may prove to be an effective alternative to neonatal VZIG alone
(11,18).

OTHER REPORTED USES OF ACYCLOVIR IN PREGNANCY

There are several anecdotal reports of acyclovir being used effectively to
suppress frequently recurring herpetic whitlow in nonpregnant patients
(69). There is one report of oral acyclovir 200 mg five times a day being
used to treat a severe episode of herpetic whitlow occurring at approximately 37 weeks' gestation (70).

SUMMARY

There are as yet no established indications for the use of acyclovir in pregnancy. However, at present, the most reasonable and appropriate use of
acyclovir in pregnancy is for life-threatening maternal infections such as
disseminated maternal HSV infection and varicella pneumonia. Less secure is its use for otherwise uncomplicated primary genital HSV infections
in pregnancy. In this circumstance treatment is instituted for possible fetal
benefit by averting the adverse pregnancy outcomes such as prematurity
and intrauterine growth retardation attributable to the primary genital
herpes. Least secure and the most problematic use is as primary or ad-
junctive therapy for uncomplicated varicella infections during pregnancy

and as prophylaxis against a genital HSV recurrence near term. In the latter instance, acyclovir would be used to avert the maternal morbidity attendant to cesarean section for the recurrent HSV genital lesion at the onset of labor.

REFERENCES

1. Corey, L., Fife, K. H., Benedetti, J. K., Winter, C. A., Fahnlander, A., Connor, J. D., Hintz, M. A., and Holmes, K. K. (1983). Intravenous acyclovir for the treatment of primary genital herpes. *Ann. Intern. Med.* 98:914-921.
2. Mertz, G. J., Critchlow, C. W., Benedetti, J. K., Reichman, R. C., Dolin, R., Connor, J., Redfield, D. C., Savoia, M. C., Richman, D. D., Tyrrell, D. L., Miedzinski, L., Portnoy, J., Keeney, R. E., and Corey, L. (1984). Double-blind placebo-controlled trial of oral acyclovir in first-episode genital herpes simplex virus infection. *JAMA* 252:1147-1151.
3. Douglas, J. M., Critchlow, C., Benedetti, J., Mertz, G. H., Connor, J. D., Hintz, M. A., Fahnlander, A., Remington, M., Winter, C., and Corey, L. (1984). A double-blind study of oral acyclovir for suppression of recurrences of genital herpes simplex virus infection. *N. Engl. J. Med.* 310:1551-1556.
4. Whitley, R. J., Alford, C. A., Hirsch, M. S., Schooley, R.T., Luby, J. P., Aoki, F. Y., Hanley, D., Nahmias, A. J., and Soong, S. (1986). Vidarabine versus acyclovir therapy in herpes simplex encephalitis. *N. Engl. J. Med.* 3 1 4 : 114-119.
5. Balfour, H. H., Bean, B., Laskin, C. L., Ambinder, R. J., Meyers, J. D., Wade, J. C., Zaia, J. A., Aeppli, D., Kirk, L. E., Segreti, A. C., Kenney, R. E., and Burroughs Wellcome Collaborative Acyclovir Study Group. (1983). Acyclovir halts progression of herpes zoster in immunocompromised patients. *N. Engl. J. Med.* 308:1448-1453.
6. Hann, I. M., Prentice, H. G., Blacklock, H. A., Ross, M. G. R., Bridgen, D., Rosling, A. E., Burke, C., Crawford, D. H., Brumfitt, W., and Hoffbrand, A. V. (1983). Acyclovir prophylaxis against herpes virus infections in severely immunocompromised patients; randomized double blind trial. *Br. Med. J.* 287:384-388.
7. Serota, F. T., Starr, S. E., Bryan, C. K., Koch, P. A., Plotkin, S. A., and August, C. S. (1982). Acyclovir treatment of herpes zoster infections. *JAMA* 247:2131-2135.
8. Mitchell, C. D., Bean, B., Gentry, S. R., Groth, K. E., Boen, J. R., and Balfour, H. H. (1981). Acyclovir therapy for mucocutaneous herpes simplex infections in immunocompromised patients. *Lancet* 1:1389-1392.
9. Offit, P. A., Starr, S. E., Zolnick, P., and Plotkin, S. A. (1982). Acyclovir therapy in neonatal herpes simplex virus infection. *Pediatr. Infect. Dis.* 1: 253-255.

10. Arvin, A. M. (1988). Antiviral treatment of herpes simplex infection in neonates and pregnant women. *J. Am. Acad. Dermatol.* 18:200-203.
11. Brown, Z. A., Corey, L., Unadkat, J., Schumann, L., Arvin, A., Hensleigh, P., Prober, C., Bryson, Y., and Connor, J. (1987). Pharmacokinetics of ACV in the term human pregnancy and neonate. Abstract, 27th Interscience Conference on Antimicrobial Agents and Chemotherapy, 4-7 Oct., 1987, New York.
12. Van Dyke, R. B., Connor, J. D., Wyborny, C., Hintz, M., and Keeney, R. E. D. (1982). Pharmacokinetics of orally administered acyclovir in patients with herpes progenitalis. *Am. J. Med.* 73:172-175.
13. Freinkel, L., Brown, Z. A., Corey, L., Unadkat, J., Schumann, L., Arvin, A., Hensleigh, P., Prober, C., Bryson, Y., and Connor, J. (1988). Pharmacokinetics of ACV in the term human pregnancy and neonate: A second dosage. Abstract, 28th Interscience Conference on Antimicrobial Agents and Chemotherapy, 23-26 Oct., 1988, Los Angeles.
14. Lau, R. J., Emergy, M. G., and Galinsky, R. E. (1987). Unexpected accumulation of acyclovir in breast milk with estimation of infant exposure. *Obstet. Gynecol.* 69:468-470.
15. Meyer, L. J., De Miranda, P., Sheth, N., and Spruance, S. (1988). Acyclovir in human breast milk. *Am. J. Obstet. Gynecol.* 158:586-588.
16. Lagrew, D. C., Furlow, T. G., Hager, D., and Yarrish, R. L. (1984). Disseminated herpes simplex virus infection in pregnancy: Successful treatment with acyclovir. *JAMA* 252:2058-2059.
17. Kingsley, S. (1986). Foetal and neonatal exposure to acyclovir. Second World Congress on Sexually Transmitted Diseases, Paris, 25-28 June, 1986 (abstract).
18. Moore, H. L., Szczech, G. M., Rodwell, D. E., Kapp, R. W., De Miranda, P., and Tucker, W. E. (1983). Preclinical toxicology studies with acyclovir: Teratologic, reproductive and neonatal tests. *Fundam. Appl. Toxicol.* 3: 560-568.
19. Clive, D., Turner, N. T., Hozier, J., Baston, A. G., and Tucker, W. E. (1983). Preclinical toxicology studies with acyclovir: Genitic toxicity tests. *Fundam. Appl. Toxicol.* 3:587-602.
20. Andrews, E. B. (1987). Acyclovir in pregnancy registry: An observational epidemiological approach. The Wellcome International Antiviral Symposium, 2-4 Dec. 1987, Monte Carlo.
21. Corey, L., Adams, H. G., Brown, A. Z., and Holmes, K. K. (1983). Genital herpes simplex virus infections: Clinical manifestations, course, and complications. *Ann. Intern. Med.* 98:958-972.
22. Brown, Z. A., Vontver, L. A., Benedetti, J., Critchlow, C. W., Sells, C. J., Berry, S., and Corey, L. (1987). Effects on infants of a first episode of genital herpes during pregnancy. *N. Engl. J. Med.* 317:1246-1251.
23. Nahmias, A. J., Josey, W. E., Naib, Z. M., Freeman, M. G., Fernandez, R. J., and Wheeler, J. H. (1971). Perinatal risk associated with maternal genital herpes simplex virus infection. *Am. J. Obstet. Gynecol.* 110:825-837.

24. Bujko, M., Sulovic, V., and Dotlic, R. (1986). Herpes virus hominis (HVH) infection in women with preterm labor. *J. Perinat. Med.* 14:319-324.
25. Whitley, R., Nahmias, A. J., Visintine, A. M., Fleming, C. L., and Alford, C. A. (1980). The natural history of herpes simplex virus infection of mother and newborn. *Pediatrics* 66:489-494.
26. Hutto, C., Arvin, A., Jacobs, R., Steele, R., Stagno, S., Lyrene, R. J., Willett, L., Powell, D., Andersen, R., Werthammer, J., Ratcliff, G., Nahmias, A., Christy, C., and Whitely, R. (1987). Intrauterine herpes simplex virus infections. *J. Pediatr.* 110:97-101.
27. Benden, R. W., Perez, F., and Ray, M. B. (1987). Herpes simplex virus: Fetal and decidual infection. *Pediatr. Pathol.* 7:63-70.
28. Granat, M., Morag, A., Margalioth, E. J., Leviner, E., and Ornoy, A. (1986). Fetal outcome following primary herpetic gingivostomatitis in early pregnancy. *Isr. J. Med. Sci.* 22:455-459.
29. Curbelo, V., Bejar, R., Benirschke, K., and Gluck, L. (1981). Premature labor: Prostaglandin precursors in human placental membranes. *Obstet. Gynecol.* 57:473-478.
30. Baker, D. A., and Thomas, J. (1985). The effect of prostaglandin E_2 on the initial immune response to herpes simplex virus infection. *Am. J. Obstet. Gynecol.* 151:586-590.
31. Baker, D. A., Thomas, J., Epstein, J., Possilico, D., and Stone, M. (1982). The effect of prostaglandins on the multiplication and cell-to-cell spread of herpes simplex virus type 2 in vitro. *Am. J. Obstet. Gynecol.* 144:346-349.
32. Sullivan-Bolyai, J. Z., Hull, H. F., Wilson, C., Smith, A., and Corey, L. (1986). Presentations of neonatal herpes simplex virus infections: Implications for a change in therapeutic strategy. *Pediatr. Infect. Dis.* 5:308-314.
33. Brown, Z. A., Vontver, L. A., Benedetti, J. K., Critchlow, C. W., Hickok, D. E., Sells, C. J., Berry, S., and Corey, L. (1985). Genital herpes in pregnancy: Risk factors associated with recurrences and asymptomatic viral shedding. *Am. J. Obstet. Gynecol.* 153:24-30.
34. Utley, K., Bromberger, P., Wagner, L., and Schneider, H. (1987). Management of primary herpes in pregnancy complicated by ruptured membranes and extreme prematurity: Case report. *Am. J. Obstet. Gynecol.* 69:471-473.
35. Bernstein, D. I., Lovett, M. A., and Bryson, Y. J. (1984). The effects of acyclovir on antibodyr esponse to herpes simplex virus in primary genital infections. *J. Infect. Dis.* 150:7-13.
36. Prober, C. G., Sullender, W. M., Yasukawa, L. L., Au, D. S., Yeager, A. S., and Arvin, A. M. (1987). Low risk of herpes simplex infections in neonates exposed to the virus at the time of vaginal delivery to mothers with recurrent genital herpes simplex virus infections. *N. Engl. J. Med.* 316:240-244.
37. Ashley, R. L., and Corey, L. (1984). Effect of acyclovir treatment of primary genital herpes on the antibody response to herpes simplex virus. *J. Clin. Invest.* 73:681-688.

38. Hain, J., Doshi, N., and Harger, J. H. (1980). Ascending transcervical herpes simplex infection with intact fetal membranes. *Obstet. Gynecol.* 56:106-107.
39. Nahmias, A. J., Keyserling, H. L., and Kerrick, G. M. (1983). Neonatal herpes simplex virus infections. In Remington, J. S., and Klein, J. O. (eds.): *Diseases of the Fetus and Newborn Infant.* Philadelphia, W.B. Saunders, pp. 636-678.
40. Berger, S. A., Weinberg, M., Treves, T., Sorkin, P., Geller, E., Yedwab, G., Tomer, A., Rabey, M., and Michaeli, D. (1986). Herpes encephalitis during pregnancy: Failure of acyclovir and adenine arabinoside to prevent neonatal herpes. *Isr. J. Med. Sci.* 22:41-44.
41. Sridama, V., Pacini, T., Yang, S., Moawad, A., Reilly, M., and De Groot, L. J. (1982). Decreased levels of helper T cells: A possible cause of immunodeficiency of pregnancy. *N. Engl. J. Med.* 307:352-356.
42. Bailey, K., Herrod, H. G., Younger, R., and Shaver, D. (1985). Functional aspects of T-lymphocyte subsets in pregnancy. *Obstet. Gynecol.* 66:211-214.
43. Gonik, B., Loo, L. S., West, S., and Kohl, S. (1987). Natural killer cell cytotoxicity and antibody-dependent cellular cytotoxicity to herpes simplex virus-infected cells in human pregnancy. *Am. J. Reprod. Immunol. Microbiol.* 13:23-26.
44. Weinberg, E. D. (1984). Pregnancy-associated depression of cell-mediated immunity. *Rev. Infect. Dis.* 6:814-831.
45. Weinberg, E. D. (1987). Pregnancy associated immune suppression: Risks and mechanisms. *Microbiol. Pathogenesis* 3:393-397.
46. Goyert, G. L., Bottoms, S. F., and Sokol, R. J. (1985). Anicteric presentation of fatal herpetic hepatitis in pregnancy. *Obstet. Gynecol.* 65:585.
47. Rubin, M. H., Ward, D. M., and Painter, J. (1985). Fulminant hepatic failure caused by genital herpes in a healthy person. *JAMA* 253:1299-1301.
48. Lagrew, D. C., Furlow, T. G., Hager, W. D., and Yarrish, R. L. (1984). Disseminated herpes simplex virus infection in pregnancy: Successful treatment with acyclovir. *JAMA* 252:2058-2059.
49. Hankey, G. J., Bucens, M. R., and Chambers, J. S. W. (1987). Herpes simplex encephalitis in third trimester of pregnancy: Successful outcome for mother and child. *Neurology* 37:1534-1537.
50. Chazotte, C., Andersen, F., and Cohen, W. R. (1987). Disseminated herpes simplex infection in an immunocompromised pregnancy: Treatment with intravenous acyclovir. *Am. J. Perinat.* 4:363-364.
51. Sullivan-Bolyai, J., Hull, H. F., Wilson, C., and Corey, L. (1983). Neonatal herpes simplex virus infection in King County, Washington. Increasing incidence and epidemiologic correlates. *JAMA* 250:3059-3062.
52. Daling, J. R., and Wolfe, M. E. (1984). The role of decision and cost analysis in the treatment of pregnant women with recurrent genital herpes. *JAMA* 251:2828.

53. Ciraru-Vigneron, N., Nguyen Tan Lung, R., Blondeau, M. A., Brunner, C., and Barrier, J. (1987). Prescribing acyclovir in late pregnancy: A new protocol for the prevention of herpes in the at-risk neonate. *Presse Med* 16:128.
54. Preblud, S. R., and D'Angelo, L. J. (1979). Chickenpox in the United States, 1972-1977. *J. Infect. Dis.* 140:257-260.
55. Gershon, A. A., Raker, R., Steinberg, S., Topf-Olstien, B., and Drusin, L. (1976). Antibody to varicella-zoster virus in parturient women and their offspring during the first year of life. *Pediatrics* 58:692-696.
56. CDC. (1984). *MMWR* 33:85-88.
57. Young, N. A., and Gerson, A. A. (1983). Chickenpox, measles and mumps. In Remington, J. S., and Klein, J. O. (eds.): *Diseases of the Fetus and Newborn Infant.* Philadelphia: W.B. Saunders, pp. 37427.
58. Harris, R. E., and Rhoades, E. R. (1985). Varicella pneumonia complicating pregnancy: Report of a case and review of the literature. *Obstet. Gynecol.* 25:734-740.
59. Paryani, S. G., and Arvin, A. M. (1986). Intrauterine infection with varicella zoster virus after maternal varicella. *N. Engl. J. Med.* 314:1541-1546.
60. Glaser, J. B., Luftus, J., Ferragamo, V., Mootbar, H., and Castellano, M. (1986). Varicella-zoster infection in pregnancy: Letter to the editor. *N. Engl. J. Med.* 315:1416.
61. Hankins, G. D. V., Gilstrap, L. C., and Patterson, A. R. (1987). Acyclovir treatment of varicella pneumonia in pregnancy. *Crit. Care Med.* 15:336-337.
62. Eder, S. E., Apuzzio, J. J., and Weiss, G. (1988). Varicella pneumonia during pregnancy. Treatment of two cases with acyclovir. *Am. J. Perinat.* 5: 16-18.
63. Leen, C. L. S., Mandal, B. K., and Ellis, M. E. (1987). Acyclovir and pregnancy. *Br. Med. J.* 294:308.
64. Boyd, K., and Walker, E. (1988). Use of acyclovir to treat chickenpox in pregnancy. *Br. Med. J.* 296:393-394.
65. Landsberger, E. J., Hager, W. D., and Grossman, J. H. (1986). Successful management of varicella pneumonia complicating pregnancy. A report of three cases. *J. Reprod. Med.* 31:311-314.
66. Al-Nakib, W., Al-Kandari, S., El-Khalik, D. M. A., et al. (1983). A randomized controlled study of intravenous acyclovir, Zovirax, against placebo in adults with chickenpox. *J. Infect. Dis.* 6(suppl):49.
67. Preblud, S. R., Cochi, S. L., and Orenstein, W. A. (1986). Varicella-zoster infection in pregnancy. *N. Engl. J. Med.* 315:416-417.
68. Holland, P., Isaacs, D., and Moxon, E. R. (1986). Fetal neonatal varicella infection. *Lancet* 2:1156.
69. Laskin, O. L. (1985). Acyclovir and suppression of frequently recurring herpetic whitlow. *Ann. Intern. Med.* 102:494-495.
70. Tschen, E. H., and Baack, B. (1987). Treatment of herpetic whitlow in pregnancy with acyclovir. *J. Am. Acad. Dermatol.* 17:1059-1060.

10
Neonatal Herpes Simplex Virus Infections

Steven T. Baldwin and Richard J. Whitley *School of Medicine,
University of Alabama at Birmingham, Birmingham, Alabama*

INTRODUCTION

The first cases of neonatal herpes simplex virus (HSV) infection were reported by Batignani and Haas in the mid-1930s (1,2). Since then, HSVs have come to be recognized as an important cause of infection during pregnancy and the neonatal period. Infections due to these viruses are now known to produce a vast and variable spectrum of maternal, fetal, and neonatal disease. Perinatal HSV infections also are now well respected for the serious morbidity and significant mortality they often produce.

In the past, attempts to reduce the frequency and improve the outcome of these infections were very limited owing to the poor understanding of many virologic, epidemiologic, clinical, therapeutic, and preventive issues. Recently, much better understanding of many of these relevant issues has been achieved and has stimulated the current development and application of much more insightful strategies to try to reduce the terrible impact of these infections.

THE VIRUS

Two types of HSV, type 1 and type 2, commonly infect humans (3). Type 1 and type 2 HSVs are very closely related but distinct viruses. Both of these viruses are composed of a central core concentrically surrounded by three different layers (15,16). The core contains nucleoproteins and the viral genome. The inner concentric layer, or capsid, is an icosahedral structure made of 162 protein capsomeres. The tegument is an amorphous layer tightly adherent to the capsid. The envelope is the outer layer and is formed from lipids, glycoproteins, and polyamines.

The complete virions of each type are morphologically identical. They are approximately 150-200 nm in diameter and contain approximately 100 megadaltons of DNA (4). The genome of both types of viruses is composed of two pieces of covalently linked linear double-stranded DNA called the long (L) and short (S) regions. It is interesting that four equally frequent isomeric arrangements of the L and S regions are naturally present in DNA isolated from all strains of these viruses, but the significance of this finding remains unknown (5,6,15).

Over 70 different HSV polypeptides have been identified including DNA polymerase, thymidine kinase, and several glycoproteins (7). The glycoproteins are of particular interest because they appear to mediate viral infectivity and to elicit host responses (8). Glycoproteins from type 1 and type 2 viruses are often indistinguishable, but a few are unique. While the role of most viral polypeptides remains unknown, the role of several of the glycoproteins is becoming clearer (8,11).

Glycoprotein B (gB) is required for viral infectivity. Glycoprotein C (gC) binds to the C3b component of complement. A deletion in this glycoprotein appears to increase the neurovirulence of the virus (9). Antigenic differences in gC also can be used to distinguish type 1 from type 2 virus (10). Glycoprotein D (gD) is related to infectivity and is the most potent inducer of neutralizing antibodies. Glycoprotein E (gE) binds to the Fc portion of IgG, and glycoprotein G (gG) determines the specific antibody response which distinguishes between HSV type 1 and type 2 infections (8,11,101). The role of the newly recognized glycoprotein, gI, is unknown (17).

Considerable DNA homology (about 50%) and glycoprotein (antigenic) cross-reactivity exist between type 1 and type 2 HSVs (8,11-14). Nevertheless, restriction enzyme DNA analysis and type-specific glycoprotein assays using monoclonal antibodies both permit accurate typing of virus isolates (241,242). Restriction enzyme DNA analysis also accurately differentiates strains of either type of virus (18).

Both types of virus replicate in the same manner. A virus initiates its replicative cycle by attaching to a host cell using its envelope glycoproteins. Viral DNA is then introduced into the host cell and induces the production of the viral enzymes, regulatory proteins, and structural proteins necessary to divert host cell functions to the formation of new virions. The viral DNA is repeatedly replicated and coupled with newly formed capsids in the host cell nucleus. Forming virions are thought to acquire their outer envelopes during evagination through the host cell nuclear membrane. Host cell lysis then releases the progeny virions to reiterate this replicative process in other cells.

Both types of virus have been shown to produce primary, latent, and recurrent infections. Primary infection with either type occurs when a host is first exposed to virus of that type. Latent infection develops during the primary infection and is characterized by the lifelong presence of dormant viral DNA in the host. Latent infections are notably unaffected by current antiviral drugs, which require active viral replication to be effective.

Sometimes latent virus spontaneously reactivates via an unknown mechanism. This produces a recurrent infection. Reactivation may occur at variable intervals despite the presence of preexisting specific humoral and cell-mediated immunity against the virus (18,19). Recurrences are associated at times with changes in body temperature, physical or emotional stress, exposure to ultraviolet light, tissue damage, or immune suppression (18-21). Endonuclease restriction analysis techniques have demonstrated that the same strain of virus isolated during a primary infection is invariably isolated during subsequent recurrences in the same individual (22,23). This strongly supports the concept that reactivation of latent endogenous virus is the mechanism of recurrent infections. Only very rarely does an individual become superinfected with a second exogenous strain of the same type of HSV (24,25). This is termed reinfection and most commonly occurs in immunosuppressed individuals with repeated exposure to multiple strains of the virus (18).

Active infections with either type of HSV generally produce cytopathic and cytolytic changes in infected cells. Shortly after a cell is infected, the viral replicative cycle leads to extensive chromosomal damage and the appearance of intranuclear inclusion bodies in the host cell. Early (Feulgen-positive) bodies are basophilic and are thought to represent viral DNA, while Cowdry type A bodies are eosinophilic and are formed by an unknown mechanism. Involved cells usually become swollen and subsequently undergo cytolysis. Sometimes infected cells are transformed into multinucleated giant cells. It is important to note that these events occur only in cells in which active viral replication is taking place since these changes are not produced by latent infections (18).

Both types of HSV are very infectious and exhibit a tropism for ectodermally derived host tissues. This tropism appears to have an important role in the expression of recurrent infections. After transmission to a susceptible host, virus quickly begins to replicate at the site of infection. Local sensory or autonomic nerve fibers become involved and carry the virus or viral elements to their corresponding sensory or autonomic ganglia via their retrograde axonal transport mechanism (26-29). The virus replicates in the ganglia for several days and then becomes latent (26,28,30). The infected nerve ganglia appear to serve as a locus for latent virus and consequently as a source of virus capable of producing recurrent infections (26,31-42). Anterograde transport of reactivated virus along the same sensory or autonomic nerve fibers presumably accounts for the tendency for recurrent infections to localize to the site of the antecedent primary infection.

The biochemical mechanisms governing latency and reactivation are still not clear. Some evidence suggests that the virus-specific enzyme, thymidine kinase, may be necessary for the establishment of latency or may be required for viral reactivation since mutant viruses lacking thymidine kinase replicate well but infrequently become latent (44,45). Interestingly, thymidine kinase is found in all wild-type isolates of HSV types 1 and 2 (19).

The virus-host interactions responsible for viral reactivation also remain unclear. Individuals with more severe primary infections have been noted to have an increased risk of recurrent infections (18). Yet, it remains unknown why some infected individuals do not experience recurrent infections while other hosts experience mutliple recurrences.

EPIDEMIOLOGY

General

Both types of HSV infections occur throughout the world. Infection is primarily restricted to humans, although other susceptible species are recognized. Since humans are the sole natural source of these viruses, transmission is generally effected by direct person-to-person transfer of virus. Transmission of virus usually requires close or intimate personal contact with an infected individual who is shedding the virus, since the virus is relatively unstable in the environment. Most commonly, mucosal surfaces or abraded skin is the portal of entry and the site of initial infection (18, 19,46-50).

Characteristically, primary infections with HSV type 1 tend to occur in childhood and are localized to the oropharynx. Type 1 infections may be transmitted through direct contact with infectious secretions or respiratory droplets. Asymptomatic infection appears to be the rule. Clinical manifestations, when present, include the gingivostomatitis seen in young children and the pharyngitis or mononucleosislike syndrome seen in young adults. Recurrent type 1 oropharyngeal herpes infections occur in an estimated 10-20% of infected individuals. Acquisition of type 1 infection tends to occur earlier and more frequently when poor socioeconomic conditions are present (18,19,46,47).

Herpes simplex virus type 2 infections are generally acquired via direct contact with infectious secretions during sexual activity. As a result, primary type 2 infections tend not to occur until the onset of sexual activity and usually involve the genital area. Many infected individuals do not experience clinical disease. When present, clinical manifestations are mostly mucocutaneous lesions. Recurrences are commonplace, and promiscuity, low socioeconomic status, and onset of sexual activity at an early age are risk factors for infection (18,19,46,47,51-53).

It is true that the majority of HSV infections "above the belt" are due to type 1 virus while those infections occurring "below the belt" are predominantly due to type 2 virus (18,55). Nevertheless, it should be emphasized that both type 1 and type 2 virus can infect the oropharynx and the genital tract. From 8% to 50% of genital herpes infections have been reported to be due to type 1 virus (54). Orogenital sexual practices may account for many of these cases.

The true incidence and prevalence of HSV infections remain unknown, but some pertinent data have been compiled. For type 1 virus, a progressively increasing rate of seropositivity occurs with age such that by adulthood anywhere from 30% to 40% to over 90% of individuals are seropositive (18,47,56-61). Estimated seropositivity rates for type 2 virus have varied from 10-20% in high-socioeconomic status groups to 35% in middle-socioeconomic status groups to 50-60% in low-socioeconomic status groups (18,51-53,57,61-64).

Gestational Infections

Herpes simplex virus infections that occur during pregnancy can sometimes produce serious maternal disease or adversely affect the pregnancy. Very rarely, primary HSV infections of pregnant women will disseminate and produce fulminant, life-threatening disease in the mother. According to one review, disseminated maternal infections typically occur during the third trimester, but cases occurring earlier in pregnancy have been noted

(65,66). Such cases may result from either oral or genital infections and are usually characterized by the presence of visceral disease (65,67-79). These infections are associated with a very high maternal mortality rate (43% in one review) (65).

Fetal mortality is also very common with these infections and usually results from the effects of maternal disease rather than direct infection of the fetus with the virus (67,78). Surviving fetuses usually do not have evidence of viral infection at delivery (65,67-69,71-76,78-80). However, apparent transplacental infection of the fetus during maternal disseminated herpes infection has been reported (77). Culture and/or cytological examination of amniotic fluid has been advocated to assess for possible fetal infection in these cases but may not be reliably predictive since uninfected neonates have been noted to have amniotic fluid cultures yielding HSV and cytological examinations revealing intranuclear inclusion bodies prior to birth (68,81,82). Anecdotal reports of the use of antiviral drug therapy for disseminated maternal herpes infections have noted successful and unsuccessful outcomes (77-80). Nevertheless, systemic antiviral therapy remains the only therapy with activity against the virus and therefore should be used with the intent of reducing maternal morbidity and mortality.

Nondisseminated herpes infections are a much more common problem during pregnancy. Oropharyngeal herpes infections have not been associated with significant problems during pregnancy, but genital herpes infections have definitely been associated with adverse pregnancy outcomes and adverse neonatal outcomes due to infection of the fetal before or during birth. It is therefore important to understand the epidemiology of genital herpes infections.

In the United States, an estimated 300,000-750,000 primary and 30 million recurrent cases of genital herpes occur annually (18,66,83). Cases of genital herpes have been increasing rapidly in several study populations during the past few years (18,47,64,84-86). It is therefore not surprising that genital herpes infections are a relatively common and increasingly frequent complication during pregnancy.

Socioeconomic status, age, past sexual history, and possibly other variables affect the prevalence of genital herpes. Genital herpes infections appear to be relatively more common in Caucasians than in other ethnic groups and appear to constitute a disproportionately large percentage of all sexually transmitted diseases among middle-class and upper-class patients (64,87,88).

Genital infections due to HSV type 1 and type 2 are clinically indistinguishable. Type 2 viruses are responsible for the majority of cases, but

type 1 infections account for an appreciable number of cases and are becoming more frequent in some studies (89-91,97,103).

Genital herpes infections are often transmitted unknowingly. Most
adults are unaware of past HSV genital infections (100,101). Only one
third of individuals who transmit the virus are aware that they have genital herpes despite an obvious clinical history of genital herpes in two thirds
of these same individuals (96). Herpetic lesions are frequently overlooked,
not directly visible, or mistakenly attributed to some other cause. Virus
can be transmitted unknowingly during the asymptomatic infections that
account for up to 50-70% of genital herpes infections (57). Genital herpes can probably also be transmitted during the episodes of asymptomatic
low-titer viral shedding that are known to variably occur between recurrent infections in individuals with genital herpes (64,92,93). Type 1 genital
herpes infections may be acquired unknowingly by individuals who engage
in orogenital sex since 2% of adults asymptomatically shed HSV in saliva
(94-96).

The distinction between primary and recurrent genital herpes infections is epidemiologically important but often not easily made clinically.
Primary as well as recurrent infections may or may not produce symptoms, but primary infections are symptomatic much more often than recurrent infections. Primary infections are associated with prolonged clinical manifestations, frequent signs of viremia, extremely frequent cervical
involvement, and high-titer viral shedding for relatively long periods of
time. Recurrent genital herpes infections are frequently asymptomatic,
have relatively mild and brief (average 8-12 days) clinical findings if any,
have modestly frequent cervical involvement, and have low-titer viral shedding for a short (average 4 days) period of time (18,64,97,98,117,183,243).

Genital herpes infections recur frequently. Fifty percent of individuals
with type 1 and 80% of those with type 2 primary genital herpes will experience a recurrent infection within 12 months of their primary infection (104,105). Individuals who have symptomatic recurrences average
five to eight recurrences each year (106). The titer of virus shed during
recurrent infections (10^2 to 10^3) is much lower than the titer of virus shed
during primary infections ($> 10^6$) (18). During recurrences, virus is shed
in greatest concentration during the first 24 h following onset, and shedding usually ceases within 5 days (107). Cervicitis is much less common
during recurrent infections than during primary infections. Virus can be
isolated from the cervix of 12-20% of women during recurrences compared to 70-90% of women during a first episode of genital herpes (92,
105,108,109).

Cervical involvement during recurrent infections usually produces minimal or no visible lesions (64). Asymptomatic shedding of virus from the genital tract can be variably detected between active recurrences in individuals with recurrent genital herpes. Asymptomatic viral shedding most commonly occurs at the usual lesion sites and not the cervix (110,121). The frequency of detection of asymptomatic viral shedding depends primarily on the frequency with which serial examinations are performed (64,110). Patients with known recurrent genital herpes have been shown to shed virus in the absence of lesions as much as 10% of the time (111). The duration of asymptomatic shedding appears to average 1 to 2 days (110,244). It should be remembered that the rate and nature of recurrences of genital herpes usually vary considerably over time in individual patients.

Primary genital herpes infections during pregnancy are probably uncommon. One recent study found only two cases of primary genital herpes among almost 7,000 unselected consecutive women evaluated at delivery (102). On the other hand, a relatively large percentage of pregnant women have serological evidence of previous genital herpes. In one study, 36% of pregnant women were seropositive for HSV type 2 antibodies (99). Ten percent to 35% seropositivity rates have been noted by others (18, 101,102).

It remains unclear whether the pregnant state itself modifies the activity, course, or recurrence rate of genital herpes infections. Some studies have suggested somewhat higher recurrence rates or somewhat longer disease durations for genital herpes in pregnant women (112-115). Other studies have shown no differences in the frequency of recurrences, rate of cervicitis, or duration of lesions in pregnant and nonpregnant women (116-118). Different factors were controlled for in these studies and may account for some of the variations observed. If pregnancy does in fact influence genital herpes infections, then the effect is not particularly striking clinically.

Herpes simplex virus can be isolated from the genital tract sometime during gestation in approximately 1% of all pregnancies (18,68,99,112, 115,119). As in nonpregnant women, viral shedding noted during pregnancy is predomimently due to recurrent infection or asymptomatic intercurrent shedding and uncommonly due to primary genital herpes infection. Primary genital herpes infections occurring during pregnancy have not been specifically studied. On the other hand, recurrent infections have been examined in several studies.

Only about 4% of unselected pregnant women give a history of genital herpes or exposure to genital herpes according to one large recent study

(102). The seroprevalence of HSV type 2 antibodies was approximately 20% in this same study. Another study similarly found that only 20% of pregnant women with serological evidence of past genital herpes give a history of genital herpes or exposure to genital herpes (101). It is therefore obvious that historical screening alone will not identify most pregnant women with previous episodes of genital herpes.

Among groups of pregnant women selected for a past history of genital herpes, about 75-85% of the women experience at least one clinical recurrence during their pregnancy (110,116-118). The average is three recurrences each (116-118). Virus can be isolated from lesions 50-75% of the time and from cervical cultures 1-12% of the time (110,116-118). Asymptomatic viral shedding between recurrences is detected by 0.5-3.0% of cervical cultures from pregnant women with a past history of genital herpes (93,99,110,116-118,120,121). A total of 2.3-14% of pregnant women with a history of genital herpes can be demonstrated to asymptomatically shed virus at least once during gestation (110,116,118). The frequency of viral shedding detected has not been shown to vary during the course of pregnancy, and viral shedding during the latter weeks of gestation has not been shown to predict viral shedding at the time of delivery (110,117, 123).

Herpes simplex virus can be cultured from the genital tract at delivery in 1% of women with a known history of genital herpes but in only 0.01-0.39% of unselected pregnant women (18,93,99,102,110,116,124,125). Interestingly, in one of the studies, unselected women with virus isolated at the time of delivery had HSV type 2 isolated in all instances, had an 86% seropositivity rate for past HSV type 2 infection, but had only a 7% rate of past genital herpes infection by history (102).

Maternal genital infections during pregnancy may significantly affect fetal outcome in some instances. Women who experience a primary genital infection early in pregnancy have been noted to have a significantly increased rate of spontaneous abortion (18,67,112,114,126-130). A spontaneous abortion rate of 25% has been reported when primary genital herpes infection occurs prior to week 20 of gestation, but only small numbers of women were followed in this study, so this figure may be too high (112).

Both hematogenous and ascending routes of infection may be important in the pathogenesis of spontaneous abortions associated with primary genital herpes infections (18,64). It has also been suggested that primary genital infections occurring during the first 20 weeks of gestation may be associated with stillbirths and congenital malformations, particularly

hydranencephaly and chorioretinitis as a consequence of fetal infection
(18,67,112,130). Primary genital herpes infections that occur later in pregnancy do not appear to be associated with fetal loss but have been associated with premature labor in some instances (18,67,112,114,117,131).
One study also noted a 35% incidence of low birth weight among infants
whose mothers had a primary genital herpes infection after week 23 of
gestation (112). Recurrent genital herpes infections have not been associated with spontaneous abortions. Although recurrent genital infections
during the last trimester of pregnancy have been reported by some studies
to be associated with increased rates of preterm delivery, some prospective studies have not confirmed this finding (18,67,112,116-118,131,132).

Fetal and Neonatal Infections

The incidence of neonatal herpes is generally thought to range from 1 in
2,000 to 1 in 5,000 live births per year, but rates as low as 1 in 20,000 live
births per year have been suggested (18,64,133-137). Therefore, an estimated 700-1,000 of the 3.5 million infants delivered each year in the United
States have neonatal herpes. The rate of neonatal herpes infection is significantly higher in some areas and is paradoxically extremely low in countries where genital herpes infections are very common (18,135,138,139).
The incidence of neonatal herpes appears to be increasing in the United
States as genital herpes becomes ever more common (18,135,140). However, the number of cases of neonatal herpes occurring each year remains
very small compared to the estimated 10,000-200,000 pregnant women
each year with genital herpes sometime during their pregnancy and the
estimated 3,500-14,000 pregnant women each year with herpes virus iso-
lable at delivery (18,116-118,125,131,133,141-145).

It is now recognized that HSV infections may be transmitted to the
fetus or neonate in utero, during birth, or postnatally. Intrauterine transmission may apparently occur transplacentally or transcervically. Intrapartum transmission requires direct contact with infectious virus present
in the maternal genital tract. Importantly, most neonatal herpes infections result from this mode of transmission. Postnatal infections result
from direct contact with infectious material from a family member, a care
giver, or another individual.

Congenital HSV infections are rare and have not been well studied
(18,66,67,75,77,89,123,130,132,133,135,146-175,182). The distinction between congenital and neonatal herpes infections may be very difficult to
make, but babies who manifest signs of HSV infection at birth or shortly

thereafter (usually defined to be within 48 h of birth) and who subsequently have herpesvirus isolated from culture specimens are generally presumed to have congenital herpes infection (18,66,133,176). This definition is problematic, however. The times of onset of clinical manifestations in neonates infected in utero and neonates infected during birth may overlap. Also, cursory examinations may easily overlook subtle findings, delay diagnosis, and lead to erroneous classification of a congenital infection as a neonatal infection. Some congenitally infected babies have no clinical manifestations until late in the neonatal period or early in infancy, when they are found to have stigmata of subacute or chronic HSV infection obviously of such duration as could only plausibly be produced by an intrauterine infection. These latter cases as well as those congenitally infected babies with a clinical onset at a few days of age can sometimes be anticipated if examination of the placenta demonstrates evidence of viral disease, which stresses the importance of examining the placenta (18,66, 133,153-155,164).

Congenital herpes infections are estimated to occur at a rate of 1 in every 300,000 deliveries and are thought to account for approximately 5% of all babies with herpes infection during the neonatal period according to data collected by the NIAID Collaborative Antiviral Study Group (18,66,67,135,148,171). Intrauterine herpes infections are known to occur at any time during gestation and may be due to type 1 or, more often, type 2 virus (18,66,148). Both primary and recurrent maternal herpes infections can produce infection of the fetus (66,148). Transplacental and transcervical routes of infection have been proposed. Hematogenous transplacental transmission appears to be a rare complication of maternal herpes viremia (66,150). When chorioamnionitis is absent, transplacental transmission is evidenced by finding virus or intranuclear inclusion bodies in the abortus, placenta, and/or endometrium following spontaneous abortion or by finding disseminated herpes infection of the newborn at birth (18,66,77,79,133,150,154,164,175,177). An ascending route of infection has been surmised when chorioamnionitis is present or when isolated mucocutaneous disease of the infant is noted at birth (18,66,130,132,133, 148-152,156,160,161,163,178,179). It is important to remember that iatrogenic transcervical infection of the fetus can occur during instrumentation of the maternal genital tract (66,180,181).

The factors that govern in utero transmission of HSV infections remain unknown (66,148). Factors that determine the sites and severity of fetal disease also remain unclear.

The distinction between congenitally and neonatally infected infants is important because significant differences possibly exist between these two groups with regard to morbidity, mortality, response to therapy, and amenability to preventive strategies. One might especially predict a significant difference in outcome for congenitally infected infants since their infections are often present for a variable, but often significant, period of time in utero during which they remain undiagnosed and untreated unlike their neonatally infected counterparts who are observable and treatable from the moment of infection.

Intrapartum neonatal herpes infections are considerably more common than congenital herpes infections. The importance of mother-to-infant transmission of virus during birth is supported by the finding that neonatal herpes infections are predominantly caused by HSV type 2 as are maternal genital herpes infections (18,133,136). Further confirmation of the importance of intrapartum transmission of virus results from strain typing studies using endonuclease restriction enzyme DNA analysis. Mother-to-infant transmission was confirmed by the isolation of identical strains of virus from the mother's genital tract and from the neonate since only epidemiologically related strains of virus are identical (18).

It is now known that almost all neonatal herpes infections are acquired during birth as a result of direct contact with virus being shed in the maternal genital tract (18,97,124,132,133,135,136,183,189). Intrapartum neonatal herpes infections may be caused by type 1 or type 2 HSV and may follow exposure to primary or recurrent genital herpes (18). Seventy-five percent or more of intrapartum neonatal herpes infections are caused by type 2 viruses (122,132). About 50% occur following exposure of the infant to a primary genital herpes infection at the time of delivery (18, 122,140). Mothers of infected infants are most commonly primagravidas (73%), white (63%), and young (mean age 21 years) (132). Only infants exposed to herpesvirus at the time of labor and delivery are at risk to develop intrapartum neonatal herpes infection. It should be noted that most exposed infants do not subsequently develop neonatal herpes.

The epidemiology of intrapartum neonatal herpes infections centers on two major concerns. The first is the infant's risk of intrapartum exposure to HSV. This is an all-or-none risk. The second major concern is the exposed infant's subsequent risk of infection with HSV. This risk is a continuous function.

Clearly, the infant's risk of exposure to infectious virus depends first and foremost on whether or not virus is present in the mother's birth canal at the time of labor and delivery. Unfortunately, history and physical examination are unable to predict or identify most women who are virus positive at the time of delivery (18,101,102,110,122-124,132,133,136,184,

188). Most mothers of infected newborns are completely unaware that they have genital herpes (101,124,132). Over 40% of pregnant women with cytologically diagnosed genital herpes are asymptomatic (112). Among mothers of infants with neonatal herpes, over 70% report no history or evidence of recurrent lesions indicative of genital herpes during their pregnancy, and over 85% deny the presence of genital herpes in their sexual partners (101,122-124,132,133).

Whitley et al. recently noted that 20% of mothers of infected infants give a history of genital herpes during their current or previous pregnancy but that only about 5% report any recurrences during their current pregnancy (122). All of the women in this study who had a history of recurrent genital herpes reported their sexual partners also had genital herpes (122). Most important of all, mothers of babies with neonatal herpes often have no history or physical findings suggestive of genital herpes at the time of labor and delivery (18,102,122-124,132,136,184,188). Sixty percent to 80% of mothers of infected infants give no history of genital herpes or exposure to genital herpes and have no symptoms or signs of genital herpes at the time of delivery (18,101,122,123,132,133,184). Twenty-five percent of mothers of infected infants have a fever of indeterminant cause at delivery, but only 10% have genital herpes lesions (122).

Cultures for herpesvirus are the only accurate and reliable means to detect HSV in the genital tract at the time of labor and delivery. Unfortunately, cultures often require a few days to be interpretable and are therefore not useful for making management decisions in most cases. Serial antepartum cultures from women with recurrent herpes do not predict the presence of herpes virus at delivery and are expensive (110).

When virus is present in the birth canal at the time of labor and delivery, the route of delivery can influence whether the infant becomes exposed to the virus. Vaginal delivery results in exposure of the infant to the virus in these cases. On the other hand, cesarean section bypasses the virus-containing genital tract and thereby allows the infant to potentially avoid contact with infectious virus (112). Cesarean section effectively but not completely eliminates fetal exposure to virus in the maternal genital tract when the protective barrier formed by the amniotic membranes remains intact until the time of operative delivery (18,112,122,132,133,191, 192). If the amniotic membranes are ruptured or broached by the virus prior to surgery, then the fetus may be exposed to virus or vaginal secretions containing virus. This presumably explains the much decreased effectiveness of cesarean section for the prevention of neonatal herpes reported when rupture of membranes occurs more than a few hours prior to surgery (112).

The risk of neonatal herpes infection following intrapartum exposure to herpes virus appears to depend on the nature of the infant's exposure to the virus. This risk can be appreciable in some instances. Factors that increase the infant's contact with the virus increase the risk of neonatal herpes, and factors that decrease the infant's contact with the virus decrease the risk of neonatal herpes (18,97,133,136,185,188). The duration of exposure to the virus, anatomic considerations, and the quantity of virus present during exposure all appear to be important determinants of risk for infection for the infant.

The amniotic membranes are usually a very effective barrier between the fetus and virus in the maternal genital tract. Therefore, the amount of time between rupture of the membranes and birth is usually an accurate index of the duration of the infant's exposure to infectious virus. This explains the increased risk of intrapartum neonatal herpes associated with prolonged rupture of the membranes (18,97,112,133,136,185).

Several anatomical considerations may be important risk factors for intrapartum transmission of neonatal herpes infection. The anatomic site of maternal viral shedding or virus-positive lesions is thought to be very important. Shedding or lesions involving the cervix portend possibly greater risk than lesions involving the external genitalia or the perineum (18,136). This is because the fetus is in much closer proximity to the cervix during labor, must pass through the cervix during birth, and is directly exposed to vaginal secretions that likely contain virus when cervical but not necessarily when perineal involvement with genital herpes occurs. The presence of multiple versus single maternal herpes lesions may be another anatomic risk factor (18,136). The simultaneous presence of multiple versus single virus-containing lesions may increase the infant's chance of contacting a virus-positive lesion. The total amount of virus in vaginal secretions produced by multiple concomitant lesions may also be greater than that produced by a single lesion.

The fetal skin is an important anatomical barrier to the virus. Transmission of HSV is enhanced when the skin barrier is abraded, damaged, or lacerated (18,133,136,181,186,187). Therefore, instrumentation of the vagina, fetal scalp electrodes, and any other factors that interfere with fetal skin integrity may increase the risk of intrapartum neonatal herpes infection.

The amniotic membranes are an important anatomical barrier, too. They protect the fetus when intact. Frequent vaginal examinations during labor and delivery may be another anatomic risk factor. Frequent vaginal examinations may contaminate vaginal secretions with virus from perineal herpes lesions, rupture herpes vesicles, release virus into the maternal genital tract, interfere with amniotic membrane or fetal skin integrity, and transport virus-containing secretions into direct contact with the fetus. Probably the most important anatomic issue is the use of cesarean section to bypass maternal genital herpes and thereby avoid fetal intrapartum exposure to the virus altogether (18,133,136).

The quantity of virus to which an infant is exposed appears to be a particularly important determinant of risk for intrapartum neonatal herpes infection. Infants exposed to genital herpes during birth have a progressively increasing risk of neonatal herpes as the titer of virus present during exposure increases (18,133,136,183). Therefore, primary genital herpes is associated with the greatest risk since it produces virus in very high titer. Recurrent genital herpes lesions and intercurrent episodes of asymptomatic shedding are associated with lower risk than primary lesions since they produce virus in lower titer (18,102,107,112,124,133,136,183, 188,189). The increased risk of neonatal herpes infection in association with primary genital herpes is probably also attributable in part to the frequent and severe cervical involvement that almost always occurs with primary genital herpes infections (18,112,113,133,136,183).

Several studies have attempted to quantify the risk of intrapartum neonatal herpes infection when a genital herpes infection complicates delivery. One study noted the risk of neonatal herpes for vaginally delivered infants to be 33% for infants of mothers with primary genital herpes after week 33 of gestation, 3% for infants of mothers with recurrent genital herpes after week 32 of gestation, and 42% for infants of mothers with virus-positive lesions at the time of delivery (112). Other studies have shown neonatal herpes to occur in approximately 50% of babies vaginally delivered to mothers with primary genital herpes lesions present at the time of delivery (18,97,102,107,118,133,136,137,142,143,145,188,189). The same studies have shown mothers with recurrent genital herpes lesions present at delivery to have about a 5% chance of transmitting herpes infection to their vaginally delivered neonates and have also shown the risk to increase to 30-40% if virus is present in the birth canal at the time of delivery (18, 97,102,107,118,133,136,137,142,143,145,188,189). Recent studies have continued to confirm the very high risk associated with primary genital herpes at delivery but have questioned the previously reported risk associated with recurrent genital herpes at delivery (101,102,110,136,188-190). A recent study at the University of Alabama at Birmingham noted that only 1 out of 40 (2.5%) babies developed neonatal herpes following vaginal delivery to virus-positive mothers (190). Another recent study found no herpes infections among 34 neonates who were born vaginally to mothers with virus-positive recurrent genital herpes present at the time of delivery (188). The risk of neonatal herpes for infants exposed at birth to intercurrent asymptomatic viral shedding versus recurrent genital herpes lesions has not been studied (18,136). Interestingly, no mother studied has been noted to deliver a second infected neonate (122).

Postnatal HSV infections of the neonate can be acquired from several sources (18,107,133,136,193-200,208). Infants have become infected following contact with virus from maternal genital, oral, or breast lesions (18,107,124,133,136,193,196-199). The isolation of HSV type 2 from an infected infant is often a clue suggesting mother-to-infant transmission of infection (18). Oral herpes infections of the father, other family members, caretakers, or other individuals are another potential source of infection for neonates (18,107,124,133,135,136,200). The potential for exposure of the neonate to oral herpes is significant since cold sores occur in 16-46% of adults and asymptomatic shedding of virus in saliva occurs in 2% of adults (18,94,201,202).

Nosocomial transmission of neonatal herpes from other babies and from hospital personnel has also been reported but appears to be rare despite the frequency of herpes infections in hospital personnel (18,107, 133,136,194,195,203). Nongenital herpetic lesions are reported to occur in 15-34% of hospital personnel (204-206). At least 1% of all hospital personnel have been noted to have cold sores during any given week (205, 207). Likewise, cold sores are common in nursery personnel (204,206, 208). Great variations in infection control policies for nurseries exist (18), but it is likely that good hand washing and education of staff regarding nosocomial infections are largely responsible for the rarity of nosocomial herpes infections in nurseries (18). It is economically costly and of questionable benefit to isolate personnel with cold sores from the nursery (18, 107,206). However, personnel with herpetic whitlow should definitely not perform patient care (18,107).

Putative sources of virus causing postnatally acquired HSV infection of the newborn can now be confirmed using endonuclease restriction enzyme DNA analysis. The strain of virus isolated from the infant and from the putative source can be characterized using this technique. Identical strains of virus will be isolated from the infant and the putative source only if they are epidemiologically related. Otherwise, different strains will be identified (18,22,47,136,194,203,209-211,246).

Approximately 10-15% of neonatal herpes infections are estimated to be postnatally acquired (18,122). Postnatal herpes infections may be relatively more common than previously suspected since the number of HSV type 1 neonatal infections reported is disproportionately greater than the number of HSV type 1 genital infections being reported (18,122). The latest NIAID Antiviral Study Group data show that type 1 virus infections may now account for 30% of all cases of neonatal herpes but only 5-15% of cases of genital herpes (122). The incidence of postnatally acquired neonatal herpes infections affects the overall incidence of neonatal herpes and, more importantly, may have significant ramifications for studies of prophylactic and preventive strategies for neonatal herpes.

PATHOGENESIS AND PATHOLOGY

Congenital HSV infections probably arise from transplacental transmission of the virus in some cases and from transcervical transmission of the virus in others (18,66). Maternal viremia with herpesvirus is a prerequisite for transplacental transmission. Viremia with HSV does occur but is detected only infrequently and with difficulty (18,47,64,133,212). Viremia has been documented in two women with genital herpes (213). Viremia is also believed to account for the systemic symptoms and the occasional development of distant disease in association with localized herpes infections, particularly primary genital herpes infections (18,47,64,133).

When transplacental transmission occurs, maternal virus reaching the placenta gains direct access to the fetal bloodstream and is transported to the fetal tissues by the fetal circulation. One can alternatively envision that maternal virus reaching the placenta may produce placentitis and then directly spread to produce chorioamnionitis and a subsequent fetal infection. Whether or not this latter progression does occur is unknown.

Transcervical transmission of congenital herpes occurs when maternal virus ascends through the cervix and directly infects the amniotic membranes and the fetus. It is unknown whether virus spread directly to the placenta from infected amniotic membranes can hematogenously infect the fetus. It should be remembered that the pattern of fetal disease may not be a reliable clue to pathogenesis because transcervically acquired mucocutaneous disease can disseminate to involve other sites and hematogenously acquired disease may potentially localized to mucocutaneous sites and thereby mimic the other.

The foregoing discussion suggests that it may be very difficult to distinguish between transplacental and transcervical and combined modes of transmission when studying future cases of congenital herpes. The potential for iatrogenically introduced fetal infections should always be kept in mind whenever amniocentesis, chorionic villous biopsy, and transcervical or fetal surgery is performed (66,180). It is unknown whether differences in the mode of acquisition of congenital herpes have clinical, therapeutic, or prognostic significance.

Intrapartum neonatal herpes infections arise from direct contact of the infant with the virus during labor and delivery. Infection may result when virus-containing secretions are aspirated into the infant's pharynx or respiratory tract or when the virus comes into contact with the infant's eyes, scalp, skin, or umbilical cord (18,133,136). It should also be remembered that the pathogenetic mechanisms that produce congenital herpes probably do not cease to operate until the fetus is delivered. Therefore, it is possible that some cases of neonatal herpes attributed to intrapartum infection may actually represent late congenital infections (18,66,136). Iatrogenic factors that facilitate intrapartum transmission of neonatal herpes such as fetal scalp electrodes should also be remembered and avoided as much as possible.

Postnatal neonatal herpes infections appear to result from direct contact with infectious oral secretions from other individuals; from direct contact with virus present on the hands of hospital personnel, care givers, or other individuals; or from direct contact with a virus-containing breast lesion during nursing (18,133,136,193). Consequently, mucocutaneous surfaces of the infant are the portal of entry for postnatal infections.

Following onset of viral replication at the portal of entry, HSV infection can spread to involve other sites in the fetus or neonate through direct spread to adjacent sites, hematogenous spread, and possibly transneuronal spread (18,133,136,214). At the cellular level, herpesvirus infection causes cessation of synthesis of host cell DNA and proteins and formation of progeny virus. As a result of viral replication intranuclear inclusion bodies, chromatin clumping, and nucleolar dissolution become apparent. The host cell becomes swollen and dies. Multinucleated giant cells are occasionally formed also (18).

Histologically, involved tissues usually show extensive hemorrhagic necrosis, clumping of chromatin, dissolution of nucleoli, formation of multinucleated giant cells, and ultimately a lymphocytic inflammatory response, often with lymphocytic perivascular cuffing (18). Grossly, infected tissues may demonstrate small punctate yellow to gray areas of focal necrosis or other findings or organ dysfunction and cell death commensurate with the severity and the location of the disease present (18). Virus can be isolated from tissues that show obvious viral disease and sometimes from tissues that do not manifest any gross or microscopic signs of viral infection (18,133).

CLINICAL MANIFESTATIONS

Congenital Infections

Congenital HSV infections can produce a vast spectrum of disease. Disease due to congenital herpes can cause damage and dysfunction of any one or more host tissues and organs. Disease manifestations can range from subtle to florid and at times may be clinically indistinguishable from the manifestations of congenital disease produced by other infectious agents.

Fetal infection with HSV can occur at any time during gestation. The time of onset of fetal infection is usually impossible to ascertain precisely. Maternal signs of herpes infection during pregnancy, if present, may suggest the time of fetal infection. Alternatively, the fetal age at the time of infection can sometimes be very crudely estimated by taking the difference between the postconceptual age when clinical disease is noted and the clinically estimated disease duration necessary to produce the findings noted.

Congenital herpes is usually not recognized until after birth. Infants who acquire herpes infections early in gestation can therefore have infections present for a considerable period of time before treatment is initiated. These infants may be at particular risk for a poor outcome.

Intrauterine infections with herpesvirus, especially those that occur early in gestation, can affect the duration of pregnancy and can interfere with normal fetal growth and development. Preterm birth of infected infants is frequent (66,148). Congenitally infected babies commonly have intrauterine and postnatal growth retardation. Congenital malformations may occur also (66,135,147,149,150,156,158-160,170,173). Congenital malformations appear to result from viral-induced tissue destruction rather than developmental dysfunction (18,133,136).

Babies with congenital herpes can manifest one of several patterns of disease; babies may have (a) disease localized to the skin, eye, and/or mouth; (b) disease of the central nervous system with or without skin, eye, and/or mouth involvement; or (c) disseminated disease involving other organs and possibly including the skin, eye, mouth, and/or central nervous system. Classifying infants with congenital herpes according to these patterns of disease reveals that approximately 10-20% have limited mucocutaneous disease, 5-10% have eye disease only, 50% have central nervous system disease with skin and eye involvement, and about 30% have disseminated disease (18,66,123,133,148). This method of classification is important for therapeutic and prognostic purposes.

Skin involvement at or shortly after birth is common but not universal; 70% of cases of congenital herpes present with skin vesicles, but about

20% of cases never develop skin lesions (66). Skin manifestations commonly include vesicles and their scars but can also include bullous and erythematous maculopapular lesions, areas of aplastic skin, denuded skin, and extensive scarring (18,66,133,147-161,163,165-168,170-172,174,175). Extramedullary hematopoiesis involving the skin may be seen (247). Skin lesions have a tendency to occur at traumatized sites such as fetal scalp monitor sites (18,66,132,133,168). Recurrences of skin lesions may occur at a variable frequency for months to years (66). Recurrent skin lesions often occur at the sites of previous skin lesions and sometimes at previously uninvolved sites but generally do not progress to disease at other sites (66, 148,149,152,155,157,160,161,163,165).

Central nervous system disease is commonplace in infants with congenital herpes. Findings may include microcephaly, hydranencephaly, intracranial calcifications, hydrocephalus, porencephalic cysts, subependymal cysts, blindness, deafness, and mental retardation (18,66,67,130,133, 135,147-150,153,156,158-160,162-165,168-171,173,175). Microcephaly and hydranencephaly are particularly common (66,148). It is unknown whether later-appearing neurologic abnormalities such as developmental retardation, abnormalities of tone or cerebral palsy, strabismus, and others are directly or indirectly attributable to congenital herpes (66,163,165).

Ophthalmologic disease most commonly manifests as chorioretinitis. Other ocular disease findings include keratoconjunctivitis, corneal ulcerations, anterior uveitis, cataracts, vitritis, optic atrophy, nystagmus, strabismus, microophthalmia, and retinal dysplasia (66,147-149,152,155-158, 160,165,166,170-173). Ocular disease may be asymmetric in any given patient.

Disseminated disease following intrauterine herpes infection can involve any site. Most commonly the liver and the adrenal glands are involved. Other sites that have been reported to be affected in infants with congenital herpes are the larynx, trachea, lungs, esophagus, stomach, small intestine, large intestine, spleen, kidneys, pancreas, and heart (66, 130,147-151,153,156,159,160,162,164,168,169). Clinical manifestations correspond to the location and severity of disease. In addition, systemic signs of fever, acidosis, apnea, lethargy, poor suck, and poor feeding may be seen (66,162). Hyperbilirubinemia and respiratory distress may also be attributable to disseminated congenital herpes (66). Thrombocytopenia, disseminated intravascular coagulopathy, and gastrointestinal bleeding have been noted in some cases (66). Various congenital anomalies and bone disease have also been associated with disseminated infections (66, 75,147,152,161).

It should be remembered that skin, eye, mouth, and/or central nervous system disease may accompany disseminated disease. The mortality with disseminated congenital herpes is very high and is usually due to severe prematurity, respiratory failure, hepatic failure, cardiovascular collapse, or combinations of these factors. Other nonspecific manifestations have been reported in association with congenital herpes (66). Respiratory distress is frequently noted, but it is usually unclear whether lung immaturity or herpes infection is the cause. Likewise, it is unclear whether congenital herpes plays a pathogenetic role in causing the varied abnormalities that are occasionally noted such as abnormal facies, dysmorphic digits, inguinal hernias, and patent ductus arteriosis (66). It is unknown whether asymptomatic congenital herpes infections can occur.

Neonatal Infections

The clinical manifestations of neonatal herpes infections reiterate the manifestations seen with congenital herpes infections in most ways. Neonatal herpes can produce a broad range of disease in the newborn. Clinical signs can first appear anytime during the neonatal period (107). Disease can occur in a great variety of locations and can vary greatly in severity. Manifestations of neonatal herpes can be identical to those seen with other types of infections in the neonate, particularly bacterial sepsis (18,132, 133,136,184). Neonatal herpes can also interfere with postnatal growth and development.

A notable dissimilarity between congenital herpes and neonatal herpes is the manner in which each presents clinically. Congenital infections may present with disease at a more advanced stage than neonatal infections. Congenital herpes infections may remain clinically silent in utero for considerable periods of time and then present at birth with manifestations of disease at an advanced stage. On the other hand, infants with neonatal herpes infections are clinically observable throughout their entire course and may present more often with manifestations of early-stage disease.

Congenital and neonatal herpes infections usually present at different times during the neonatal period. Manifestations of congenital herpes infections are usually apparent immediately or shortly after birth. Neonatal infections usually do not become apparent until after a latent period of several days following birth. Congenital infections may sometimes present with some manifestations that are not seen with neonatal infections. Only congenital herpes can affect fetal growth and development. Therefore, intrauterine growth retardation and congenital deformities can only be attributable to congenital herpes infections.

The differentiation between congenital and neonatal herpes is useful because it emphasizes potential differences in their pathogenesis, clinical presentation, response to therapy, prognosis, and amenability to certain preventive measures. The distinction is not always clear-cut. Perinatal herpes infections are acquired over a continuum of time; intrauterine herpes infections merge into intrapartum herpes infections around the time of labor and delivery. Some infants who are believed to have neonatal herpes may actually have congenital herpes acquired very late in gestation. Other infants have been noted to have mucocutaneous herpes lesions at birth in association with prolonged rupture of membranes for many days to a few weeks. Such infants meet the criteria for a diagnosis of congenital herpes but are probably best regarded as cases of intrapartum neonatal herpes infections with an in utero incubation period (18).

Neonatal herpes infections due to HSV type 1 and type 2 are clinically indistinguishable. Isolation of HSV type 1 from an infected neonate may be suggestive of a postnatally acquired herpes infection (18). Importantly, the percentage of neonatal herpes infections caused by type 1 virus is increasing (122). This has prompted concern that postnatal acquisition of neonatal herpes infection is a significant problem.

Several reports have noted an increased incidence of preterm birth and low birth weight among infants with neonatal herpes (18,107,123, 124,132,133,136,215). About 50% of infected infants were preterm, and about 40% weighed less than 2,500 g at birth (123,132). A very recent study has noted a significant decline in the rate of preterm birth and the percent of low-birth-weight infants among newborns with neonatal herpes (122). Currently, about 25% of infected infants are preterm (122). No difference in disease severity or outcome has been noted between preterm and term infants with neonatal herpes (132). It remains unclear why neonatal herpes is associated with an increased rate of preterm birth or why this association is becoming less pronounced.

The presenting symptoms and signs of neonatal herpes are usually nonspecific. As a result, significant delays in diagnosis and treatment of neonatal herpes frequently occur (18,122,133,216). Clinical manifestations have been reported to precede diagnosis and onset of antiviral therapy by an average of 6-7 days and most recently by about 5 days (122, 216). Delayed diagnosis and treatment of neonatal herpes are associated with disease progression and hence a poor outcome (18,122,133).

Clinical classification of infants with neonatal herpes permits therapeutic and outcome comparisons and is based on the infant's pattern of disease. It should be noted that the system for classifying cases of neo-natal herpes has been revised to more accurately reflect therapeutic and prognostic issues (18). Babies with neonatal herpes should be categorized according to the presence of (a) skin, eye, and/or mouth disease; (b) central nervous system disease with or without skin, eye, and/or mouth disease; or (c) disseminated disease that may or may not additionally produce skin, eye, mouth, and/or central nervous system disease.

Among infants with neonatal herpes, reports have indicated that approximately 20% of cases have localized skin, eye, and/or mouth disease only; approximately 30% have localized central nervous system disease; and approximately 50% have disseminated disease (18,122,123,133, 136,215). This distribution appears to have changed during the past few years (122). Most recently, it has been noted that approximately 45% have skin, eye, and/or mouth disease only; approximately 35% have localized central nervous system disease; and approximately 20% have disseminated disease (122). The significant decrease in the frequency of disseminated disease and the corresponding increase in the frequency of skin, eye, and/or mouth disease is noteworthy. These changes probably reflect a slower rate of progression from skin, eye, and/or mouth disease to disseminated disease than in the past due to earlier recognition and earlier antiviral treatment of more recent cases of neonatal herpes (122).

Infants with neonatal herpes localized to the skin, eye, and/or mouth usually present at about 10-11 days of age (18). Skin lesions are particularly prevalent in these infants. About 80% of infants with this pattern of disease will have skin lesions noted (18,122). [Incidentally, about 80% of all infants with neonatal herpes will develop skin lesions sometime during their course, and about 15% of all infected infants will have disease confined just to the skin (18).] Skin lesions are typically discrete, 1- to 2-mm vesicles with an erythematous base. More rarely, erythematous maculo-papules, bullae, petechiae, or denuded skin are noted. Crops and clusters of vesicles are relatively common and occasionally form bullae. Clusters of vesicles often initially appear on the skin of the presenting part of the infant during birth, probably because this part of the skin has the longest and most direct contact with the virus during labor and delivery.

Skin lesions also have a predilection for traumatized skin, particularly fetal scalp electrode sites (18,132,133,136,181,186,187). Over time, skin lesions often spread to involve multiple distant areas of the skin. Babies occasionally have only one or two isolated vesicles as their sole manifestation of skin disease. Rarely, zosteriform eruptions occur (18, 217). Skin vesicles frequently recur periodically for months or years (18, 133,136,165). Recurrences occur whether or not antiviral therapy is administered. Skin lesions often recur at sites of previous skin lesions but can sometimes involve a new area of skin. Recurrent skin lesions do not progress to form disease elsewhere.

Neonatal herpes commonly invovles the eye, too. Eye disease can present later on as keratoconjunctivitis, microophthalmia, retinal dysplasia, or chorioretinitis (18,133,166,218). Ocular disease is unilateral in one third of patients. Bilateral disease is often asymmetric. Eye disease is the sole manifestation of disease in about 15% of all infants with neonatal herpes (18,133,184). Type 1 or type 2 HSV may be responsible for neonatal eye disease (18,133,157,219,220). Neonatal herpes infections involving the eye are notworthy for their ability to produce severe ocular damage even when treated (18). Keratoconjunctivitis can progress to chorioretinitis or retinal detachments (18). Cataracts due to neonatal herpes have been noted at long-term follow-up in very rare infants (221). The mechanism whereby HSV produces progressive ocular disease remains unknown.

About 10-30% of all infants with neonatal herpes can be demonstrated to have oropharyngeal involvement, but isolated involvement of the mouth is rare (18). Lesions of the oral mucosa or tongue may be the initial manifestations of neonatal herpes in some infants. Oral lesions usually appear as small shallow ulcers with an erythematous margin. Studies correlating the isolation of virus from the oral cavity with clinical lesions have not been done.

Infants with neonatal herpes restricted to the skin, eye, and/or mouth have a low mortality rate (< 10%) but are at significant risk for serious morbidity, especially if eye disease is present (18,122). Approximately 30% of infants with this pattern of disease eventually develop evidence of severe neurological impairment (18,122,132,133,222).

Neurological deficits may be mild or severe in nature and may be immediate or delayed in onset. Severe vision problems or blindness due to eye disease is especially devastating. It is also very disheartening that some infants with apparently localized skin, eye, and/or mouth disease have normal neurological development and functioning until 6-12 months of age and then develop long-term neurological impairments such as spastic quadriplegia, microcephaly, or blindness (18). The pathogenesis of the neurological problems in infants with skin, eye, and/or mouth disease is not understood. All of these children require very careful long-term follow-up for visual, auditory, neurological, and developmental problems.

Central nervous system (CNS) disease can result from neonatal herpes that is localized to the CNS or that is disseminated and involves the

CNS. The pathogenesis of CNS disease is believed to differ for localized and disseminated infections. Localized CNS infections possibly result from retrograde axonal transport of the virus from its portal of entry into the CNS. CNS involvement during disseminated herpes infections probably results from hematogenous passage of the virus into the CNS.

These pathogenetic differences are supported by observed differences between localized and disseminated infections involving the CNS. First, localized infections usually become apparent at an older age than to disseminated infections (16-17 days versus 9-10 days). This is as expected, since intraneuronal spread of virus is slower than hematogenous spread of virus. Second, transplacentally acquired maternal neutralizing antibodies are frequently present in infants with localized but not disseminated infections. Neutralizing antibodies may protect against blood-borne virus but should not affect intraneuronal virus.

Central nervous system disease is common among infants with neonatal herpes. About 30% of all babies with neonatal herpes have localized CNS disease, and about 65-70% of infants with disseminated disease also have CNS involvement (18). These two groups combined represent about 60% of all infants with neonatal herpes.

The initial manifestations of CNS infections with herpesvirus may include constitutional signs such as lethargy, irritability, poor sucking, poor feeding, vomiting, and temperature instability (18,133,136). Neurological signs may also be noted initially and may include bulging of the fontanelle, focal or generalized seizures, tremors, coma, opisthotonus, decerebrate posturing, and pyramidal tract signs (18,133,136). Signs of skin, eye, and/or mouth disease may precede or accompany CNS disease in many but not all cases. It is very important to realize that only 60% of infants with localized CNS disease have skin lesions anytime during their course (18,57,124,162,184). Babies with disseminated disease may initially present with evidence of disease at other or additional sites. Babies with disseminated disease also very frequently have skin vesicles at presentation and often have a fulminant stormy course from the outset (18).

Laboratory studies may initially or additionally suggest HSV infection of the CNS. CNS disease is frequently first indicated by abnormal results of cerebrospinal fluid (CSF) analysis. CSF pleiocytosis and proteinosis (up to 500-1,000 mg/dl) are usually seen when CNS involvement is present. Serial CSF analyses usually show progressively increasing proteinosis. Unfortunately, only 25-40% of infants with CNS disease have positive CSF cultures for HSV (18). Occasionally CNS involvement is suggested by other neurodiagnostic tests. Electroencephalography and computerized tomographic scanning of the head may sometimes suggest the diagnosis. Rarely, infants have no clinical manifestations and completely normal CSF findings but are discovered to have CNS involvement when herpesvirus is isolated from a brain biopsy specimen (18).

Localized CNS disease is associated with a 50% mortality rate when untreated (18,132,133,136). Death from localized CNS disease usually results from brainstem involvement. Long-term morbidity is very common and often severe and devastating when neonatal herpes involves the CNS (18,124,133,162). Most of these infants are damaged. Many will develop microcephaly, spasticity, learning disabilities, visual impairment or blindness, hydranencephaly, porencephalic cysts, or chorioretinitis.

Up to 50% of infants with CNS disease develop some degree of psychomotor retardation (18). Infants with localized and disseminated infections involving the CNS have the same spectrum of clinical findings and long-term problems. It should be remembered that even infants with very subtle clinical or CSF abnormalities initially can ultimately develop severe neurological or developmental deficits (18,222). It is unclear whether CNS disease can be progressive after the initial viral infection resolves, as can occur with eye disease and possibly other forms of disease due to neonatal herpes (18,122,133,215,223).

Babies with disseminated neonatal herpes usually are recognized at 9-10 days of age after symptoms or signs of infection have been present for a few days. Presenting manifestations of disseminated neonatal herpes may be constitutional or may be a reflection of disease in involved organs (18,129,132,133,136,184,224). Frequently noted constitutional findings include lethargy, temperature instability, irritability, poor sucking, poor feeding, and vomiting. Skin vesicles are very frequently the first recognized sign of disseminated infection. The presence of skin vesicles and constitutional signs is almost pathognomonic of disseminated herpes, but it is imperative to remember that over 20% of infants with disseminated neonatal herpes do not develop skin vesicles (18,122,162). Other presenting manifestations of disseminated neonatal herpes include respiratory distress, jaundice, hepatosplenomegaly, seizures, cyanosis, bleeding diatheses, disseminated intravascular coagulopathy, and shock. Disseminated neonatal herpes not infrequently mimics neonatal sepsis and therefore should be included in the differential diagnosis of any "septic-appearing" neonate.

Disseminated neonatal herpes may produce disease in any one or more organs. The liver and adrenal glands are most commonly involved, but disease may also occur in the larynx, trachae, lungs, esophagus, stomach, small intestine, large intestine, spleen, kidneys, pancreas, or heart (18, 129,133,136,184,218,225-227). Sixty percent to 75% of infants with disseminated herpes have CNS involvement (18). Skin, eye, and/or mouth lesions are found in approximately 80% of these infants (18).

The clinical manifestations of disseminated neonatal herpes infections generally correspond to the severity and location of disease. Systemic findings may include temperature instability, acidosis, apnea, lethargy, poor feeding, and shock. Jaundice, respiratory distress, or bleeding due to thrombocytopenia or disseminated intravascular coagulopathy may be prominent findings also.

Untreated, disseminated neonatal herpes is associated with a mortality rate exceeding 80% (132,133). Death is usually attributable to respiratory failure caused by herpes pneumonitis, bleeding, or cardiovascular collapse. Infants that survive are almost always impaired, often severely (18,132,133).

Very rare infants have been reported to have neonatal HSV infections without apparent disease (133,228). HSV infection confirmed by isolation of the virus from culture specimens has been reported in two infants without demonstrable disease, but it should be remembered that these infants may have had very subtle disease that was not detected because initial and follow-up evaluations were too insensitive or because the length of follow-up was too short (18). Disease-free neonatal herpes must be exceedingly rare if it occurs at all, since no cases have been noted among over 1,000 infants with neonatal herpes reported by multiple centers across the United States (18). Therefore, all neonates with herpes infections should be expected to develop disease and should always be treated with antiviral medication to prevent potentially devastating outcomes (18,229,230).

DIAGNOSIS

Herpes simplex virus infection of the newborn is usually first suggested by clinical findings and ultimately confirmed by isolation of the virus from infected babies. Unfortunately, the clinical features of herpes infections of infants are mostly nonspecific. Infected babies frequently have clinical findings that are similar or identical to those seen with other infectious and noninfectious conditions. Diagnosis of infected infants therefore requires that a high index of suspicion always be maintained.

The first clinical manifestations of herpes infections in babies can appear anytime during the neonatal period, but most infected babies do not develop any clinical findings until several days of age. Therefore, many infected infants appear to be normal when discharged from the nursery. The initial manifestations seen in infected babies are very variable. They may include mucocutaneous lesions, ocular lesions, neurological signs, constitutional signs, or findings of dysfunction of other organs. About one third of cases present with skin, eye, and/or mouth findings; one third present with systemic or CNS findings before skin, eye, and/or mouth findings appear; and about one third of cases present with systemic or CNS findings and never develop skin, eye, and/or mouth findings (107). Congenital abnormalities or intrauterine growth retardation may also be initial manifestations of congenital herpes infections (66).

Mucocutaneous lesions are the first manifestation of herpes infections relatively commonly. Skin vesicles should always immediately suggest herpes infection of the newborn. Ulcerative lesions of the mouth are also suggestive. Several alternative causes of vesicular and pustular skin lesions in neonates can sometimes be confused with herpes lesions. These may include varicella-zoster virus, cytomegalovirus, enteroviruses, erythema toxicum, bullous impetigo, transient pustular melanosis of the newborn, neonatal acne, miliaria, epidermolysis bullosa, acrodermatitis enteropathica, sucking bullae, traumatic ulcers, incontinentia pigmenti, histiocytosis X, scabies, and syphilis (18,133).

Viral cultures can distinguish herpes lesions from other viral lesions and other dermatological diseases. Erythema toxicum is readily identified by demonstrating the presence of eosinophils within skin lesions. Serological tests and other cultures can exclude other perinatal infections. Cytological examination of scrapings from herpes lesions may be very suggestive of herpes infection but cannot reliably establish or exclude a diagnosis of herpes in the newborn.

Neonatal conjunctivitis due to herpesvirus can be mistakenly attributed to chemical or bacterial causes. Viral and bacterial cultures and Gram stain permit proper diagnosis. Herpetic keratitis may demonstrate a characteristic dendritic pattern but may sometimes resemble congenital glaucoma. Chorioretinitis due to herpesvirus is clinically indistinguishable from chorioretinitis due to cytomegalovirus and toxoplasmosis, but viral cultures and serological tests can differentiate these entities. Cataracts due to herpesvirus should be differentiated from those due to rubella and other causes (133,221,248).

The diagnosis of herpes infection of the CNS in neonates can be extremely difficult. Concomitant skin vesicles may be a revealing clue, but it must be emphasized that about 40% of babies with herpetic CNS disease do not have a vesicular rash at the time of their clinical presentation

(18). Herpes infection should be a considered diagnosis in all neonates with clinical manifestations of meningoencephalitis. CSF findings that further suggest herpes infection include pleiocytosis, progressively increasing proteinosis, sterile bacterial culture, and absence of bacteria on Gram stain. Viral culture of the CSF yields the virus less than half the time when herpetic disease is actually present and therefore cannot be used to exclude the diagnosis.

Other neurodiagnostic tests such as electroencephalography, cranial ultrasound, and cranial computerized tomographic scanning may also suggest herpetic CNS disease or may help to exclude other causes of disease such as intracranial hemorrhage. Herpes infection of the CNS can also mimic metabolic disorders and other infections. Sometimes brain biopsy and culture are required to demonstrate herpes encephalitis (18, 132,152).

Herpes infections of the newborn should be included in the differential diagnosis whenever an infant is noted to have temperature instability or appears "septic." Appropriate bacterial and viral cultures can identify infectious causes of these findings. Metabolic disorders, necrotizing enterocolitis, intracranial hemorrhage, and cardiac disorders can also produce similar clinical findings. It should be remembered that occasional infants may have concomitant infections with HSV and a bacterial organism, particularly group B streptococcus, *Staphylococcus aureus*, or *E. coli*.

Rigorous and aggressive diagnostic efforts are imperative whenever an infant manifests signs suggestive of HSV infection. Isolation of the virus in culture should be the basis for definitive diagnosis of infected infants. Skin lesions, the conjunctivae, the nasopharynx and oropharynx, and the CSF should all be cultured. Urine and stool cultures may also potentially yield the virus. Culture of brain biopsy specimens and any other tissue specimens should also be done. Duodenal aspirates obtained through a transpyloric tube may be the only site from which virus can be isolated when herpetic hepatitis is present (230). Serial cultures may be necessary to isolate the virus. Specimens for viral culture can be placed in transport media and shipped on ice if a diagnostic virology laboratory is not located nearby (18,249).

Whenever evaluating a baby for herpes infection, it is important not to overlook the maternal history and physical examination. Specific inquiries should be made for any evidence of herpes infection of the mother or her sexual partners before or during the pregnancy, during labor and delivery, or following delivery. The obstetrical records of the pregnancy and the delivery should be reviewed. Examination of the mother and any putative source contacts may reveal evidence of herpes infection. All of these efforts can sometimes provide an important clue to the correct diagnosis. It should be emphasized that these efforts are most often nonproductive. Rarely, careful examination of the placenta and membranes provides an early clue to the presence of congenital herpes.

Cytologic examination and monoclonal antibody staining techniques may allow presumptive diagnosis of herpes infections of babies while awaiting the results of viral cultures. Cytologic examination of cells from the mother's cervix or genital tract lesions or from the infant's skin, conjunctival, corneal, and/or mouth lesions may be useful. Specimens for cytologic studies can be smeared on a slide and fixed in cold ethanol for transport to the laboratory. Giemsa and Wright (Tzank) unlike Papanicolaou smears are unlikely to demonstrate intranuclear inclusion bodies (18,133,250).

HSV infection is suggested by the identification of intranuclear inclusion bodies and multinucleated giant cells. Cytology has a sensitivity of about 60-70% for the demonstration of herpes infection of the newborn (18,133,136,145,250-252). Monoclonal antibody staining of specimens obtained from potential herpes lesions may provide a rapid presumptive diagnosis (18,47,136,242). Other monoclonal antibody assays are being developed and have been useful in preliminary studies. The use of electron microscopy to identify virus in clinical specimens has also been reported (47).

Infants with herpes infections should be initially and serially evaluated to determine the severity and location of disease. This is extremely important for therapeutic and prognostic reasons. Measurements of hepatic enzymes, bilirubin, blood cell counts, and bleeding parameters may be useful. CSF analysis, cranial computerized tomographic scanning, electroencephalography, chest roentgenography, and abdominal ultrasonography or roentgenography should be used judiciously to properly assess and to serially follow infected babies. Chest roentgenograms characteristically show a diffuse interstitial pattern when herpetic pneumonitis is present. Pneumonitis typically becomes hemorrhagic. Abdominal roentgenograms not infrequently reveal pneumatosis intestinalis when herpetic enterocolitis is present. Ophthalmologic consultation should be obtained for initial and serial follow-up evaluations of the eyes.

Serologic testing of the newborn is not usually beneficial. Many seroassays do not distinguish transplacental IgG maternal antibodies from the endogenous antibodies of the infant and often do not accurately distinguish antibodies induced by type 1 virus from those induced by type 2 virus (18, 110,133,136). Neonatal IgM antibodies appear 2-3 weeks into the course of neonatal herpes (136). Typing of viral isolates is available in some virology laboratories. Viral typing does not have any clinical importance since both types of the virus produce the same disease manifestations and are equally responsive to currently used antiviral drugs. Viral typing may sometimes have epidemiological importance, however.

THERAPY

The development of safe and effective antiviral drugs for the treatment of HSV infections of the newborn has greatly reduced the morbidity and mortality of these infections. Two drugs, vidarabine and acyclovir, are currently available for the treatment of neonatal herpes infections (215, 231). Vidarabine (adenine arabinoside; ara-A) is a nucleoside analog that nonspecifically inhibits both cellular and viral replication. Collaborative studies have shown vidarabine-treated infants to have much lower mortality rates than untreated infants. Mortality rates declined with the use of vidarabine from 90% to 70% of infants with disseminated disease, from 75% to 40% of infants with CNS disease (localized and disseminated infections), and from 50% to 15% of infants with localized CNS disease (123,215).

In these same studies, vidarabine-treated infants also had significantly lower morbidity rates than untreated infants. The rate of neurological impairment at 1 year of age declined with the use of vidarabine from 90% to 75% of infants with CNS disease (localized and disseminated infections) and from 30% to 10% of infants with skin, eye, and/or mouth disease (123,215). Vidarabine is administered intravenously at a dose of 15-30 mg/kg/day and is infused continuously for 12 h daily for a total of 10-14 days. No significant acute toxicity occurs with this regimen. It is recommended to use a dose of 30 mg/kg/day because significantly fewer babies have progression of their disease using this dose than the lower dose (5% vs. 20%) (123,184,215).

Some infected infants may require a longer duration of therapy than normally used (18). About 2% of treated infants have a recurrence of their infection with resultant CNS disease (18,107,123,215). It is unclear whether these infants have a true recurrence or merely progression of their infections (18). Infants with recurrences should be retreated. Viral resistance to vidarabine does not seem to be a factor when recurrences are noted (18,107,136).

Acyclovir (cycloguanosine) is a nucleoside analog that is specifically active against herpesviruses. Acyclovir is activated by viral thymidine kinase. Once activated, acyclovir competitively inhibits HSV DNA polymerase and thus inhibits viral replication (18,232). Acyclovir has not been as extensively studied as vidarabine for neonatal herpes. Reports of the use of acyclovir to treat neonatal herpes are limited (152,155,239).

Comparison studies of acyclovir versus vidarabine for neonatal herpes have not yet been completed. Preliminary results of these comparison studies suggest that there is no significant difference in outcome or toxicity for one drug compared to the other (18,231). Acyclovir has been shown to be superior to vidarabine for treatment of herpes encephalitis in children and adults, however (238,253). Acyclovir is administered intravenously at a dose of 30 mg/kg/day divided into three doses for infusion over 1 h at 8-h intervals. Acyclovir generally has no significant toxicity when given in this manner (18,234,240). Acyclovir has been effectively used in adults with genital herpes, patients with herpes encephalitis, and immunocompromixed patients with herpes infections (18,233-239,253). The potential of acyclovir treatment to produce resistant strains of virus or to lead to more severe recurrences by suppressing the initial immune response to the virus needs further study (47,239).

All infants with HSV infections should be promptly started on antiviral therapy. Early identification and treatment of infected babies halts the natural progression of the infection and results in substantial reductions in morbidity and mortality (18,123,136,184,215). Untreated infants with neonatal herpes have over a 70% chance of having skin, eye, and/or mouth disease progress to localized CNS disease or disseminated disease (132,133). The risk for a poor or fatal outcome is greatly increased when neonatal herpes progresses to involve the CNS or becomes disseminated even when antiviral drugs are given. Patient outcome is best when antiviral therapy is started early in the course of herpes infections of the neonate.

The most recent data available indicate that overall mortality of neonatal herpes is about 20% (122). The reduction in mortality in this report compared to earlier reports appears to be primarily due to earlier recognition and treatment of neonatal herpes. Treated babies have recently been receiving antiviral therapy an average of 3 days earlier in their course than was noted in the past (122). Importantly, a delay of 4-5 days is being noted between the onset of disease and the start of treatment for most infected babies (122). This suggests that if antiviral therapy can be started even earlier in these infants, further significant reductions in morbidity and mortality may be possible.

All infected infants should receive parenteral antiviral medicine. Infants with eye disease should be treated additionally with topical antiviral therapy (18,47,136). Several antiviral drugs come in an ophthalmological form. Very little information is available regarding the activity, safety, and toxicity of each of these preparations. Viroptic (trifluorothymidine) has been shown to have the greatest antiviral activity in older patients and is the treatment of choice for ocular herpes infections. Vidarabine and Stoxil (idoxuridine) are less active but have been used for longer periods of time and have a better-defined safety profile.

It is very important to monitor infants serially during treatment for evidence of disease progression. Such monitoring should focus particularly on the eyes, CNS, liver, and bone marrow. Patients should also be monitored for signs of drug toxicity. Blood cell counts, hepatic function tests, and renal function tests should be serially assessed. The potential for long-term adverse effects from antiviral drugs remains to be defined. There may be a potential for these drugs to cause mutagenic or teratogenic problem much later in life since these drugs interfere with DNA replication (18). It is also unknown whether the virus can potentially develop resistance to these drugs (18). No significant problems with resistant strains of HSV have been reported.

Antiviral medications are the only therapy available that is directly active against the virus. However, it is important not to overlook the role of supportive therapy for infected infants. These infants are often very ill and may require intensive support for various life-threatening problems including respiratory failure, disseminated intravascular coagulopathy, shock, and metabolic imbalances. Close attention to general supportive measures, such as mechanical ventilation, treatment for shock, blood component therapy, control of seizures, maintenance of fluid and electrolyte balance, correction of metabolic problems, maintenance of nutrition, and treatment of other infections significantly improves outcome. No other therapeutic interventions have been demonstrated to be of benefit for newborns with neonatal herpes. No vaccine is available.

Supportive counseling for the parents is often very important for optimal adaptation of the parents to the stresses imposed by an infant with HSV infection. Feelings of guilt, marital strains, and the stresses of coping with and caring for an infected infant may be severe and often require intervention. It is important for the clinician to address and to be sensitive to the issues of the parents. Parents should be provided information regarding HSV infections of the newborn in general, planned evaluations and treatments, anticipated risks, necessary follow-up, and possible future issues for their child. Infants require long-term follow-up after their acute infection resolves. Neurodevelopment, vision, and hearing should be monitored closely. Early intervention should occur for any problems identified. The use of suppressive antiviral therapy to prevent progressive eye disease needs to be studied.

It should always be remembered that infants with acute or recurrent infections with herpesvirus are a potential source of virus that can infect others. This may be a significant problem particularly if the affected infant attends day care or comes into contact with pregnant women or neonates. Covering active lesions helps to prevent transmission of the virus to susceptible individuals (107).

PREVENTION

Prevention of HSV infections of the fetus and neonate is extremely important. Prevention of herpes infections is the only effective way to eliminate the morbidity and mortality produced by these infections. Two general preventive strategies are available: measures can prevent herpetic disease in infants by preventing exposure of the fetus or neonate to the virus or by preventing exposed infants from developing herpes infections.

Efforts directed at preventing fetal and neonatal exposure to the virus begin with measures to prevent herpes infections of women of childbearing age in general and pregnant women in particular. These women should be made aware of the risks for themselves and for their babies associated with sexually transmitted diseases (STDs), particularly herpes and human immunodeficiency virus infections. Education and counseling can increase awareness of the increased risk of herpes infection and other STDs associated with promiscuity, casual sex, sex during adolescence, and sex with partners at high risk for having herpes or STDs. The use of condoms and the maintenance of monogamous relationships may reduce the risk for acquiring herpes and other infections. Pregnant women should be specifically informed of the potential for fetal or neonatal damage associated with STDs and should be encouraged to seek evaluation whenever symptoms of these infections are present.

Preventive efforts should focus particularly on pregnant women who have had genital herpes in the past or who develop genital herpes during their pregnancy. The babies of these women have a higher risk for herpes infections. Currently there are no specific recommendations possible for preventing fetal herpes infections when maternal herpes infections occur during gestation.

Measures to interdict in utero transmission of the virus to the fetus have not been studied. The use of antiviral medications for this purpose is not recommended because pharmacokinetic, toxicity, and effectiveness studies have not been performed. The rate of intrauterine transmission of herpesvirus to the fetus appears to be very low since congenital herpes only seems to occur about once in every 200,000-300,000 births (18,66). There is also insufficient information to be able to accurately assess the fetus for the presence of congenital herpes infection or to treat and monitor the fetus in utero for presumed congenital herpes infection. In utero antiviral therapy of fetuses presumed to be infected has been anecdotally reported but remains experimental (66,77-80).

Preventive efforts that protect the infant from exposure to the virus during labor and delivery prevent intrapartum neonatal herpes infections. Such efforts are especially important because most cases of neonatal herpes result from intrapartum transmission of the virus. Ideally, pregnant women could be checked for the presence of HSV in their genital tract at the time of labor and delivery. Women without detectable virus could be delivered routinely since their infants have no risk for exposure to the virus. Methods to protect the infant from exposure to the virus could then be selectively directed at those with virus detected at delivery.

Unfortunately, the lack of a rapid, accurate method to detect the presence of herpesvirus in the maternal genital tract during labor and delivery severely constrains selective utilization of preventive measures. History and physical examination identify only a minority of pregnant women who are virus positive at delivery (18,101,102,110,122-124,132,133,136, 184,188). Viral cultures of specimens from the maternal genital tract during labor and delivery are very accurate but usually are not rapid enough to be clinically useful for this purpose. As a result, an alternative approach has been recommended. Women at risk (those with a previous episode of genital herpes) are serially monitored clinically and virologically in an attempt to predict which women are likely to be virus positive at the time of delivery (116-118,131,133,142,143,145,254). This approach has been widely espoused and implemented.

Most protocols have recommended weekly clinical and virological evaluations of women at risk beginning at about 32-34 weeks of gestation. Women with no evidence of genital herpes at their last weekly prenatal evaluation and a normal clinical examination at delivery are considered unlikely to be virus positive and are delivered routinely. Women with clinical findings or a positive herpes culture from their last weekly prenatal evaluation are considered to be potentially virus positive and are targeted for preventive interventions to protect the infant from intrapartum exposure to the virus (116,117,131,133,145).

There are several problems with this approach. Primary genital herpes infections at delivery cannot be anticipated. Women at risk cannot be easily identified because most women with recurrent herpes have no suggestive history or findings (18,101,102,110,122-124,132,133,136,184,188). Clinically silent recurrences or viral shedding occurring after the last prenatal visit but before delivery can potentially infect the infant (110).

This approach is also costly (245). Very recently, this approach has been also shown to be unsatisfactory for predicting virus positivity at delivery for women with known recurrent genital herpes (110,188). Serial cultures may be useful to document cessation of viral shedding from lesions occurring shortly before delivery. Many cesarean deliveries can be avoided in this manner (110,117).

Cesarean section is the only preventive measure that has been shown to protect the infant from intrapartum exposure to herpesvirus in the maternal genital tract (18,116,117,131,133,136,145). Cesarean section is effective when the membranes are intact or are ruptured less than 4 h prior to delivery (133). The effectiveness of cesarean section for the prevention of neonatal herpes diminishes when the membranes have been ruptured for longer than 4 hs.

The increased risks for the mother and the infant as well as the increased cost and hospitalization associated with cesarean section make selective utilization of cesarean section for prevention of neonatal herpes highly desirable. At present, all women with clinical evidence of genital herpes at the time of labor and delivery should be delivered by cesarean section if the membranes are intact or are ruptured for less than 4 h. Cesarean section is also frequently performed for women with clinical genital herpes at delivery whose membranes are ruptured for more than 4 h. This is of probable but unknown benefit since the relative benefit of cesarean section for prevention of neonatal herpes as a function of the duration of ruptured membranes has not been studied.

Decisions regarding the use of cesarean section for prevention of neonatal herpes for women without clinical manifestations but at risk for the presence of genital herpes at delivery are much less clear. Infants of women who are virus positive at delivery and who have a known history of recurrent genital herpes appear to have a very low risk ($< 5\%$) for neonatal herpes when delivered vaginally (18,101,107,133,188). On the other hand, infants of mothers with primary genital herpes at the time of delivery have a high risk for neonatal herpes if delivered vaginally (18,101, 133). Prenatal testing of mothers for HSV type 2 specific antibodies is now possible and may be very useful for risk-benefit decisions regarding cesarean section for prevention of neonatal herpes (18,101,188,189). Indications for cesarean section should therefore be individualized in such circumstances. Every effort should be made to protect the integrity of the membranes until surgery. It should also be emphasized that cesarean section does not always prove effective; infants rarely can develop neonatal herpes despite cesarean delivery with intact membranes (18,132,193). Hopefuly, rapid detection assays will become available in the very near future so that these problems can be overcome.

Methods to prevent postnatal exposure of neonates to HSV should not be overlooked. Since direct contact of the infant with the virus is the mode of transmission for postnatal herpes infections, preventive measures should protect the infant from direct contacts with the virus. Good hand washing and covering of infectious lesions by care givers the virus. A frequent issue is the prevention of infant exposures when the mother had herpes lesions. Mothers with orolabial herpes, genital herpes, and herpetic lesions at other sites (i.e., breast lesions, herpetic whitlow, etc.) may expose their infants to the virus. Precautions taken by the mother to prevent direct contact of her infant with her lesions as well as careful hand washing should prevent postnatal infection of the infant (107). Isolation of the mother from her infant is generally unnecessary. Breast feeding should only be proscribed if breast lesions are present (18,107). Babies of mothers with herpes infections do not require isolation unless they are infected. Uninfected babies should be discharged from the nursery on time. Infected mothers should be carefully educated regarding preventive measures they should follow.

Hospital personnel should protect themselves from direct contact with the lesions of infected mothers, also. Similar preventive measures should be practiced by fathers, other relatives, care givers, and other individuals having contact with the infant whenever they have herpes lesions. In general, no other preventive measures are normally necessary for nonhospital personnel (107).

Nosocomial exposures of babies to the virus can be prevented by proper hand-washing techniques, avoidance of direct contact of the infant with infectious lesions or secretions of the staff personnel and other patients, and proper staff education programs focused on prevention of nosocomial infections. Infected babies should be isolated. Contact isolation should be used for infected mothers. Hospital personnel with herpes infections do not generally need to be isolated from the nursery. Personnel with herpetic whitlow are an exception, since even gloves may not prevent exposures to the virus (107). Masks should be worn by nursery personnel with orolabial herpes lesions. At the time of discharge of the baby, it is important for nursery personnel to educate parents regarding their role in preventing postnatal herpes infection of their baby. Undue parental anxiety should be recognized and addressed. Sometimes an infant is nevertheless exposed to the virus, and parents should be told to seek immediate medical advice should they notice signs of possible herpes infection of their baby.

Preventing exposure of the infant to the virus is the initial strategy currently employed to prevent HSV infections of the infant. Recently more and more attention is being focused on the issues surrounding preventive management of exposed infants. Sometimes an infant is inadvertently or uncontrollably exposed to the virus during delivery. Preventive measures could conceivably prevent exposed infants from going on to develop herpes infection. The use of antiviral medications in this context has not been studied adequately. Currently, it appears that infants exposed to recurrent genital herpes during delivery are at very low risk for the development of neonatal herpes, so prophylactic antiviral therapy is not recommended for these infants (110,188,190). On the other hand, infants exposed to a primary genital herpes infection at birth have an appreciable risk for developing neonatal herpes and may benefit from prophylactic antiviral therapy. Prenatal serologic testing of the mother may help distinguish primary infections.

Other factors may influence the infant's risk for developing infection following intrapartum exposure such as the presence of skin lacerations, the use of fetal scalp electrodes, the duration of ruptured membranes, and possibly other factors. Prophylactic antiviral therapy is not recommended. Hopefully, controlled trials will soon clarify the role of prophylactic antiviral therapy, if any, for preventing neonatal herpes in exposed infants.

Exposed infants who develop signs of neonatal herpes should be given anticipatory antiviral therapy. This is analogous to the use of antibiotics for the expectant treatment of bacterial infections in the nursery. For this reason it is usually prudent to obtain cultures from the maternal genital tract and from the infant at the time of delivery. If the cultures are positive and the infant develops symptoms, then a presumptive diagnosis can be made, additional cultures of the infant can be obtained, and expectant antiviral therapy can be initiated (110).

The use of antiviral therapy of the mother before delivery to prevent genital herpes from occurring at delivery has not been studied. The efficacy and the risks of this approach deserve very careful study before any consideration should be given to its use (18,110).

The use of antiviral therapy of the mother immediately prior to delivery or of the infant following birth as an alternative to cesarean section has not been studied and is not recommended.

REFERENCES

1. Batignani, A. (1934). Conjunctivite da virus erpetico in neonato. *Boll. Ocul.* 13:1217.
2. Haas, M. (1935). Hepatoadrenal necrosis with intranuclear inclusion bodies: Report of a case. *Am. J. Pathol.* 11:127.
3. Nahmias, A. J., and Dowdle, W. (1968). Antigenic and biologic differences in herpesvirus hominis. *Prog. Med. Virol.* 10:110.
4. Kieff, E. D., Bachendheimer, S. L., and Roizman, B. (1971). Size, comparison, and structure of the DNA of subtypes 1 and 2 of herpes simplex virus. *J. Virol.* 8:125.
5. Hayward, G. S., Jacob, R. J., Wadsworth, S. C., et al. (1975). Anatomy of herpes simplex virus DNA: Evidence for four populations of molecules that differ in the relative orientation of their long and short segments. *Proc. Natl. Acad. Sci. USA* 72:4243.
6. Sheldrick, P., and Berthelot, N. (1975). Inverted repetitions in the chromosome of herpes simplex virus. *Cold Spring Harbor Symp. Quant. Biol.* 39:667.
7. Honess, R. W., and Roizman, B. (1973). Proteins specified by herpes simplex virus. Identification and relative molar rates of synthesis of structural and nonstructural herpesvirus polypeptides in the infected cell. *J. Virol.* 12:1346.
8. Spear, P. G. (1984). Glycoproteins specified by herpes simplex virus. In Roizman, B. (ed.): *The Herpesviruses*, Vol. 3. New York, Plenum, p. 315.
9. Centifanto-Fitzgerald, Y. M., Yamaguchi, T., Kaufman, H. E., et al. (1982). Ocular disease pattern induced by herpes simplex virus is genetically determined by a specific region of the viral DNA. *J. Exp. Med.* 155:475.
10. Roizman, B. (1980). Structural and functional organization of herpes simplex virus genomes. In Rapp, F. (ed.): *Oncogenic Herpesviruses*, Vol. 1. Boca Raton, FL, CRC Press, p. 19.
11. Corey, L., and Spear, P. (1986). Infections with herpes simplex viruses. *N. Engl. J. Med.* 314:686-691, 749.
12. Roizman, B., Norrild, B., Chan, C., et al. (1984). Identification of a herpes simplex virus 2 glycoprotein lacking a known type 1 counterpart. *Virology* 133:242.
13. Ludwig, H. O., et al. (1972). Studies on the relatedness of herpesviruses through DNA-DNA hybridization. *Virology* 49:95.
14. Kieff, E. D., et al. (1972). Genetic relatedness of type 1 and type 2 herpes simplex viruses. *J. Virol.* 9:738.
15. Roizman, B. (1979). The organization of the herpes simplex virus genomes. *Annu. Rev. Genet.* 13:25.

16. Nahmias, A. J., and Norrild, B. (1979). Herpes simplex viruses 1 and 2: Basic and clinical aspects. *Dis. A Month* 25:5.
17. Longnecker, R., Chatterjee, S., Whitley, R. J., et al. (1987). Identification of a novel herpes simplex virus 1 glycoprotein gene within a gene cluster dispensable for growth in cell culture. *Proc. Natl. Acad. Sci. USA* 84:4303.
18. Whitley, R. J. (in press). Herpes simplex virus infections. In Remington, J. S., and Klein, J. O. (eds.): *Infectious Diseases of the Fetus and Newborn Infant*, 3d Ed.
19. Rapp, F. (1984). Herpes simplex viruses. In Holmes, K. K., Mardh, P.-A., Sparling, P. F., et al. (eds.): *Sexually Transmitted Diseases*. New York, McGraw-Hill, pp. 438-449.
20. O'Neill, F. J. (1977). Prolongation of herpes simplex virus latency in cultured human cells by temperature elevation. *J. Virol.* 24:41.
21. Colberg-Poley, A. M., et al. (1979). Experimental HSV latency using phosphonoacetic acid. *Proc. Soc. Exp. Biol. Med.* 162:235.
22. Buchman, T. G., Roizman, B., and Nahmias, A. J. (1979). Demonstration of exogenous genital reinfection with herpes simplex virus type 2 by restriction endonuclease fingerprinting of viral DNA. *J. Infect. Dis.* 140:195.
23. Buchman, T. G., Roizman, B., and Nahmias, A. J. (1980). Structure of herpes simplex virus DNA and application to molecular epidemiology. *Ann. N.Y. Acad. Sci.* 354:279.
24. Schmidt, O. W., Fife, K. H., and Corey, L. (1984). Reinfection is an uncommon occurrence in patients with symptomatic recurrent genital herpes. *J. Infect. Dis.* 149:645.
25. Lakeman, A. D., Nahmias, A. J., and Whitley, R. J. (1986). Analysis of DNA from recurrent genital herpes simplex virus isolates by restriction endonuclease digestion. *Sex. Trans. Dis.* 13:61.
26. Hill, T. J. (1985). Herpes simplex virus latency. In Roizman, B. (ed.): *The Herpesviruses*, Vol. 3. New York, Plenum, p. 175.
27. Kristensson, K., Lycke, E., and Sjostrand, J. (1971). Spread of herpes simplex virus in peripheral nerves. *Acta Neuropathol.* 17:44.
28. Hill, T. J., Field, H. J., and Roome, A. P. C. (1972). Intraaxonal location of herpes simplex virus particles. *J. Gen. Virol.* 15:253.
29. Cook, M. L., and Stevens, J. G. (1973). Pathogenesis of herpetic neuritis and ganglionitis in mice: Evidence of intraaxonal transport of infection. *Infect. Immun.* 7:272.
30. Cook, M. L., and Stevens, J. G. (1976). Latent herpetic infections following experimental viremia. *J. Gen. Virol.* 31:75.
31. Stevens, J. G., and Cook, M. L. (1971). Latent herpes simplex virus in spinal ganglia of mice. *Science* 173:843.
32. Cabrera, C. V., Wohlenberg, C., and Openshaw, H. (1978). Herpes simplex virus DNA sequences in the CNS of latently infected mice. *Nature* 298:1068.
33. Fraser, N. W., Lawrence, W. C., Wroblewska, Z., et al. (1981). Herpes simplex virus type 1 DNA in human brain tissue. *Proc. Natl. Acad. Sci. USA* 78:6451.

34. Rock, D. L., and Fraser, N. W. (1983). Detection of HSV-1 genome in central nervous system pf latently infected mice. *Nature* 302:523.
35. Baringer, J. R. (1974). Recovery of herpes simplex virus from human sacral ganglions. *N. Engl. J. Med.* 291:828.
36. Baringer, J. R., and Swoveland, P. (1973). Recovery of herpes simplex virus from human trigeminal ganglions. *N. Engl. J. Med.* 288:648.
37. Warren, K. G., Brown, S. M., Wroblewska, Z., et al. (1978). Isolation of latent herpes simplex virus from the superior cervical and vagus ganglions of human beings. *N. Engl. J. Med.* 298:1068.
38. Sequiera, L. W., Jennings, L. C., Carrasso, L. H., et al. (1979). Detection of herpes simplex virus genome in brain tissue. *Lancet* 2:609.
39. Galloway, D. A., Fenoglio, C., Shevchuk, M., et al. (1979). Detection of herpes simplex RNA in human sensory ganglia. *Virology* 95:265.
40. Carton, C. A., and Kilbourne, E. D. (1952). Activation of latent herpes simplex by trigeminal sensory-root section. *N. Engl. J. Med.* 246:172.
41. Pazin, G. J., Ho, M., and Jannetta, P. J. (1978). Herpes simplex reactivation after trigeminal nerve root decompression. *J. Infect. Dis.* 138:405.
42. Pazin, G. J., Armstrong, J. A., Tarr, G. C., et al. (1979). Prevention of reactivation of herpes simplex virus infection by human leukocyte interferon after operation on the trigeminal root. *N. Engl. J. Med.* 301:225.
43. Stevens, J. G. (1978). Latent characteristics of selected herpesviruses. *Adv. Cancer Res.* 26:227.
44. Tenser, R., et al. (1979). Trigeminal ganglion infection by thymidine kinase-negative mutants of herpes simplex virus. *Science* 205:915.
45. Tenser, R. B., and Dunstan, M. E. (1979). Herpes simplex virus thymidine kinase expression in infection of the trigeminal ganglion. *Virology* 99:417.
46. Douglas, R. G. (1985). Herpes simplex virus infections. In Wyngaarden, J. B., and Smith, L. H. (eds.): *Textbook of Medicine*, 17th Ed. Philadelphia, W. B. Saunders, pp. 1714-1716.
47. Kohl, S. (1987). Postnatal herpes simplex virus infection. In Feigin, R. D., and Cherry, J. D. (eds.): *Textbook of Pediatric Infectious Diseases*. Philadelphia, W. B. Saunders, pp. 1577-1601.
48. Nahmias, A. J., and Josey, W. E. (1982). Epidemiology of herpes simplex viruses 1 and 2. In Evans, A. S. (ed.): *Viral Infections of Humans: Epidemiology and Control*. New York, Plenum, pp. 351-372.
49. Nerurkar, L. S., West, F., May, M., et al. (1983). Survival of herpes simplex virus in water specimens collected from hot tubs in spa facilities and on plastic surfaces. *J.A.M.A.* 250:3081-3083.
50. Turner, R., Shehab, Z., Osborne, K., et al. (1982). Shedding and survival of herpes simplex virus from "fever blisters." *Pediatrics* 70:547-549.
51. Duenas, A., Adma, E., Melnick, J. L., et al. (1972). Herpesvirus type 2 in a prostitute population. *Am. J. Epidemiol.* 95:483-489.
52. Rawls, W. E., Gardner, H. L., Flanders, R. W., et al. (1971). Genital herpes in two social groups. *Am. J. Obstet. Gynecol.* 110:682-689.

53. Stavraky, K. M., Rawls, W. E., Chiavetta, J., et al. (1983). Sexual and socio-economic factors affecting the risk of past infections with herpes simplex virus type 2. *Am. J. Epidemiol.* 118:109-121.
54. Overall, J. C. Jr. (1984). Dermatologic viral diseases. In Galasso, G. J., Merigan, T. C., and Buchanan, R. A. (eds.): *Antiviral Agents and Viral Diseases of Man*, 2d Ed. New York, Raven Press, pp. 247-312.
55. Dowdle, W. R., Nahmias, A. J., Harwell, R. W., et al. (1967). Association of antigenic type of herpesvirus hominis with site of viral recovery. *J. Immunol.* 99:774-780.
56. Wu, E., Sayre, J., Wiesmeier, E., et al. (1984). A prospective seroepidemiological survey of herpes simplex (HSV) infections in a college population. *Pediatr. Res.* 18:289A.
57. Nahmias, A. J., and Roizman, B. (1973). Herpes simplex virus. *N. Engl. J. Med.* 289:667, 719, 781.
58. McClung, H., Seth, P., and Rawls, W. E. (1976). Relative concentrations in human sera of antibodies to cross-reacting and specific antigens of herpes simplex virus types 1 and 2. *Am. J. Epidemiol.* 104:192.
59. Smith, I. W., Peutherer, J. F., and McCallum, F. O. (1967). The incidence of herpesvirus hominis antibodies in the population. *J. Hyg. (Lond.)* 65:395.
60. Wentworth, B. B., and Alexander, E. R. (1971). Seroepidemiology of infections due to members of the herpesvirus group. *Am. J. Epidemiol.* 94:496.
61. Nahmias, A. J., Josey, W. E., Naib, Z. M., et al. (1970). Antibodies to herpesvirus hominis types 1 and 2 in humans. *Am. J. Epidemiol.* 91:539.
62. Nahmias, A. J., Keyserling, H., Bain, R., et al. (1985). Prevalence of herpes simplex virus (HSV) type-specific antibodies in USA prepaid group medical practice population. Abstract, Sixth International Meeting of the International Society for STD Research, London.
63. Mann, S. L., Meyers, J. D., Holmes, K. L., et al. (1984). Prevalence and incidence of herpesvirus infections among homosexually active men. *J. Infect. Dis.* 149:1026.
64. Corey, L. (1984). Genital herpes. In Holmes, K. K., Mardh, P.-A., Sparling, P. F., et al. (eds.): *Sexually Transmitted Diseases*. New York, McGraw-Hill, pp. 449-474.
65. Peacock, J. E. Jr., and Sarubbi, F. A. (1983). Disseminated herpes simplex virus infection during pregnancy. *Obstet. Gynecol.* 61(Suppl.):13S-18S.
66. Baldwin, S., Benfield, M., and Whitley, R. J. (in press). Intrauterine HSV infection. *J. Teratol.*
67. Stagno, S., and Whitley, R. J. (1985). Herpesvirus infections of pregnancy. II. Herpes simplex virus and varicella-zoster virus infections. *N. Engl. J. Med.* 313:1327-1329.
68. Hillard, P., Seeds, J., and Cefalo, R. (1982). Disseminated hperes simplex in pregnancy: Two cases and a review. *Obstet. Gynecol. Surv.* 37:449-453.
69. Goyert, G. L., Bottoms, S. F., and Sokol, R. J. (1985). Anicteric presentation of fatal herpetic hepatitis in pregnancy. *Obstet. Gynecol.* 65:585-588.

70. Wertheim, R. A., Brooks, B. J., Rodriguez, F. H., et al. (1983). Fatal herpetic hepatitis in pregnancy. *Obstet. Gynecol.* 62(Suppl.):38-42.
71. Anderson, J. M., and Nicholls, N. W. N. (1972). Herpes encephalitis in pregnancy. (Letters.) *Br. Med. J.* 1:632.
72. Goyette, R. E., Donowho, E. M., Hieger, L. R., et al. (1974). Fulminant herpes virus hominis hepatitis during pregnancy. *Obstet. Gynecol.* 43:191-196.
73. Flewett, T. H., Parker, R. G. F., and Philip, W. M. (1969). Acute hepatitis due to herpes simplex virus in an adult. *J. Clin. Pathol.* 22:60-66.
74. Young, E. J., Killam, A. P., and Greene, J. F. (1974). Disseminated herpes virus infection. Association with primary genital herpes in pregnancy. *JAMA* 235:2731-2733.
75. Kobberman, T., Clark, L., and Griffith, W. T. (1980). Maternal death secondary to disseminated herpes virus hominis. *Am. J. Obstet. Gynecol.* 137: 742-743.
76. Hensleigh, P. A., Glover, D. B., and Cannon, M. (1979). Systemic herpes virus hominis in pregnancy. *J. Reprod. Med.* 22:171-176.
77. Berger, S. A., Weinberg, M., Treves, T., et al. (1986). Herpes encephalitis during pregnancy: Failure of acyclovir and adenine arabinoside to prevent neonatal herpes. *Isr. J. Med. Sci.* 22:41-44.
78. Lagrew, D. C., Furlow, T. C., Hager, D., et al. (1984). Disseminated herpes simplex virus infection in pregnancy. Successful treatment with acyclovir. *JAMA* 252:2058-2059.
79. Greffe, B. S., Dooley, S. L., Deddish, R. B., et al. (1986). Transplacental passage of acyclovir. *J. Pediatr.* 100:1020-1021.
80. Grover, L., Kane, J., Karvitz, J., et al. (1985). Systemic acyclovir in pregnancy: A case report. *Obstet. Gynecol.* 65:284-287.
81. Zervoidakis, I. A., Silverman, F., Senterfit, L. B., et al. (1980). Herpes simplex in the amniotic fluid of an uninfected fetus. *Obstet. Gynecol.* 55:165.
82. Black, B. S. B., and Goodner, D. M. (1979). False positive amniotic fluid cytology in a parturient with active herpes at term. *Obstet. Gynecol.* 54:658.
83. Centers for Disease Control. (1982). Genital herpes infections—United States, 1966-1979. *M.M.W.R.* 31:137-139.
84. MacDougall, M. L. (1975). Genital herpes simplex in the female, 1968 to 1973. *N.Z. Med. J.* 82:333.
85. Srinannaboon, S. (1979). Cytologic study of herpes simplex virus infection and dysplasia in the female genital tract. *J. Med. Assoc. Thai.* 62:201.
86. Britto, E., et al. (1976). Herpes simplex virus infection of the female genital tract. *Univ. Mich. Med. Bull.* 42:152.
87. Centers for Disease Control. (1981). *STD Fact Sheet*, 35th Ed. Atlanta, U.S. Department of Health and Human Services, Public Health Service, pp. 5-12.
88. Sumaya, C. V., et al. (1980). Genital infections with herpes simplex virus in university student populations. *Sex. Transm. Dis.* 7:16.
89. Kawana, T., et al. (1976). Clinical and virological studies on genital herpes. *Lancet* 2:964.
90. Smith, E., et al. (1976). Virologic studies in genital herpes. *Lancet* 2:1089.

91. Kalinyak, J. E., et al. (1977). Incidence and distribution of herpes simplex virus types 1 and 2 from genital lesions in college women. *J. Med. Virol.* 1: 175.

92. Corey, L., et al. (1978). Cellular immune response in genital herpes simplex virus infection. *N. Engl. J. Med.* 299:986.

93. Rattray, M. C., et al. (1978). Recurrent genital herpes among women: Symptomatic versus asymptomatic viral shedding. *Br. J. Vener. Dis.* 54:262.

94. Douglas, R. J. Jr., and Couch, R. B. (1970). A prospective study of chronic herpes simplex virus infection and recurrrent herpes labialis in humans. *J. Immunol.* 104:289.

95. Embil, J. A., et al. (1981). Concurrent oral and genital infection with an identical strain of herpes simplex virus type 1. *Sex. Transm. Dis.* 8:70.

96. Mertz, G. J., et al. (1981). Sexual transmission of initial genital herpes (HSV): Implications for prevention. Abstract 622, Twenty-first Interscience Conference on Antimicrobial Agents and Chemotherapy, Chicago, Ill.

97. Corey, L., Adams, H. G., Brown, Z. A., et al. (1983). Genital herpes simplex virus infections: Clinical manifestations, course, and complications. *Ann. Intern. Med.* 98:958.

98. Corey, L. (1982). The diagnosis and treatment of genital herpes. *JAMA* 248:1041.

99. Bolognese, R. J., et al. (1976). Herpesvirus hominis type II infections in asymptomatic pregnant women. *Obstet. Gynecol.* 48:507.

100. Coleman, R. M., Pereira, L., Bailey, P. D., et al. (1983). Determination of herpes simplex virus type-specific antibodies by enzyme-linked immunosorbent assay. *J. Clin. Microbiol.* 18:287-291.

101. Sullender, W. M., Yasukawa, L. L., Schwartz, M., et al. (1988). Type-specific antibodies to herpes simplex virus type 2 (HSV-2) glycoprotein G in pregnant women, infants exposed to maternal HSV-2 infection at delivery, and infants with neonatal herpes. *J. Infect. Dis.* 157:164-171.

102. Prober, C. G., Hensleigh, P. A., Boucher, F. D., et al. (1988). Use of routine viral cultures at delivery to identify neonates exposed to herpes simplex virus. *N. Engl. J. Med.* 318:887-891.

103. Nahmias, A. J., Whitley, R. J., Visintine, A. N., et al. (1982). Herpes simplex virus encephalitis: Laboratory evaluations and their diagnostic significance. *J. Infect. Dis.* 145:829-836.

104. Reeves, W. C., et al. (1981). Risk of recurrence after first episodes of genital herpes: Relation to HSV type and antibody response. *N. Engl. J. Med.* 305:315.

105. Corey, L., et al. (1983). Clinical course of genital herpes simplex infection in men and women. *Ann. Intern. Med.* 98:973.

106. Knox, S. R., et al. (1982). Demography of patients with genital herpes simplex virus infections. *Sex. Transm. Dis.* 9:15.

107. Whitley, R. J. (in press). Herpes simplex virus. In Fields, B. N., Knipe, D. M., Chanock, R., Hirsch, M., Melnick, J., Monath, T., and Roizman, B. (eds.): *Virology*, 2nd ed. New York, Raven Press.

108. Adams, H. G., et al. (1976). Genital herpetic infection in men and women: Clinical course and effect of topical application of adenine arabinoside. *J. Infect. Dis.* 133:A151.
109. Barton, I. G., et al. (1981). Association of HSV-1 with cervical infection. *Lancet* 2:1108.
110. Arvin, A. M., Hensleigh, P. A., Prober, C. G., et al. (1986). Failure of antepartum maternal cultures to predict the infant's risk of exposure to herpes simplex virus at delivery. *N. Engl. J. Med.* 315:796-800.
111. Adam, E., Kaufman, R. H., Mirkovic, R. H., et al. (1979). Persistence of virus shedding in asymptomatic women after recovery from herpes genitalis. *Obstet. Gynecol.* 54:171-173.
112. Nahmias, A. J., Josey, W. E., Naib, Z. M., et al. (1971). Perinatal risk associated with maternal genital herpes simplex virus infection. *Am. J. Obstet. Gynecol.* 110:825-837.
113. Ng, A. B. P., Reagan, J. W., and Yen, S. S. C. (1970). Herpes genitalis. *Obstet. Gynecol.* 36:645-651.
114. Naib, Z. M., et al. (1970). Association of maternal genital herpetic infection with spontaneous abortion. *Obstet. Gynecol.* 35:260.
115. Nahmias, A. J., et al. (1972). Significance of herpes simplex virus infection during pregnancy. *Clin. Obstet. Gynecol.* 15:929.
116. Vontver, L. A., Hickok, D. E., Brown, Z., et al. (1982). Recurrent genital herpes simplex virus infection in pregnancy: Infant outcome and frequency of asymptomatic recurrences. *Am. J. Obstet. Gynecol.* 143:75-84.
117. Harger, J. H., Pazin, G. J., Armstrong, J. A., et al. (1983). Characteristics and management of pregnancy in women with genital herpes simplex virus infection. *Am. J. Obstet. Gynecol.* 145:784-791.
118. Wittek, A. E., Yeager, A. S., Au, D. S., et al. (1984). Asymptomatic shedding of herpes simplex virus from the cervix and lesion site during pregnancy: Correlation of antepartum shedding with shedding at delivery. *Am. J. Dis. Child.* 138:439-442.
119. Knox, G. E., Pass, R. F., Reynolds, D. W., et al. (1979). Comparative prevalence of subclinical cytomegalovirus and herpes simplex virus infections in the genital and urinary tracts of low-income, urban women. *J. Infect. Dis.* 140:419-422.
120. Jacob, A. J., Epstein, J., Madden, D. L., et al. (1984). Genital herpes infection in pregnant women near term. *Obstet. Gynecol.* 63:480-484.
121. Brown, Z. A., Vontver, L. A., Benedetti, J., et al. (1985). Genital herpes in pregnancy: Risk factors associated with recurrences and asymptomatic viral shedding. *Am. J. Obstet. Gynecol.* 153:24-30.
122. Whitley, R. J., Corey, L., Arvin, A., et al. (1988). Changing presentation of herpes simplex virus infection in neonates. *J. Infect. Dis.* 158:109-116.
123. Whitley, R. J., Yeager, A., Kartus, P., et al. (1983). Neonatal herpes simplex virus infection: Follow-up evaluation of vidarabine therapy. *Pediatrics* 72:778.

124. Yeager, A. S., and Arvin, A. M. (1984). Reasons for the absence of a history of recurrent genital infections in mothers of neonates infected with herpes simplex virus. *Pediatrics* 73:188-193.
125. Tejani, N., Klein, S. W., and Kaplan, M. (1979). Subclinical herpes simplex genitalis infections in the preinatal period. *Am. J. Obstet. Gynecol.* 135:547.
126. Altshuler, G. (1974). Pathogenesis of congenital herpesvirus infection. *Am. J. Dis. Child.* 127:427.
127. Altshuler, G. (1977). Placentitis with a new light on an old TORCH. *Obstet. Gynecol. Annu.* 6:197.
128. Hain, J., et al. (1980). Ascending transcervical herpes simplex infection with intact fetal membranes. *Obstet. Gynecol.* 56:106.
129. Hanshaw, J. B., Dudgeon, J. A., and Marshall, W. C. (1985). *Viral Diseases of the Fetus and Newborn.* Philadelphia, W. B. Saunders, pp. 1-308.
130. Florman, A. L., Gershon, A. A., Blackett, P. R., et al. (1973). Intrauterine infection with herpes simplex virus: Resultant congenital malformations. *JAMA* 225:129-132.
131. Grossman, J. H. III, Wallen, W. C., and Sever, J. L. (1981). Management of genital herpes simplex virus infection during pregnancy. *Obstet. Gynecol.* 58:1-4.
132. Whitley, R. J., Nahmias, A. J., Visintine, A. M., et al. (1980). The natural history of herpes simplex virus infection of mother and newborn. *Pediatrics* 66:489-494.
133. Nahmias, A. J., Keyserling, H. L., and Kerrick, G. M. (1983). Herpes simplex. In Remington, J. S., and Klein, J. O. (eds.): *Infectious Diseases of the Fetus and Newborn Infant,* 2d Ed. Philadelphia, W. B. Saunders, pp. 636-678.
134. Nahmias, A. J. (1974). The TORCH complex. *Hosp. Pract.* 9:65.
135. Sullivan-Bolyai, J. Z., Hull, H. F., Wilson, C., et al. (1983). Neonatal herpes simplex virus infection in King County, Washington: Increasing incidence and epidemiologic correlates. *JAMA* 250:3059-3062.
136. Overall, J. C. Jr. (1987). Viral infections of the fetus and the neonate. In Feigin, R. D., and Cherry, J. D. (eds.): *Textbook of Pediatric Infectious Diseases,* 2d Ed. Philadelphia, W. B. Saunders, pp. 966-1007.
137. Baley, J. E. (1987). Viral infections. In Fanaroff, A. A., and Martin, R. J. (eds.): *Neonatal-Perinatal Medicine,* 4th Ed. St. Louis, C. V. Mosby, pp. 799-817.
138. Adam, E., Sharma, S. D., Zeigler, O., et al. (1972). Seroepidemiologic studies of herpesvirus type 2 and carcinoma of the cervix. II. Uganda. *J.N.C.I.* 48:65.
139. Templeton, A. C. (1970). Generalized herpes simplex in malnourished children. *J. Clin. Pathol.* 23:24.
140. Brunham, R. C., Holmes, K. K., and Eschenbach, D. (1984). Sexually transmitted diseases in pregnancy. In Holmes, K. K., Mardh, P.-A., Sparling,

P. F., et al. (eds.): *Sexually Transmitted Diseases*. New York, McGraw-Hill, pp. 782-816.

141. South, M. A., and Rawls, W. E. (1970). Treatment of neonatal herpesvirus infection. *J. Pediatr.* 76:497-498.

142. Scher, J., Bottone, E., Desmond, E., et al. (1982). The incidence and outcome of asymptomatic herpes simplex genitalis in an obstetric population. *Am. J. Obstet. Gynecol.* 144:906-909.

143. Monif, G. R. G., and Hardt, N. S. (1983). Management of herpetic vulvovaginitis in pregnancy. *Semin. Perinatol.* 7:16-21.

144. Grossman, J. H. III. (1982). Herpes simplex virus (HSV) infections. *Clin. Obstet. Gynecol.* 25:555-561.

145. Boehm, F. H., Estes, W., Wright, P. F., et al. (1981). Management of genital herpes simplex virus infection occurring during pregnancy. *Am. J. Obstet. Gynecol.* 141:735-740.

146. Walpole, I. R., and Grauaug, A. (1979). Intra-uterine infection with herpes simplex virus and observed radiological changes. *Aust. Paediatr. J.* 15:123.

147. Chalhub, E. G., Baenziger, J., Feigin, R. D., et al. (1977). Congenital herpes simplex type II infection with extensive hepatic calcification, bone lesions and cataracts: Complete postmortem examination. *Dev. Med. Child Neurol.* 19:527-533.

148. Hutto, C., Arvin, A., Jacobs, R., et al. (1987). Intrauterine herpes simplex virus infections. *J. Pediatr.* 110:97-101.

149. South, M. A., Tompkins, W. A. F., Morris, R., et al. (1969). Congenital malformation of the central nervous system associated with genital type (type 2) herpesvirus. *J. Pediatr.* 75:13-18.

150. Sieber, O. F. Jr., Fulginitti, V. A., Brazie, J., et al. (1966). In utero infection of the fetus by herpes simplex virus. *J. Pediatr.* 69:30-34.

151. Strawn, E. Y., and Scrimenti, R. J. (1973). Intrauterine herpes simplex infection. *Am. J. Obstet. Gynecol.* 115:581-582.

152. Honig, P. J., and Brown, D. (1982). Congenital herpes simplex virus infection initially resembling epidermolysis bullosa. *J. Pediatr.* 101:958-959.

153. Monif, G. R. G., Kellner, K. R., and Donnelly, W. H. Jr. (1985). Congenital herpes simplex type II infection. *Am. J. Obstet. Gynecol.* 152:1000-1002.

154. Gagnon, R. A. (1968). Transplacental inoculation of fetal herpes simplex in the newborn. *Obstet. Gynecol.* 31:682-684.

155. Offit, P. A., Starr, S. E., Zolnick, P., et al. (1982). Acyclovir therapy in neonatal herpes simplex virus infection. *Pediatr. Infect. Dis.* 1:253-255.

156. Dublin, A. B., and Merten, D. F. (1977). Computed tomography in the evaluation of herpes simplex encephalitis. *Radiology* 125:133-134.

157. Nahmias, A. J., Visintine, A. M., Caldwell, D. R., et al. (1976). Eye infections with herpes simplex virus in neonates. *Surv. Ophthalmol.* 21:100-105.

158. Reynolds, J. D., Griebel, M., Mallory, S., et al. (1986). Congenital herpes simplex retinitis. *Am. J. Ophthalmol.* 102:33-36.

159. Karesh, J. W., Kapur, S., and McDonald, M. (1983). Herpes simplex virus and congenital malformations. *South. Med. J.* 76:1561-1563.
160. Komorous, J. M., Wheeler, C. E., Briggaman, R. A., et al. (1977). Intrauterine herpes simplex infections. *Arch. Dermatol.* 113:918-922.
161. Montgomery, J. R., Flanders, R. W., and Yow, M. D. (1973). Congenital anomalies and herpesvirus infection. *Am. J. Dis. Child.* 126:364-366.
162. Arvin, A. M., Yeager, A. S., Bruhn, F. W., et al. (1982). Neonatal herpes simplex infection in the absence of mucocutaneous lesions. *J. Pediatr.* 100: 715-721.
163. Mitchell, J. E., and McCall, F. C. (1963). Transplacental infection by herpes simplex virus. *Am. J. Dis. Child.* 106:207-209.
164. Witzelben, C. L., and Driscoll, S. G. (1965). Possible transplacental transmission of herpes simplex infection. *Pediatrics* 36:192-199.
165. Hovig, D. E., Hodgman, J. E., Mathies, A. W. Jr., et al. (1968). Herpesvirus hominis (simplex) infection. *Am. J. Dis. Child.* 115:438-444.
166. Hagler, W. S., Walters, P. V., and Nahmias, A. J. (1969). Ocular involvement in neonatal herpes simplex virus infection. *Arch. Ophthalmol.* 82: 169-176.
167. Tomer, A., and Harel, A. (1983). Congenital absence of scalp skin and herpes simplex virus. A case report. *Isr. J. Med. Sci.* 19:950-951.
168. Merritt, T. A., and Anderson, V. M. (1983). Icterus, encephalopathy, and galloping neonatal pneumonia. *Am. J. Dis. Child.* 137:1001-1007.
169. Amortegui, A. J., MacPherson, T. A., and Harger, J. H. (1984). A cluster of neonatal herpes simplex infections without mucocutaneous manifestations. *Pediatrics* 73:194-198.
170. Schaffer, A. J. (1965). *Diseases of the Newborn*, 2d Ed. Philadelphia, W. B. Saunders, p. 733.
171. Pettay, O. (1979). Intrauterine and perinatal viral infections. A review of experiences and remaining problems. *Ann. Clin. Res.* 11:258-266.
172. Schaffer, D. B. (1981). Eye findings in intrauterine infections. *Clin. Perinatol.* 8:415-443.
173. Sullender, W. M., Miller, J. L., Yasukawa, L. L., et al. (1987). Humoral and cell-mediated immunity in neonates with herpes simplex virus infection. *J. Infect. Dis.* 155:28-37.
174. Hayward, A. R., Herberger, M. J., Groothuis, J., et al. (1984). Specific immunity after congenital or neonatal infection with cytomegalovirus or herpes simplex virus. *J. Immunol.* 133:2469-2473.
175. Goldsmith, M. F. (1984). Possible herpesvirus role in abortion studied. *JAMA* 251:3067-3070.
176. Abrahams, C. A. (1966). Isolation of herpes simplex from a mother and aborted fetus. *Ghana Med. J.* 5:41.
177. Garcia, A. (1970). Maternal herpes simplex infection causing abortion: Histopathological study of the placenta. *Hospital* 78:1266.

178. Lapinleimu, K., Cantell, K., Koskimies, O., et al. (1974). Association between maternal herpesvirus infections and congenital malformations. *Lancet* 1:1127-1129.

179. Shackelford, G. D., and Kirks, D. R. (1977). Neonatal hepatic calcification secondary to transplacental infection. *Radiology* 122:753-757.

180. Merchese, C. A. (1984). Biopsy of chorionic villi for prenatal diagnosis. (Letter.) *Acta Obstet. Gynecol. Scand.* 63:737.

181. Parvey, L. S., and Ch'ien, L. T. (1980). Neonatal herpes simplex virus infection introduced by fetal monitor scalp electrode. *Pediatrics* 65:1150.

182. Blackett, P. R., et al. (1973). Intrauterine infection with herpes simplex virus: Resultant congenital malformations. *J.A.M.A.* 225:129.

183. Corey, L., and Spear, P. G. (1986). Infections with herpes simplex viruses. *N. Engl. J. Med.* 314:686-691.

184. Whitley, R. J., and Hutto, C. (1985). Neonatal herpes simplex virus infections. *Pediatr. Rev.* 7:119-126.

185. Jenista, J. A. (1983). Perinatal herpesvirus infections. *Semin. Perinatol.* 7: 9-15.

186. Echeverra, P., Miller, G., Campbell, A. G. M., et al. (1973). Scalp vesicles within the first week of life: A clue to early diagnosis of herpes neonatorum. *J. Pediatr.* 83:1062-1064.

187. Kaye, E. M., and Dooling, E. C. (1981). Neonatal herpes simplex meningoencephalitis associated with fetal monitor scalp electrodes. *Neurology* 31: 1046-1047.

188. Prober, C. G., Sullender, W. M., Yasukawa, L. L., et al. (1987). Low risk of herpes simplex virus infections in neonates exposed to the virus at the time of delivery to mothers with recurrent genital herpes simplex virus infections. *N. Engl. J. Med.* 316:240-244.

189. Brown, Z. A., Vontver, L. A., Benedetti, J., et al. (1987). Effects on infants of a first episode of genital herpes during pregnancy. *N. Engl. J. Med.* 317:1246-1251.

190. Overall, J. C. Jr., Whitley, R. J., Yeager, A. S., et al. (1984). Prophylactic or anticipatory antiviral therapy for newborns exposed to herpes simplex infection. *Pediatr. Infect. Dis.* 3:193-195.

191. Stone, K. M., Brooks, C. A., Guinan, M. E., et al. (1985). Neonatal herpes—results of one year's surveillance. Abstract 515, Interscience Conference on Antimicrobial Agents and Chemotherapy, Minneapolis, Minn.

192. Light, I. J., and Linnemann, C. C. Jr. (1974). Neonatal herpes simplex infection following delivery by cesarean section. *Obstet. Gynecol.* 44:496-499.

193. Light, I. J. (1979). Postnatal acquisition of herpes simplex virus by the newborn infant: A review of the literature. *Pediatrics* 63:480-482.

194. Linnemann, C. C., Light, I. J., Buchman, T. G., et al. (1978). Transmission of herpes simplex virus type 1 in a nursery for the newborn: Identification of viral isoaltes by DNA "fingerprinting." *Lancet* 1:964-966.

195. Hammerberg, O., Watts, J., Chernesky, M., et al. (1983). An outbreak of herpes simplex virus type 1 in an intensive care nursery. *Pediatr. Infect. Dis.* 2:290-294.
196. Sullivan-Bollyai, J. Z., Fife, K. H., Jacobs, R. F., et al. (1983). Disseminated neonatal herpes simplex virus type 1 from a maternal breast lesion. *Pediatrics* 71:455-457.
197. Dunkle, L. M., Schmidt, R. R., and O'Connor, D. M. (1979). Neonatal herpes simplex infection possibly acquired via maternal breast milk. *Pediatrics* 63:250-251.
198. Kibrick, S. (1979). Herpes simplex virus in breast milk. *Pediatrics* 64:390.
199. Yeager, A. S., Ashley, R. L., and Corey, L. (1983). Transmission of herpes simplex virus from father to neonate. *J. Pediatr.* 103:905.
200. Douglas, J. M., Schmidt, O., and Corey, L. (1983). Acquisition of neonatal HSV-1 infection from a paternal source contact. *J. Pediatr.* 103:908-910.
201. Rawls, W. E., and Campione-Piccardo, J. (1981). Epidemiology of herpes simplex virus type 1 and type 2 infections. In Nahmias, A. J., Dowdle, W., and Schinazi, R. (eds.): *The Human Herpesviruses: An Interdisciplinary Perspective.* New York, Elsevier North Holland, p. 137.
202. Nahmias, A. J., and Josey, W. E. (1982). Epidemiology of herpes simplex viruses 1 and 2. In Evans, A. (ed.): *Viral Infections of Humans*, 2d Ed. New York, Plenum Press, p. 351.
203. Van Dyke, R. B., and Spector, S. A. (1984). Transmission of herpes simplex virus type 1 to a newborn infant during endotracheal suctioning for meconium aspiration. *Pediatr. Infect. Dis.* 3:153-156.
204. Hatherly, L. I., Hayes, K., and Jack, I. (1980). Herpesvirus in an obstetric hospital. II. Asymptomatic virus excretion in staff members. *Med. J. Aust.* 2:273-275.
205. Schreiner, R., Kleinman, M., and Gresham, E. (1979). Maternal oral herpes: Isolation policy. *Pediatrics* 63:247.
206. Hatherly, L. I., Hayes, K., and Jack, I. (1980). Herpesvirus in an obstetric hospital. I. Herpetic eruptions. *Med. J. Aust.* 2:205-208.
207. Hatherly, L. I., Hayes, K., and Jack, I. (1980). Herpesvirus in an obstetric hospital. III. Prevalence of antibodies in patients and staff. *Med. J. Aust.* 2:325-328.
208. Francis, D. P., Herrman, K. L., MacMahon, J. R., et al. (1975). Nosocomial and maternally acquired herpesvirus hominis infections. A report of four fatal cases in neonates. *Am. J. Dis. Child.* 129:889-893.
209. Roizman, B., and Buchman, T. (1979). The molecular epidemiology of herpes simplex viruses. *Hosp. Pract.* 14:95-104.
210. Buchman, T. G., Roizman, B., Adams, G., et al. (1978). Restriction endonuclease fingerprinting of herpes simplex virus DNA: A novel epidemiological tool applied to a nosocomial outbreak. *J. Infect. Dis.* 138:488-498.

211. Hammer, S. M., Buchman, T. G., D'Angelo, L. J., et al. (1980). Temporal cluster of herpes simplex encephalitis: Investigation by restriction endonuclease cleavage of viral DNA. *J. Infect. Dis.* 141:436-440.

212. Halperin, S. A., Shehab, Z., Thacker, D., et al. (1983). Absence of viremia in primary herpetic gingivostomatitis. *Pediatr. Infect. Dis.* 2:452-453.

213. Craig, C. P., and Nahmias, A. J. (1973). Different patterns of neurologic involvement with herpes simplex virus types 1 and 2: Isolation of herpes simplex virus type 2 from the buffy coat of two adults with meningitis. *J. Infect. Dis.* 127:365-372.

214. Kern, E. R., Overall, J. C. Jr., and Glasgow, L. A. (1973). Herpesvirus hominis infection in newborn mice. I. An experimental model and therapy with iododeoxyuridine. *J. Infect. Dis.* 128:290-299.

215. Whitley, R. J., Nahmias, A. J., Soong, S.-J., et al. (1980). Vidarabine therapy of neonatal herpes simplex virus infection. *Pediatrics* 66:495-501.

216. Sullivan-Bollyai, J. Z., Hull, H. F., Wilson, C., et al. (1986). Presentation of neonatal herpes simplex virus infections: Implications for a change in therapeutic strategy. *Pediatr. Infect. Dis.* 5:309-314.

217. Music, S. T., Fine, E. M., and Togo, Y. (1971). Zoster-like disease in the newborn due to herpes simplex virus. *N. Engl. J. Med.* 284:24-26.

218. Haynes, R. E., Azimi, P. H., and Cramblett, H. G. (1968). Fatal herpesvirus hominis (herpes simplex virus) infections in children. Clinical, pathologic, and virologic characteristics. *J.A.M.A.* 206:312-319.

219. Nahmias, A. J., and Hagler, W. (1972). Ocular manifestations of herpes simplex in the newborn. *Int. Ophthalmol. Clin.* 12:191.

220. Reersted, P., and Hansen, B. (1979). Chorioretinitis of the newborn with herpes simplex type 1: Report of a case. *Acta Ophthalmol.* 57:1096.

221. Cibis, A., and Burde, R. M. (1971). Herpes simplex virus induced congenital cataracts. *Arch. Ophthalmol.* 85:220.

222. Mizrahi, E. M., and Tharp, B. R. (1981). A unique electroencephalogram pattern in neonatal herpes simplex virus encephalitis. *Neurology* 31:164.

223. Gutman, L. T., Wilfert, C. M., and Eppes, S. (1986). Herpes simplex virus encephalitis in children: Analysis of cerebrospinal fluid and progressive neurodevelopmental deterioration. *J. Infect. Dis.* 154:415.

224. Hanshaw, J. B. (1973). Herpesvirus hominis infections in the fetus and the newborn. *Am. J. Dis. Child.* 126:546-555.

225. Catalano, L. W. Jr., Safley, G. H., Museles, M., et al. (1971). Disseminated herpesvirus infection in a newborn infant. *J. Pediatr.* 79:393-400.

226. Miller, D. R., Hanshaw, J. B., O'Leary, D. S., et al. (1970). Fatal disseminated herpes simplex virus infection and hemorrhage in the neonate. *J. Pediatr.* 76:409-415.

227. Torphy, D. E., Ray, C. G., McAlister, R., et al. (1970). Herpes simplex virus infection in infants: A spectrum of disease. *J. Pediatr.* 76:405-408.

228. Sanders, D. Y., and Cramblett, H. G. (1968). Viral infections in hospitalized neonates. *Am. J. Dis. Child.* 116:251.

229. Cherry, J. D., Soriano, F., and Jahn, C. L. (1968). Search for perinatal viral infection: A prospective, clinical virology and serologic study. *Am. J. Dis. Child.* 116:245.
230. Whitley, R. J. (1989). Personal communication.
231. Whitley, R. J., Arvin, A. M., Corey, L., et al. (1986). Vidarabine versus acyclovir therapy of neonatal herpes simplex virus, HSV, infection. *Pediatr. Res.* 20:323.
232. Elion, G. B., Furman, P. A., Fyfe, J. A., et al. (1977). Selectivity of action of an antiherpetic agent 9-(2-hydroxyethoxymethyl) guanine. *Proc. Natl. Acad. Sci. USA* 74:5716.
233. Corey, L., Benedetti, J., Critchlow, C., et al. (1983). Treatment of primary first-episode genital herpes simplex virus infections with acyclovir: Results of topical, intravenous and oral therapy. *J. Antimicrob. Chemother.* 12 (Suppl. B):79-88.
234. Bryson, Y. J., Dillon, M., Lovett, M., et al. (1983). Treatment of first episodes of genital herpes infection with oral acyclovir. A randomized double blind controlled trial in normal subjects. *N. Engl. J. Med.* 308:916-921.
235. Corey, L., Nahmias, A. J., and Guinan, M. E. (1982). A trial of topical acyclovir in genital herpes simplex virus infections. *N. Engl. J. Med.* 306: 1313-1319.
236. Saral, R., Burns, W. H., Laskin, O. L., et al. (1981). Acyclovir prophylaxis of herpes simplex virus infections: A randomized double blind controlled trial in bone marrow transplant recipients. *N. Engl. J. Med.* 305:63-67.
237. Meyers, J. D., Wade, J. C., Mitchell, C. D., et al. Multicenter collaborative trial of intravenous acyclovir for treatment of mucocutaneous herpes simplex virus infection in the immunocompromised host.
238. Whitley, R. J., Alford, C. A., Hirsch, M. S., et al. (1986). Vidarabine versus acyclovir therapy in herpes simplex encephalitis. *N. Engl. J. Med.* 314:144-149.
239. Yeager, A. S. (1982). Use of acyclovir in premature and term neonates. *Am. J. Med.* 73(Suppl. 1A):205-209.
240. Hintz, M., Connor, J. D., Spector, S. A., et al. (1982). Neonatal acyclovir pharmacokinetics in patients with herpesvirus infections. *Am. J. Med.* 73:210.
241. Gerson, M., Portnoy, J., and Hamelin, C. (1984). Reliable identification of herpes simplex viruses by DNA restriction endonuclease analysis with EcoR-1. *Sex. Transm. Dis.* 11:85-90.
242. Goldstein, L. C., Corey, L., McDougall, J. K., et al. (1983). Monoclonal antibodies to herpes simplex viruses: Use in antigenic typing and rapid diagnosis. *J. Infect. Dis.* 147:829-837.
243. Brown, Z. A., Kern, E. R., Spruance, S. L., et al. (1979). Clinical and virologic course of herpes simplex genitalis. *West. J. Med.* 130:414-421.
244. Rooney, J. F., Felsner, J. M., Ostrove, J. M., et al. (1986). Acquisition of genital herpes from an asymptomatic sexual partner. *N. Engl. J. Med.* 314: 1561-1564.

245. Binkin, N. J., Koplan, J. P., and Cates, W. Jr. (1984). Preventing neonatal herpes: The value of weekly viral cultures in pregnant women with recurrent genital herpes. *J.A.M.A.* 251:2816-2821.
246. Whitley, R. J., Lakeman, A. D., Nahmias, A. J., et al. (1982). DNA restriction enzyme analysis of herpes simplex virus isolates obtained from patients with encephalitis. *N. Engl. J. Med.* 307:1060-1062.
247. Whitley, R. J., and Baldwin, S. T. (1989). Unpublished observation.
248. Nahmias, A. J., Visintine, A., Caldwell, A., et al. (1976). Eye infections. *Surv. Ophthalmol.* 21(2):100.
249. Yeager, A. S. (1979). Storage and transport of cultures for herpes simplex virus type 2. *Am. J. Clin. Pathol.* 72:977-979.
250. Arvin, A. M., and Nahmias, A. J. (1987). Herpes simplex virus infections. In Rudolf, A. (ed.): *Textbook of Pediatrics*, 17th Ed. New York, Appleton Century Crofts, pp. 561-566.
251. Naib, Z. M., Nahmias, A. J., and Josey, W. E. (1966). Cytology and histopathology of cervical herpes simplex infection. *Cancer* 19:1026.
252. Solomon, A. R., Rasmussen, J. E., Varani, J., et al. (1984). The Tzanck smear in the diagnosis of cutaneous herpes simplex. *J.A.M.A.* 251:633-635.
253. Skoldenberg, B., Alestig, K., Burman, L., et al. (1984). Acyclovir versus vidarabine in herpes encephalitis. Randomized, multicentre study in consecutive Swedish patients. *Lancet* 2:707-711.
254. Amstey, M. S., Monif, G. R. G., Nahmias, A. J., et al. (1979). Cesarean section and genital herpes virus infection. *Obstet. Gynecol.* 53:641-642.

11
Acyclovir in Pediatrics

Ann M. Arvin *Stanford University School of Medicine, Stanford, California*

BACKGROUND

Because of their susceptibility to life-threatening herpes viral infections, immunocompromised children with herpes simplex virus (HSV) and varicella zoster virus (VZV) infections were among the first patients who were given nucleoside analogs (e.g., 5-iododeoxyuridine and cytosine arabinoside) as antiviral therapy. Over the past decade, pediatric patients have benefited significantly from the identification of other nucleoside analogs, like acyclovir, which have selective antiviral activity without the toxicity for host cells that was caused by the early antiviral drugs (1).

PREPARATIONS OF ACYCLOVIR USED IN PEDIATRIC PATIENTS

Most of the clinical experience with acyclovir in children is with the intravenous formulation (500 mg per vial). Acyclovir capsules (200 mg) can be given to older children, and an oral suspension (40 mg/ml) is now being evaluated for administration to infants and young children. The oral suspension formulation is needed for pediatric use, because mixing the contents of an acyclovir capsule with fluids or food does not allow the administration of an accurate unit dose, the drug cannot be expected to stay in uniform suspension, and the bioavailability of the capsule drug in noncapsule form is not known. While topical acyclovir can be prescribed for the indications established in older patients—e.g., recurrent HSV lesions in immunocompromised patients—its clinical efficacy has not been specifically determined in pediatric patients.

PHARMACOLOGY OF ACYCLOVIR IN PEDIATRIC PATIENTS

Children given intravenous acyclovir at a dose of 250 mg/m^2 have a mean maximum plasma concentration (C_{max}) of 10.3 ± 4.0 SD μg/ml, which is comparable to the mean C_{max} at steady state of 9.8 ± 2.6 SD μg/ml in adults given 5 mg/kg per dose; similarly, the mean C_{max} was 20.7 ± 5.0 μg/ml with a 500 mg/m^2 dose regimen in children and 20.7 ± 10.2 μg/ml with a 10 mg/kg dose in adults (2-5). The mean half-life of elimination ($T_{1/2}$) for children was 2.52 ± 1.04 SD h and 2.91 ± 0.85 SD h in adults. In contrast, neonates receiving a 10 mg/kg dose had a lower peak acyclovir concentration, mean 13.9 ± 4.2 SD μg/ml, and a longer $T_{1/2}$, mean 3.78 ± 1.21 SD h. Since more than 80% of the drug is eliminated by renal clearance, at steady state, the peak acyclovir concentration was higher in infants than in children above 1 year on the same dosage regimen. Thus, in general, the intravenous administration of acyclovir to infants and children at doses of 10 mg/kg or 250-500 mg/m^2 can be expected to produce peak plasma concentrations of approximately 10-25 μg/ml. In infants and children, as in older patients, the intravenous drug must be given as a 1-h infusion to avoid acyclovir concentrations that are potentially nephrotoxic, and the dosage must be adjusted for impaired clearance if the creatinine clearance is < 50 ml/min/1.73 m^2 (7).

The pharmacology of oral acyclovir has been evaluated less extensively in children (8). The peak plasma concentrations were 0.11-3.42 μg/ml in 10 immunocompromised children with VZV infections who were given oral acyclovir (200-mg tablets) in doses ranging from 250 to 850 mg/m^2 five times daily (9). The mean peak plasma concentration was 1.8 μg/ml in another gorup of 14 immunocompromised children who were given 600 mg/m^2 per dose (10). The pharmacokinetics of the oral suspension of acyclovir was investigated in 18 children, ages 3 weeks to 6.9 years, who had HSV or VZV infections that were not life threatening. Among children who were at least 6 months old, a dose of 600 mg/m^2 produced a C_{max} of 0.99 ± 0.38 SD μg/ml and the $T_{1/2}$ was 2.59 ± 0.78 SD h. Three infants less than 2 months of age who received 300 mg/m^2 per dose had a C_{max} of 1.88 ± 1.11 SD μg/ml and $T_{1/2}$ of 3.26 ± 0.33 SD h. These three infants had higher mean plasma concentrations at 2-8 h after the last dose than two children given the same dose who were 1-2 years old, reflecting creatinine clearances of 50 ml/min/1.73 m^2 in the infants. With the exception of the youngest infants, children treated with the oral suspension of acyclovir had lower peak plasma concentrations than those measured in adults given capsules in approximately equivalent doses; less of the dose was absorbed, and absorption occurred over a longer time interval (11).

THERAPEUTIC INDICATIONS FOR ACYCLOVIR THERAPY IN PEDIATRIC PATIENTS

Infections Caused by Herpes Simplex Type 1 and Type 2

The indications for intravneous acyclovir therapy include HSV-1 encephalitis in older children, life-threatening HSV-1 or HSV-2 infections in immunocompromised patients, and neonatal HSV-1 or HSV-2 infections. Acyclovir was superior to vidarabine for the treatment of HSV-1 encephalitis in older children and adults and should be considered the drug of choice for pediatric patients with this diagnosis (12). The dosage regimen for acyclovir therapy of HSV-1 encephalitis is 30 mg/kg/day given as 10 mg/kg every 8 h for at least 10 days. Although disseminated infection arising from mucocutaneous HSV is unusual, an immunocompromised child may occasionally develop severe primary HSV-1 infection or recurrent HSV-1 causing herpes esophagitis. The dosage regimen for these patients is 250 mg/m^2 given every 8 h. These patients should be treated for 5-7 days, depending on the clinical response. Children with severe eczema herpeticum (Kaposi's varicelliform eruption) also require treatment with this regimen of intravenous acyclovir because of the potential for dissemination. The optimal approach to antiviral therapy of neonatal HSV infections has not yet been established. Although acyclovir (30 mg/kg/day) and vidarbine (30 mg/kg/day) appear to have comparable efficacy for the treatment of infants with mucocutaneous HSV, disseminated herpes, or HSV encephalitis (13), the morbidity and mortality associated with the latter two forms of neonatal herpes are still significant. To investigate higher-dose regimens, longer treatment schedules, combination therapy, or other strategies, infants with HSV infections should be referred to tertiary care centers that are participating in the Collaborative Antiviral Study Group protocols for neonatal herpes when possible.

There are few indications for oral acyclovir therapy of HSV infections in the pediatric population. Adolescent patients who have genital herpes can be treated with acyclovir capsules based on the clinical experience in adults with primary and recurrent genital herpes. Most otherwise healthy children who develop extensive primary herpes stomatitis are too young to take acyclovir capsules. Depending on the outcome of a controlled trial that is now in progress, one potential indication for the oral suspension of acyclovir will be the early treatment of herpes stomatitis. Pediatric recipients of organ or bone marrow transplants who are HSV seropositive before transplant can be expected to benefit from oral acyclovir prophylaxis to prevent HSV reactivation (14-16). Less severely immunocompromised children who develop recurrent orolabial herpes lesions may have milder episodes of reactivation if given a short course of oral acyclovir at the onset of symptoms.

Infections Caused by Varicella Zoster Virus

Primary VZV infection, which causes varicella, is associated with a high risk of fatal infection among immunocompromised children. Intravenous acyclovir therapy reduces the risk of VZV dissemination, manifesting most often as varicella pneumonia, and therefore improves the survival of these patients (17). While clinical judgment can be excercised about whether to treat varicella in an immunocompromised child, the decision should be made early in the clinical course, preferably within the first 72 h after the appearance of the exanthem, because fatal infections have occurred with later initiation of acyclovir therapy (18). Because VZV is significantly less susceptible to inhibition by acyclovir than HSV (19), the drug must be given as 500 mg/m^2 per dose every 8 h. The reactivation of VZV, resulting in herpes zoster, is much less likely to be life threatening than varicella in immunocompromised children. Herpes zoster does not always require antiviral therapy, but intravenous acyclovir should be given to those who are at high risk for dissemination (e.g., bone marrow transplant recipients and patients in relapse) and should be considered for those with herpes zoster in the distribution of the cranial nerves—e.g., trigeminal involvement (20).

Experience with oral acyclovir therapy for VZV infections in pediatric patients is limited. The diminished susceptibility of VZV to acyclovir in vitro and the relatively low plasma concentrations achieved in children given oral acyclovir suggest that otherwise healthy children with varicella should not receive oral acyclovir until its efficacy has been established in placebo-controlled clinical investigations. Similarly, oral acyclovir therapy cannot be considered to be a substitute for intravenous acyclovir treatment of primary VZV infection in immunocompromised children.

Infections Caused by Cytomegalovirus and Epstein-Barr Virus

Acyclovir has minimal activity against CMV infection and is not indicated for the treatment of pediatric CMV infections. Acyclovir restricts EBV replication in vitro at relatively low concentrations. Nevertheless, its intravenous administration to hospitalized patients with primary EBV infection failed to modify the common symptoms of infectious mononucleosis substantially (21).

ADVERSE EFFECTS

The adverse effects of acyclovir in children are similar to those observed in adults. Some patients complain of nausea, vomiting, and headache, but these side effects rarely interfere with drug treatment. Care must be taken to ensure adequate hydration in infants and children who are receiving the drug to avoid its precipitation in the renal tubules. Many pediatric patients given acyclovir may be immunocompromised children or newborns who are also receiving other drugs that reduce renal clearance (e.g., amphotericin), thereby increasing the plasma and renal concentrations of acyclovir and the risk of nephrotoxicity. Acyclovir crystalluria has been observed in children without evidence of altered renal function (22). Excessive doses of acyclovir have been administered to infants by miscalculating the 10 mg/kg dose as 100 mg/kg. Plasma acyclovir concentrations can be reduced by hemodialysis, but, as expected because of its extensive tissue distribution, drug levels were not affected in a newborn who had exchange transfusions while receiving acyclovir (7). The extravasation of the drug into soft tissues can produce severe cutaneous lesions and is a problem in children because of the difficulty of maintaining intravenous infusions. As in other patient populations, the possible emergence of drug resistance in clinical strains of HSV and VZV requires attention as the drug is used more commonly in pediatrics. The emergence of resistant mutants has been unusual after acyclovir treatment of both HSV and VZV infections, but one reported case occurred in a child with immunodeficiency who received several courses of intravenous acyclovir for HSV infections (23). In general, the susceptibility of pediatric patients to recurrent disease—e.g., recurrent mucocutaneous HSV after neonatal herpes—can be attributed to deficiencies in the host response rather than to drug resistance (24).

REFERENCES

1. Bryson, Y. J. (1984). The use of acyclovir in children. *Pediatr. Infect. Dis.* 3: 345-348.
2. De Miranda, P., and Blum, M. R. (1983). Pharmacokinetics of acyclovir after intravenous and oral administration. *J. Antimicrob. Chemother.* 12:29-37.
3. Hintz, M., Connor, J. D. Specter, S. A., et al. (1982). Neonatal acyclovir pharmacokinetics in patients with herpes virus infections. *Am. J. Med.* 73: 210-214.
4. Blum, M. R., Liao, S. H. T., and De Miranda, P. (1982). Overview of acyclovir pharmacokinetic disposition in adults and children. *Am. J. Med.* 73: 186-192.
5. Hintz, M., Connor, J. D., Spector, S. A., et al. (1982). Neonatal acyclovir pharmacokinetics in patients with herpes virus infections. *Am. J. Med.* 73: 210-214.
6. Leitman, P. (1987). Acyclovir. In Koren, G., Prober, C. G., and Gold, R. (eds.): *Antimicrobial Therapy in Infants and Children.* New York: Marcel Dekker, pp. 577-586.
7. Englund, J. A., Fletcher, C. V., Johnson, D., et al. (1987). Effect of blood exchange on acyclovir clearance in an infant with neonatal herpes. *J. Pediatr.* 110:151-153.
8. Arvin, A. M. (1987). Oral therapy with acyclovir in infants and children. *Pediatr. Infect. Dis. J.* 6:56-58.
9. Novelli, V. M., Marshall, W. C., Yeo, J., et al. (1984). Acyclovir administered perorally in immunocompromised children with varicella-zoster infections. *J. Infect. Dis.* 149:478.
10. Novelli, V. M., Marshal, W. C., Yeo, J., et al. (1985). High-dose oral acyclovir for children at risk of disseminated herpesvirus infections. *J. Infect. Dis.* 151:372.
11. Sullender, W., Arvin, A., Diaz, P., Connor, J., Straube, R., Dankner, W., Levin, M., Weller, S., and Chapman, S. (1987). The pharmacokinetics of acyclovir suspension in children. *Antimicrob. Agents Chemother.* 31:1722-1726.
12. Whitley, R. J., Alford, C. A., Hirsch, M. S., et al. (1986). Vidarabine versus acyclovir therapy in herpes simplex encephalitis. *N. Engl. J. Med.* 314:144-149.
13. Whitley, R. J., Arvin, A. M., Corey, L., Powell, D., et al. (1986). Vidarabine versus acyclovir therapy of neonatal herpes simplex virus infection. Abstract, Society for Pediatric Research, May 1986.
14. Wade, J. C., Newton, B., Flournoy, N., et al. (1984). Oral acyclovir for prevention of herpes simplex virus reactivation after marrow transplant. *Ann. Intern. Med.* 100:823-828.
15. Straus, S. E., Seidlin, M., Takiff, H., et al. (1984). Acyclovir to suppress recurring herpes simplex virus infections in immunodeficient patients. *Ann. Intern. Med.* 100:522-524.

16. Pettersson, E., Hovi, T., Ahonen, J., et al. (1985). Prophylactic oral acyclovir after renal transplantation. 39:279-281.
17. Prober, C. G., Kirk, L. E., and Keeney, R. E. (1982). Acyclovir therapy of chickenpox in immunosuppressed children—a collaborative study. *J. Pediatr.* 101:662-665.
18. Balfour, H. H. Jr. (1984). Intravenous acyclovir therapy for varicella in immunocompromised children. *J. Pediatr.* 104:134-136.
19. Biron, K. K., and Elion, G. B. (1980). In vitro susceptibility of varicella-zoster to acyclovir. *Antimicrob. Agents Chemother.* 18:443-447.
20. Balfour, H. H., Bean, B., Laskin, O. L., Ambinder, R. J., Meyers, J. D., Wade, J. C., Zaia, J. A., Aeppli, D., Kirk, L. E., Segreti, A. C., and Keeney, R. E. (1983). Acyclovir halts progression of herpes zoster in immunocompromised patients. *N. Engl. J. Med.* 308:1448-1453.
21. Anderson, J., Britton, S., Ernberg, I., et al. (1986). Effect of acyclovir on infectious mononucleosis: A double blind placebo controlled study. *J. Infect. Dis.* 153:283-290.
22. Potter, J. L., and Krill, C. E. (1982). Acyclovir crystalluria. *Pediatr. Infect. Dis.* 5:710-712.
23. Sibrack, C. D., Gutman, L. T., Wilfert, C. M., et al. (1982). Pathogenicity of acyclovir-resistant herpes simplex virus type 1 from an immunodeficient child. *J. Infect. Dis.* 146:673-682.
24. Sullender, W. M., Miller, J. L., Yasukawa, L. L., et al. (1987). Humoral and cellular immunity in neonates with herpes simplex virus infection. *J. Infect. Dis.* 155:28-37.

12
Therapy of Encephalitis with Acyclovir

Stuart M. Goldsmith and Richard J. Whitley *School of Medicine, University of Alabama at Birmingham, Birmingham, Alabama*

HISTORY

Intranuclear inclusion bodies consistent with herpes simplex infection were first demonstrated in the brain of a patient with encephalitis by Smith et al. in 1941 (1). Since herpesvirus was isolated from this brain tissue, this case of neonatal herpes encephalitis provided important evidence that herpes simplex virus (HSV) can cause encephalitis. The first adult case of encephalitis providing similar findings—i.e., intranuclear inclusions in brain tissue and virus isolation—was described in 1944 by Zarafonetis et al. (2). The most striking pathology in this patient was found in the left temporal lobe, including perivascular cuffs of lymphocytes and numerous small hemorrhages. This temporal lobe localization has subsequently been found to be characteristic of adult herpes simplex encephalitis and differs from the involvement ofteń seen in neonates.

Over the past 15 years knowledge of the molecular biology of HSV has been expanded, particularly in the areas of the biochemistry of viral replication and associated gene products, as well as the epidemiology, natural history, and pathogenesis of HSV infections. Future emphasis can now be on improved methods of diagnosis, treatment, and prevention.

213

EPIDEMIOLOGY

Currently, herpes simplex encephalitis (HSE) is estimated to occur in approximately 1 in 250,000-500,000 individuals per year. At the University of Alabama at Birmingham School of Medicine, a medical center that accepts statewide referrals of patients with suspected HSE, the diagnosis of HSE has been proved by brain biopsy in an average of 10 patients per year over the past 10 years. Alabama has a population of 3.3 million: thus, the projected incidence of clinically evident disease is approximately 1 in 300,000 individuals. A similar incidence was found in Sweden and England and is believed to be the approximate incidence in other industrialized countries as well (3,4). In the United States, HSE is thought to account for as many as 10-20% of viral infections of the central nervous system (CNS) (5).

Herpes simplex encephalitis occurs throughout the year and in patients of all ages, with approximately one third occurring in patients less than age 20 and approximately one half in patients older than 50 (6). Caucasians account for 95% of patients with proven disease. The two sexes are equally affected (6).

BACKGROUND

Herpes simplex virus infections of the CNS are among the most severe of all human viral infections of the brain. The severity of disease, as defined by the natural history of infection, is best determined by the outcome of patients who have received no therapy or an ineffective antiviral medication such as idoxuridine or cytosine arabinoside. In such situations mortality is in excess of 70%; only approximately 2.5% of all patients with confirmed disease (9.1% of survivors) return to normal function following recovery from their illness (7-11). Since brain biopsy with the isolation of HSV from brain tissue was the method of diagnosis in these studies, it is likely that a far broader spectrum of HSV infections of the CNS actually exists; however, the methods of diagnosis must be evaluated with these reports. In fact, one British study has suggested milder forms of HSE that are associated with lower mortality and improved morbidity (12).

Although the clinical presentation, diagnosis, and outcome of patients with HSE have been considered for some time, the reported studies indicate extreme variability in the methods of diagnosis, mortality, morbidity, and the clinical course of disease. The studies performed in the United

States by the National Institute of Allergy and Infectious Diseases (NIAID) Collaborative Antiviral Study Group have helped resolve some of these issues. The clarification of many of these issues has become possible because of a uniform diagnostic approach, namely brain biopsy and subsequent isolation of HSV from brain tissue, as the means of disease confirmation. Unequivocal diagnosis often has created both practical dilemmas (13-15) and intellectual controversies (6,16,17). This procedure has not been routinely employed in therapeutic, natural history, or diagnostic investigations performed outside the United States for the prospective evaluation of patients with focal encephalitis. Through the NIAID studies, clinical presentation, the value of brain biopsy for diagnostic purposes as well as establishing alternative diagnoses that mimic HSE, and the relative value of therapy have all been identified.

DIAGNOSIS

Several aspects relating to the diagnosis of HSE merit discussion: the clinical presentation regarding the sensitivity and specificity of various clinical characteristics, the need for brain biopsy to establish the diagnosis, conditions that mimic HSE, and, finally, the prospects of noninvasive means of diagnosing this disease.

Since the NIAID Collaborative Antiviral Study Group required a positive brain biopsy for inclusion in its studies, a unique opportunity existed to evaluate clinical and neurodiagnostic characteristics of brain biopsy-positive and brain biopsy-negative patients (6). It is worth keeping in mind that all of these patients had clinical findings at outset compatible with HSE. Of the first 202 patients who were evaluated for HSE, HSV was isolated from brain tissue of only 113 patients. Only four of the remaining patients had combinations of serologic and clinical findings suggestive of HSE.

Most patients with biopsy-proven HSE present with a focal encephalopathic process, including altered mentation and decreasing levels of consciousness with focal neurologic findings, cerebrospinal fluid (CSF) pleocytosis and proteinosis, the absence of bacterial and fungal pathogens in the CSF, and focal encephalographic, computed tomographic (CT), and/or technetium brain scan findings (Table 1). The use of magnetic resonance imaging (MRI) in this scenario has not been adequately studied to date. From a comparative standpoint, however, only a higher frequency of headache and CSF pleocytosis occur in patients with proven HSE. A higher frequency of ataxia occurs in those individuals who have diseases

TABLE 1 Comparison of Findings in "Brain-Positive" and "Brain-Negative" Patients with Herpes Simplex Encephalitis

	No. (%) of patients	
	Brain positive	Brain negative
Historical findings		
Alteration of consciousness	109/112 (97)	82/84 (96)
CSF pleocytosis	107/110 (97)	71/82 (87)
Fever	101/112 (90)	68/85 (78)
Headache	89/110 (81)	56/73 (77)
Personality change	62/87 (71)	44/65 (68)
Seizures	73/109 (67)	48/81 (59)
Vomiting	51/111 (46)	38/82 (46)
Hemiparesis	33/100 (33)	19/71 (26)
Memory loss	14/59 (24)	9/47 (19)
Clinical findings at presentation		
Fever	101/110 (92)	84/79 (81)
Personality change	69/81 (85)	43/58 (74)
Dysphasia	58/76 (76)	36/54 (67)
Autonomic dysfunction	53/88 (80)	40/71 (58)
Ataxia	22/55 (40)	18/45 (40)
Hemiparesis	41/107 (38)	24/81 (30)
Seizures	43/112 (38)	40/85 (47)
Focal	28	13
Generalized	10	14
Both	5	13
Cranial nerve defects	34/105 (32)	27/81 (33)
Visual field loss	8/58 (14)	4/33 (12)
Papilledema	16/111 (14)	9/84 (11)

"Brain-positive" and "brain-negative" refer to positive or negative brain tissue culture findings. None of the differences were significant at 5% level by χ^2 tests.

that mimic HSV infection of the CNS. Nearly uniformly, patients with HSE present with fever and personality change. Seizures, whether focal or generalized, occur in only approximately two thirds of all patients with proven disease. Thus, the clinical findings of HSE are nonspecific and do not allow for empiric diagnosis of disease predicated solely on clinical presentation. This latter point should be stressed. While clinical evidence of a localized temporal lobe lesion is often thought to be HSE, under the proper circumstances a variety of other diseases can be shown to mimic this condition.

Noninvasive neurodiagnostic studies have been utilized to support a presumptive diagnosis of HSE, including the electroencephalogram, CT scan, and technetium brain scan. More recently, MRI has been utilized for diagnostic purposes, although the value of such scans remains to be established in carefully documented and controlled clinical situations. Focality of the electroencephalogram appears the most sensitive of the noninvasive neurodiagnostic procedures (18-22). Sensitivity of the electroencephalogram has been defined as approximately 84%, but, unfortunately, a specificity of 32.5% has been demonstrated in the NIAID Collaborative Antiviral Study Group trials. When these neurodiagnostic tests are used in combination, the sensitivity can be enhanced; however, the specificity of these diagnostic procedures is diminished. At the present time, none of these neurodiagnostic tests are uniformly satisfactory for diagnosing HSE. Perhaps MRI will prove to be the best neurodiagnostic test.

The most sensitive and specific means of diagnosis, at least at the present time, remains the isolation of HSV from tissue obtained at brain biopsy. While this diagnostic approach is considered controversial, brain biopsy has not been associated with undue complications either acute or chronic in nature. The frequency of acute complications secondary to brain biopsy is approximately 3%, the most common complication being poorly controlled cerebral edema at the time of brain biopsy or hemorrhage because of poor visualization of the tissue. While long-term complications have been thought to include seizure disorders as a consequence of the brain biopsy, these have been uncommon in the experience of the NIAID Collaborative Antiviral Study Group (23). It is important to recognize that temporal lobe necrosis, as encountered with HSE, is an irreversible pathologic process, so the tissue must be considered nonviable and not amenable to recovery. Furthermore, the scarred tissue itself can be a focus of epileptogenic activity.

SEROLOGY

Several strategies utilizing antibody production as a means of diagnosing HSV encephalitis have been studied. Data from the NIAID Collaborative Antiviral Study Group were analyzed for comparison of serum and CSF antibody production in this patient population (24). Neither a fourfold rise in CSF antibody nor the utilization of serum to CSF antibody ratios was adequate for diagnostic purposes except retrospectively. It is conceivable that the availability of an antigen detection assay to be utilized on CSF will replace the uniform diagnosis of HSE by brain biopsy (25).

In the most recent compilation of the NIAID Collaborative Antiviral Study Group data of 432 patients undergoing brain biopsy, 195 patients (45%) had HSE (26). Thirty-eight patients (9%) had disease amenable to other forms of therapy, including brain abscess, tuberculosis, cryptococcal infection, and brain tumor. An additional 40 patients (9%) had identified infections caused by non-HSV viruses but for which there is no current therapy, and an additional 17 patients (4%) had diseases neither of viral etiology nor treatable. The diagnosis of other treatable causes of encephalitis provides perhaps the most compelling support for brain biopsy of patients with suspected HSE. Thus, the future deployment of noninvasive diagnostic procedures must take into consideration those alternative diseases that mimic herpes simplex infection of the CNS and that require immediate medical intervention.

THERAPY

The first antiviral drug evaluated and the first for which therapeutic usefulness was suggested in the literature was idoxuridine, a compound studied in the late 1960s and early 1970s (14,27-31). In 1972, the NIAID Collaborative Antiviral Study Group, in cooperation with the Boston Interhospital Viral Study Group, demonstrated that idoxuridine was both ineffective and toxic for patients with HSE (7). Toxicity was manifested as bone marrow suppression (neutropenia and thrombocytopenia) and secondary bacterial infection. These life-threatening complications developed in patients who received purportedly effective dosages of medication; thus, the therapeutic index (ratio of efficacy to toxicity) was unacceptable. As a consequence of this study, idoxuridine was no longer considered an acceptable therapeutic agent for the management of HSE. These very early controlled studies of HSE demonstrated that uniform methods of data collection and uniform approaches to management of patients with HSE might clarify the issues leading to both earlier diagnosis and improved therapy.

Subsequent therapeutic trials defined vidarabine as a useful medication for the management of biopsy-proven HSE (8,9). In the first of a series of controlled studies of HSE which utilized a double-blind, placebo-controlled study design, vidarabine therapy decreased mortality from 70% to 28% 1 month after disease onset and to 44% 6 months later for patients with biopsy-proven disease (8). This report was predicated on a study of

28 patients, which was terminated for ethical reasons because of decreased mortality in the vidarabine recipients. This study was followed by an open and uncontrolled trial to verify mortality and define long-term morbidity (9). The follow-up study of nearly 100 patients with proved disease defined long-term mortality as 40%. Of importance, variables such as age and level of consciousness at the onset of therapy were proved to be major determinants of clinical outcome. Patients less than 30 years of age and with a more normal level of consciousness (lethargic as opposed to coma-

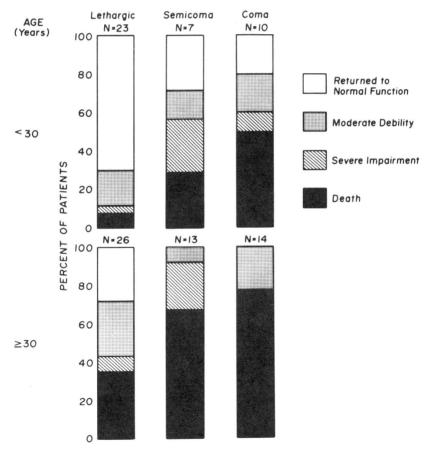

FIGURE 1   Influence of level of consciousness and age on mortality and morbidity.

tose) were more likely to return to normal function after HSE than older patients, especially those who were semicomatose or comatose, as displayed in Figure 1.

From these data, it is apparent that older patients (> 30 years of age) whether comatose or semicomatose had mortality rates that approached 70%—a figure very similar to that encountered in the placebo recipients of the previously cited studies. In patients less than 30 years of age, a more acceptable outcome was achieved, as evidenced by a mortality rate of 25% and with 40% of individuals returning to normal function. Clearly, an important lesson learned from these trials was that if therapy is to be effective, it must be instituted prior to the onset of hemorrhagic necrosis of a dominant temporal lobe as associated with deterioration in the patient's level of consciousness.

More recently, the NIAID Collaborative Antiviral Study Group has demonstrated that acyclovir is superior to vidarabine for the treatment of HSE. The design and mechanism of action of acyclovir have been discussed at some length (32). The single criterion for inclusion in the study's data

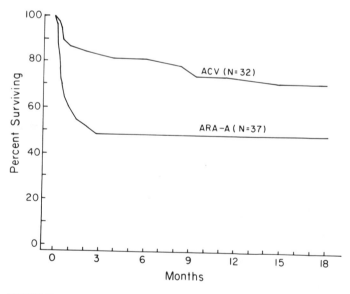

FIGURE 2 Comparison of survival in patients with biopsy-proven herpes simplex encephalitis treated with vidarabine (ARA-A) or acyclovir (ACV); $p = .008$.

base was the establishment of diagnosis by isolation of HSV from brain biopsy tissue. Notably, this criterion is somewhat different from that of a similar study performed in Sweden that also compared these two medications. The NIAID study demonstrated that acyclovir decreased mortality to 19% 6 months after therapy (33). Importantly, 38% of patients irrespective of age returned to normal function. Scandinavian investigators, led by Dr. Birgit Skoldenberg, defined a similar outcome but in a smaller group of patients whose diagnoses were established by a variety of methods (3). The two studies taken together indicate that acyclovir is superior to vidarabine for the treatment of HSE.

As displayed in Figure 2, the data from the NIAID Collaborative Antiviral Study Group indicate a mortality of 50% for 37 patients who received vidarabine compared to 19% 6 months after the onset of treatment and 24% 18 months after the onset of treatment for the acyclovir group. Late deaths in this study were not a consequence of either persistent

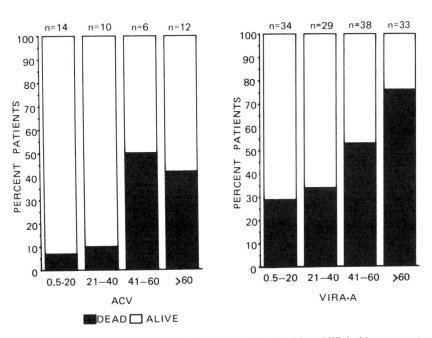

FIGURE 3   Mortality after acyclovir (ACV) or vidarabine (VIRA-A) treatment of biopsy-proven herpes simplex encephalitis, according to age.

or reactivated HSV infection of the CNS but occurred in patients who were severely impaired as a consequence of their disease.

It should be noted that the mortality rate following vidarabine therapy in this study was greater than that encountered in the original trials. A partial explanation for enhanced mortality in the vidarabine-treated group was that this group of patients consisted of older individuals who had a lower level of consciousness—both factors are known to be associated with higher mortality. When patient populations were compared according to specific age and level of consciousness, however, differences in therapeutic outcome remain significant for long-term mortality (utilizing a two-tailed test, $p = .04$) (Figs. 3, 4).

Although these graphs illustrate the difference between acyclovir and vidarabine, they also reveal the importance of age and level of consciousness on survival. For these analyses, the Glasgow coma score (GCS) was used as a more objective reflection of level of consciousness. This score rates patients according to motor, verbal, and sensory responses. Again, scores that approached normal, and younger age predicted enhanced survival. The vidarabine response with increasing GCS is less dramatic pri-

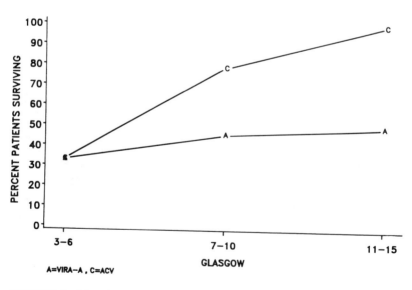

FIGURE 4   Mortality after vidarabine (VIRA-A) or acyclovir (ACV) treatment of biopsy-proven herpes simplex encephalitis, according to GCS.

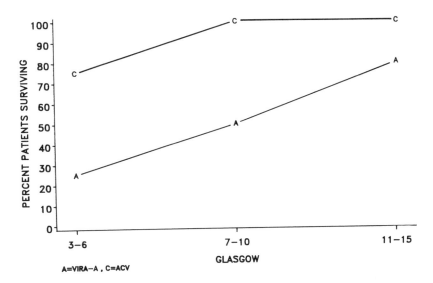

FIGURE 5 Mortality after vidarabine (VIRA-A) or acyclovir (ACV) treatment of biopsy-proven herpes simplex encephalitis for patients less than 30 years of age.

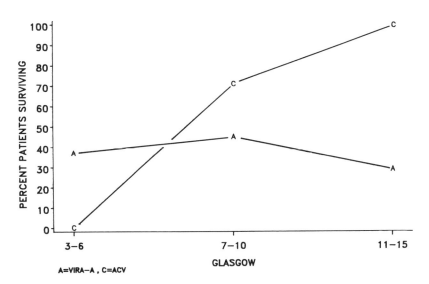

FIGURE 6 Mortality after vidarabine (VIRA-A) or acyclovir (ACV) treatment of biopsy-proven herpes simplex encephalitis for patients over 30 years of age.

marily because older patients treated with vidarabine did poorly even
with higher GCSs.

As can be seen from Figures 5 and 6, older patients treated with acyclovir and younger patients treated with vidarabine were influenced most
by GCS but for different reasons. Young patients treated with acyclovir

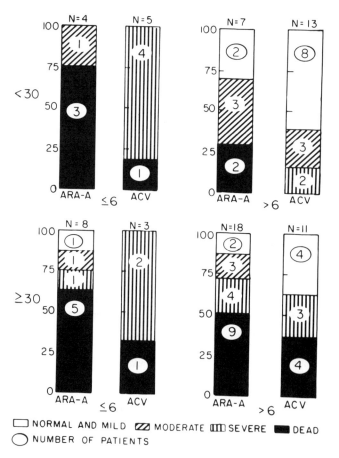

FIGURE 7 Morbidity after vidarabine (ARA-A) or acyclovir (ACV) treatment
of biopsy-proven herpes simplex encephalitis, according to age (<30 vs. >30)
and the GCS (<6 vs. >6).

had a high survival rate regardless of GCS, whereas older patients treated with vidarabine did poorly regardless of GCS. When GCS and age were assessed simultaneously, as displayed in Figure 7, a GCS ≤6 led to a poor therapeutic outcome irrespective of the agent administered or the age of the patient.

Long-term morbidity following administration of an antiviral is of particular importance. Historically, the vidarabine therapeutic studies indicated that approximately 15-20% of patients overall would develop normally following therapy of HSE on long-term follow-up. The current trial indicated that 13% of vidarabine recipients were left with no or minor sequelae whereas those with moderate or severe sequelae and dead on follow-up were 22% and 65%, respectively. For acyclovir recipients, 38% of patients were normal or with minor impairment, 9% of patients had moderate sequelae, and 53% of patients were either left with severe impairment or dead.

No patient in the current trial suffered a relapse after completion of therapy. Nevertheless, when causes of fever other than HSE were excluded, such as bacterial pneumonia, urinary tract infection, etc., the median duration of an afebrile state was only 3.1 days at the completion of 10 days of treatment. Thus, a longer afebrile state might be considered desirable, extending therapy to a minimum of 14 days. Relapse of HSE has been documented in a few patients following the administration of vidarabine (34,35); recently, relapse of HSE has been reported in a normal host after treatment with acyclovir (36). These reports of relapse also support a longer duration of treatment. Demyelination syndromes have also been identified after successful treatment of HSE (37).

In defining the therapeutic index of a compound for the management of HSE, the denominator, or toxicity, becomes an important component of the equation. As shown in Table 2, the vidarabine recipients more likely developed laboratory abnormalities during the course of treatment than the counterpart acyclovir recipients (50% vs. 25%, $p = .04$).

The most significant laboratory abnormalities encountered among vidarabine recipients were a platelet count < 100,000 (11%), an elevated serum glutamic-oxaloacetic transaminase > 250 IU (14%), and an elevated blood urea-nitrogen > 30 mg/dl (11%). In contrast, 10% of acyclovir recipients experienced an elevated BUN, and 6% developed a creatinine > 2 mg/dl. It should be emphasized that the administration of neither drug was associated with clinical evidence of toxicity and that these findings simply represented laboratory aberrations encountered during the course of management of these patients.

TABLE 2　Abnormal Laboratory Values in 69 Patients with Biopsy-Proven Herpes Simplex Encephalitis

| | Treatment group | |
| | Vidarabine | Acyclovir |
Laboratory index*	No. (%)	No. (%)
Platelets (<100,000 cells/mm³)	4 (11)	2 (6)
SGOT (>250 IU/dl)	5 (14)	1 (3)
BUN (>50 mg/dl)	4 (11)	3 (10)
White cells (<2500 cells/mm³)	2 (6)	0 (0)
Total bilirubin (>3 mg/dl)	1 (3)	0 (0)
Creatinine (>3 mg/dl)	0 (0)	2 (6)
Combinations		
SGOT + bilirubin	1 (3)	0 (0)
White cells + platelets	0 (0)	0 (0)
BUN, platelets + SGOT	1 (3)	0 (0)
Total	18 (49)	8 (25)

*SGOT denotes serum aspartate aminotransferase; BUN, blood urea nitrogen. To convert values for BUN to millimoles per liter, multiply by 0.357; to convert values for bilirubin and creatinine to micromoles per liter, multiply by 17.10 and 88.40, respectively.

These findings taken together indicate the therapeutic of choice for the management of HSE is acyclovir rather than vidarabine. While not licensed in the United States for the treatment of HSE, a New Drug Application is currently under review by the Food and Drug Administration for utilization of this compound at a dosage of 10 mg/kg q8h (total 30 mg/kg/day) for a period of 10-14 days. It is conceivable that in certain circumstances a longer period of therapy may be indicated. Clinical response and duration of fever should guide the physician in the deployment of these therapies.

FUTURE THERAPEUTIC DIRECTIONS

The current data indicate that acyclovir is the treatment of choice for biopsy-proven HSE, resulting in significantly improved morbidity and mortality; however, even in patients with a favorable GCS, mortality and morbidity remain problematic. Thus, alternative therapeutic approaches will need to be developed. It should always be kept in mind that the development of sensitive and specific noninvasive diagnostic procedures may contribute to improved outcome by avoiding delays in the onset of therapy while awaiting a biopsy. However, the value of such procedures and their standardization remain to be established. As mentioned above, a longer duration of therapy with current agents and at current doses may be beneficial. Also a trial is planned to test a higher dose of acyclovir (15 mg/kg q8h).

Another approach to the future therapy of HSE is the utilization of combination chemotherapy, which has been used for the management of malignancy and certain viral infections (38,39). Such approaches have been developed in order to decrease therapeutic failures, minimize potential for drug resistance, and potentially decrease dosages of medication to avoid toxic effects. The application of combination therapy to the treatment of viral infections has been studied in vitro as well as in animal model systems for several years (40-46). In tissue culture experiments, acyclovir and vidarabine usually have an additive effect for reduction of replication of both HSV-1 and HSV-2 in Vero cells. In studies of this nature, an antagonistic effect has not been demonstrated for these two antiviral compounds (40).

Animal model data indicate that combination chemotherapy, utilizing acyclovir and vidarabine, has at least an additive and, perhaps, a synergistic effect for decreasing mortality even when therapy is initiated *late* after infection. Similar animal model data have previously predicted the value of both acyclovir and vidarabine as single agents for treatment of HSE and support the potential utility of combination chemotherapy (45). Animal studies performed by Dr. Raymond Schinazi indicate synergy between acyclovir and vidarabine at dosages of 150 mg/kg/day of both medications with delayed therapy. For these studies, combination chemotherapy was initiated 72 h after intercerebral inoculation with HSV-2 and resulted in mortalities ranging from 20% to 50% as dosages were varied (45). However, when fluoromethylarabinosyl uracil was used alone or in combination with acyclovir or vidarabine, mortality was decreased to 0-10%. Because of the existing toxicity profile of this compound, however, it is unlikely that it will be deployed for therapeutic purposes.

Combination chemotherapy may well have potential for decreasing the development of viral resistance as well. However, while resistant viral mutants can be generated easily in tissue culture systems, the appearance of such strains has not been a major problem in experimentally infected animals or humans at the present time (47-50).

New compounds with increased activity or increased lipophilicity, thereby allowing enhanced penetration of drug into the central nervous system, are being sought but are not currently identified. Thus, future therapeutic efforts, at least initially, will use compounds currently in use but either in combination, for longer durations, or in higher doses.

CONCLUSION

The study of HSE has evolved from the descriptive stages of disease to carefully controlled studies to answer targeted questions. Treatment of individuals with this life-threatening and debilitating disease has clearly led to improved outcome and improved quality of life. Acyclovir is the current treatment of choice for HSE. Nevertheless, the significant mortality and morbidity even in treated patients indicate that improvements in the therapeutic regimens for management of this disease are mandatory.

ACKNOWLEDGMENTS

Studies performed and reported by the authors were initiated and supported by contract NO-1-AI-62554 with the Development and Applications Branch of the National Institutes of Allergy and Infectious Diseases and by grant RR-032 from the General Clinical Research Program and the State of Alabama.

REFERENCES

1. Smith, M. G., Lennette, E. H., and Reames, H. R. (1941). Isolation of the virus of herpes simplex and the demonstration of intranuclear inclusions in a case of acute encephalitis. *Am. J. Pathol.* 17:55-68.
2. Zarafonetis, C. J. D., Smodel, M. C., Adams, J. W., and Haymaker, W. (1944). Fatal herpes simplex encephalitis in man. *Am. J. Pathol.* 20(3):429-445.
3. Skoldenberg, B., Alestig, K., Burman, L., et al. (1984). Acyclovir versus vidarabine in herpes simplex encephalitis. A randomized multicentre study in consecutive Swedish patients. *Lancet* 8405:707-711.
4. Longson, M. (1975). The general nature of viral encephalitis in the United Kingdom. In: Illis, L. S. (ed.): *Viral Diseases of the Central Nervous System*. London, Bailliere Tindall, pp. 19-31.
5. Corey, L., and Spear, P. G. (1986). Infections with herpes simplex viruses. *N. Engl. J. Med.* 314:749-757.
6. Whitley, R. J., Tilles, J., Linneman, C., et al. (1982). Herpes simplex encephalitis: Clinical assessment. *JAMA* 247:317-320.

7. Boston Interhospital Virus Study Group and the NIAID Sponsored Cooperative Antiviral Clinical Study (1975). Failure of high dose 5-2-deoxyuridine in the therapy of herpes simplex virus encephalitis. *N. Engl. J. Med.* 292:600-603.
8. Whitley, R. J., Soong, S.-J., Doline, R., et al. (1977). Adenine arabinoside therapy of biopsy-proved herpes simplex encephalitis: National Institute of Allergy and Infectious Diseases Collaborative Antiviral Study. *N. Engl. J. Med.* 297:289-294.
9. Whitley, R. J., Soong, S.-J., Hirsh, M. S., et al. (1981). Herpes simplex encephalitis: Vidarabine therapy and diagnostic problems. *N. Engl. J. Med.* 304:313-318.
10. Longson, M. (1979). Le difi des encephalitis herpetiques. *Ann. Microbial.* (*Paris*) 130:5.
11. Longson, M. M., Bailey, A. S., and Klapper, P. (1980). In Waterson, A. T. (ed.): *Recent Advances in Clinical Virology*, Vol. 2. Philadelphia, Churchill Livingston, pp. 147-157.
12. Klapper, P. E., Cleator, G. M., and Longson, M. (1984). Mild forms of herpes encephalitis. *J. Neurol. Neurosurg. Psychol.* 47:1247-1250.
13. Meyer, M. H. Jr., Johnson, R. T., Crawford, I. P., Dascomb, H. E., and Rogers, N. G. (1960). Central nervous system syndromes of "viral" etiology. *Am. J. Med.* 29:334-347.
14. Rappel, M., Dubois-Dalcq, M., Sprecher, S., et al. (1971). Diagnosis and treatment of herpes encephalitis: A multidisciplinary approach. *J. Neurol. Sci.* 12:443-458.
15. Johnson, R. T., Olson, L. C., and Buescher, E. L. (1968). Herpes simplex virus infections of the nervous system. Problems in laboratory diagnosis. *Arch. Neurol.* 18:260-264.
16. Braun, P. (1980). The clinical management of suspected herpes virus encephalitis: A decision-analytic view. *Am. J. Med.* 69:895-902.
17. Braza, M., and Pauker, S. G. (1980). The decision to biopsy, treat, or wait in suspected herpes encephalitis. *Ann. Intern. Med.* 92:641-649.
18. Radermecker, J. (1956). Systematique its electrocencephalographic des encephalitis it encephalopathies. *Electroencephalogr. Clin. Neurophysiol.* 5 (Suppl.):239.
19. Upton, A., and Grumpert, J. (1970). Electroencephalography in diagnosis of herpes simplex encephalitis. *Lancet* 1:650-652.
20. Smith, J. B., Westmoreland, B. F., Reagan, T. J., and Sandok, B. A. (1975). A distinctive clinical EEG profile in herpes simplex encephalitis. *Mayo Clin. Proc.* 50:469-474.
21. Miller, J. H. D., and Coey, A. (1959). The EEG in necrotizing encephalitis. *Electroencephalogr. Clin. Neurophysiol.* 2:582-585.
22. Ch'ien, L. T., Boehm, R. M., Robinson, H., Liu, C., and Frenkel, L. D. (1977). Characteristic early electroencephalographic changes in herpes simplex encephalitis. *Arch. Neurol.* 34:361-364.

23. Soong, S. J., Caddell, G. R., Alford, C. A., Whitley, R. J., and the NIAID Collaborative Antiviral Study Group. (1986). Utilization of brain biopsy for diagnostic evaluation of patients with herpes simplex encephalitis (HSE): A statistical model. Abstract, 26th Interscience Conference on Antimicrobial Agents and Chemotherapy, New Orleans.

24. Nahmias, A. J., Whitley, R. J., Visintine, A. N., Takei, Y., Alford, C. A. Jr., and the NIAID Collaborative Antiviral Study Group. (1982). Herpes simplex virus encephalitis: Laboratory evaluations and their diagnostic significance. *J. Infect. Dis.* 145:829-836.

25. Lakeman, F. D., Koga, J., and Whitley, R. J. (1987). Detection of antigen to herpes simplex virus in cerebrospinal fluid from patients with herpes simplex encephalitis. *J. Infect. Dis.* 155:1172-1178.

26. Whitley, R. J., Cobbs, C. G., Alford, C. A. Jr., et al. (1989). Diseases which mimic herpes simplex encephalitis: Diagnosis, presentation, and outcome. *JAMA* (in press).

27. Sarubbi, F. A. Jr., Sparling, P. F., and Glezen, W. P. (1973). Herpesvirus hominis encephalitis virus isolated from brain biopsy in seven patients and results of therapy. *Arch. Neurol.* 29:268-273.

28. Nolan, D. C., Carruthers, M. M., and Lerner, A. M. (1970). Herpesvirus hominis encephalitis in Michigan. Report of thirteen cases, including six treated with idoxuridine. *N. Engl. J. Med.* 282:10-13.

29. Illis, L. S., and Merry, R. T. G. (1972). Treatment of herpes simplex encephalitis. *J. R. Coll. Physicians (Lond.)* 7:34-44.

30. Breeden, C. J., Hall, T.C., and Tyler, H. R. (1966). Herpes simplex encephalitis treated with systemic 5-iodo-2' deoxyuridine. *Ann. Intern. Med.* 65:1050-1056.

31. Nolan, D. C., Lauter, C. B., and Lerner, A. M. (1973). Idoxuridine in herpes simplex virus (type 1) encephalitis experience with 29 cases in Michigan, 1966 to 1971. *Ann. Intern. Med.* 78:243-246.

32. Gnann, J. W., Barton, N. H., and Whitley, R. J. (1983). Acyclovir—developmental aspects and clinical applications. Evaluations of new drugs. *Pharmacotherapy* 3:275-283.

33. Whitley, R. J., Alford, C. A. Jr., Hirsch, M. S., et al. (1986). Vidarabine versus acyclovir therapy of herpes simplex encephalitis. *N. Engl. J. Med.* 314:144-149.

34. Davis, L. E., and McLaren, L. C. (1983). Relapsing herpes simplex encephalitis following antiviral therapy. *Ann. Neurol.* 13:192-195.

35. Dix, R. D., Baringer, J. R., Panitch, H. S., Rosenberg, S. H., Hagedoren, J., and Whaley, J. (1983). Recurrent herpes simplex encephalitis: Recovery of virus after ara-A treatment. *Ann. Neurol.* 13:196-200.

36. VanLandingham, K. E., Mansteller, H. B., Ross, G. W., and Hayden, F. G. (1988). Relapse of herpes simplex encephalitis after conventional acyclovir therapy. *JAMA* 259:1051-1053.

37. Loenig, H., Rabinouitz, S. G., Day, E., and Miller, V. (1979). Post-infectious encephalomyelitis after successful treatment of herpes simplex encepha-

litis with adenine arabinoside-ultrastructural observations. *N. Engl. J. Med.* 300:1089-1093.

38. DeVita, V. T. Jr., Young, R. C., and Canellos, G. P. (1975). Combination versus single agent chemotherapy: A review of the basis for selection of drug treatment of cancer. *Cancer* 35:98-110.

39. Rahal, J. J. (1978). Antibiotic combinations: The clinical relevance of synergy and antagonism. *Medicine* 57:179-195.

40. Biron, K. K., and Elion, G. B. (1982). Effect of acyclovir combined with other antiherpetic agents on varicella zoster virus in vitro. *Am. J. Med.* 73: 54-57.

41. Fischer, P. H., Leed, J. J., Chen, M. S., Lin, T. S., and Prusoff, W. H. (1979). Synergistic effect of 5'-amino-5'-deoxythymidine and 5-iodo-2' deoxyuridine against herpes simplex virus infections in vitro. *Biochem. Pharmacol.* 28:3483-3486.

42. Ayisi, N. K., Gupta, V. S., Meldrum, J. B., Taneja, A. K., and Babiuk, L. A. (1980). Combination chemotherapy: Interaction of 5-methyoxymethyl-deoxyuridine with adenine arabinoside, 5-ethyldeoxyuridine, 5-iododeoxy-uridine, and phosphenoacetic acid against herpes simplex virus types 1 and 2. *Antimicrob. Agents Chemother.* 17(4):558-566.

43. Wigand, R., and Hassinger, M. (1980). Combined antiviral effect of DNA inhibitors on herpes simplex virus multiplication. *Med. Microbiol. Immunol.* 168:179-190.

44. DeClerq, E., Descamps, J., Verhelst, G., et al. (1980). Comparative efficacy of antiherpes drugs against different strains of herpes simplex virus. *J. Infect. Dis.* 141:563-574.

45. Schinazi, R. F., Peters, J., Williams, C. C., Chance, D., and Nahmias, A. J. (1982). Effect of combinations of acyclovir with vidarabine or its 5-mono-phosphate on herpes simplex viruses in cell culture and in mice. *Antimicrob. Agents Chemother.* 22:499-507.

46. Shinazi, R. F., and Nahmias, A. J. (1982). Different in vitro effects of dual combinations of anti-herpes simplex virus compounds. *Am. J. Med.* 73: 40-48.

47. Field, J. H. (1983). A perspective on resistance to acyclovir in herpes simplex virus. *J. Antimicrob. Chemother.* 12:129-135.

48. Wade, J. C., McLaren, C., and Meyers, J. D. (1983). Frequency and significance of acyclovir-resistant herpes simplex virus isolated from marrow transplant patients receiving multiple courses of treatment with acyclovir. *J. Infect. Dis.* 148:1077-1082.

49. Barry, D. W., Nusinoff-Lehrman, S., Ellis, M. N., Biron, K. K., and Furman, P. A. (1985). Viral resistance. Clinical experience. *Scand. J. Infect. Dis.* 47:155-164.

50. Svennerholm, B., Vahlne, A., Lowhagen, G. B., Widell, A., and Lycke, E. (1985). Sensitivity of HSV strains isolated before and after treatment with acyclovir. *Scand. J. Infect. Dis.* 47:149-154.

13
Acyclovir Therapy for Varicella

Sandor Feldman *University of Mississippi Medical Center, Jackson, Mississippi*

INTRODUCTION

Acyclovir (ACV), the focus of this presentation, is an acyclic purine nucleoside analog that has inhibitory activity and selectivity for herpes simplex virus (HSV) and varicella zoster virus (VZV) (1,2). The drug is activated by phosphorylation by virus-specific thymidine kinase. The triphosphorylated drug, a potent inhibitor of DNA polymerase, results in viral DNA chain termination. The selectivity of acyclovir for viral enzymes rather than mammalian enzymes is responsible in a large measure for the drug's specificity (and safety).

VZV, the etiological agent of varicella, is one of the human herpesviruses (3). The virion is about 200 nm in diameter, composed of a double-stranded DNA core and a capsid of 162 capsomeres and surrounded by an envelope containing host cell protein (4). VZV was first isolated in tissue culture by Weller in 1953 (5). The virus is cell associated, and it is best propagated in cell cultures of human origin. The cytopathic effect consists of plaques that extend to involve the entire cell monolayer. In infected cells the virus produces eosinophilic (Cowdry type A) intranuclear inclusions, characteristic of the herpesviruses. There is a single serotype of VZV, but the DNAs of different isolates have unique restriction endonuclease cleavage patterns (6).

CHICKENPOX—HISTORICAL BACKGROUND

The derivation of chickenpox has been ascribed to the word *cicer* (or *chiche*) which in English denotes the chickpea (7-9). The lesions of chick-

233

enpox were thought to resemble the small chickpea. An alternative hypothesis proposed for the derivation of the word is from the old English term for "itch," *gican*, in which the "g" is silent (10).

One of the earliest descriptions of varicella was from Rhazes, a ninth-century Persian physician, who described a mild vesicular eruption, not protective against smallpox (7). The 16th century witnessed the spread of chickenpox (and smallpox and measles) throughout Europe. Giovanni Ingrassia (1553), sometimes referred to as the Sicilian Hippocrates, first described chickenpox (*crystalli*) and differentiated it from scarlet fever (*rosania*) (8). In 1694 an English physician, Richard Morton, applied the term chickenpox to an infection that he believed was a mild form of small-pox (8). Vogel in 1765 introduced the term *varicella* to convey the impression of small, irregular-size lesions appearing in crops that he also thought was mild smallpox (8). William Heberden, in a 1767 presentation to the Royal College of Physicians in London, is credited with differentiating chickenpox from smallpox (8). This distinction was necessary, since those with the chickenpox infection might have a false sense of security about the smallpox "which might prevent them either from keeping out of the way of smallpox or from being inoculated." It wasn't until the latter half of the 19th century that the medical community fully accepted different etiologies for the two "pox" infections.

In 1873 Trousseau in his famous work on clinical medicine stated, "No physician has ever seen a patient die of chickenpox, though of course, there may be fatal issue from some complications independent of the ex-anthematous fever" (11). In 1935 Bullowa and Wishik published their experience with 2534 cases of varicella (12). Complications occurred in 5.2%, and the mortality was only 0.4%. In only two instances (encephalitis) did the complications appear to be related to dissemination of the virus. Secondary bacterial infections were the major cause for morbidity and mortality. Well before the advent of immunosuppressive therapy, with its recognized deleterious effect on the outcome of VZV infections, evidence was accumulating that the usually self-limiting childhood chick-enpox did have a more serious side. In 1927 fatal visceral dissemination was reported in 3-week-old premature twins (13). Seven years later a death from varicella was noted in an adult with leukemia (14). The following year Baron reported a fatal case in a 7-day-old full-term infant (15). During the 1940s and 1950s the list of subjects at risk for fatal infections was expanded to encompass otherwise normal, healthy adults (16) and pregnant women (17). The introduction of corticosteroids and antimetabolites into clinical medicine soon revealed that fulminant chickenpox could occur in patients treated with these therapeutic agents (18,19).

HIGH-RISK CATEGORIES

The availability of effective antiviral chemotherapeutic agents has dramatically changed the management of VZV infections. Knowledge of subjects at risk for visceral dissemination and fatalities is mandatory if the drugs are to be used judiciously. Table 1 lists conditions associated with severe varicella for which antiviral therapy is either indicated or should be considered. Although VZV may disseminate to any organ, the majority of deaths are due to pulmonary infection. Acute encephalitis (as opposed to the self-limiting postinfectious encephalitis), although much less common than pneumonitis, has also resulted in fatalities.

Neonate

In neonates there is a correlation between postnatal severity of infection and age at onset of rash. Meyer's review of perinatally acquired varicella revealed a 21% fatality rate if the infection occurred 5-10 days postpartum

TABLE 1 Patients at Risk for Severe and Fatal Varicella

Category	Relative risk
Neonate, age 5-10 days	+ + +
Cancer	+ + +
BMT	+ + +
Congenital immune deficiencies of CMI	+ + +
AIDS	+ + to + + +
Cytotoxic and/or radiation therapy	+ + to + + +
Organ transplant (other than BMT)	+ + to + + +
Pregnancy	+ + to + + +
LBW and VLBW infants	+ +
Adult	+ to + +
Severe malnutrition	+ to + +
Cystic fibrosis	+
Severe burns	+

Key: +, minimal; + +, moderate; + + +, high.

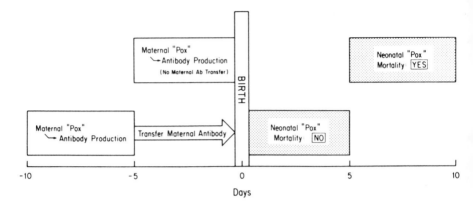

FIGURE 1 Relationship of antepartum varicella and antibody production with neonatal varicella. The time required for maternal development and transfer of antibody coincides with the 10- to 15-day incubation period of varicella. Therefore, infants less than 4 days old or whose mother had varicella more than 5 days before delivery have the modifying benefit of transplacental VZV antibody. [Reproduced with permission from Feldman and Stokes (79).]

as compared to no deaths in those developing infection within the first 4 days of life (20). A similar correlation exists if the antepartum onset of rash in the mother is considered. Deaths occurred in 31% of infants whose mothers had the rash within 4 days of delivery, but none occurred in those instances in which the mother had varicella 5-10 days before delivery. As illustrated in Figure 1, these findings can be explained by production and transplacental passage of maternal VZV antibodies (21).

Maternal varicella 5 days or more prior to delivery is adequate to produce and transfer antibodies to the fetus. Therefore, neonates with varicella in the first 4 days of life have received maternal antibodies, whereas neonates developing the infection at 5-10 days of life have not. Thus, at least in some instances, 5- to 10-day-old newborns are unable to mount an adequate immune response against the virus, are without the maternally derived antibodies, and are at risk for dissemination. Beyond 10 days of life the full-term neonate appears to have adequate defenses to have an uneventful course of varicella. By contrast, fatalities have been reported in premature infants at 3 weeks of age (13). Antiviral therapy for varicella is indicated during days 5-10 of life for full-term infants. Therapy is also warranted for premature infants during the first 3-6 weeks of life and extending to 8-12 weeks of life for infants of low birth weight and very low birth weight.

Cancer

Feldman and Lott reported 288 children with varicella and cancer in whom the overall mortality was 7% (23), a sharp contrast with the 0.4% death rate in the over 2500 apparently normal children studied by Bullowa and Wishik in 1935 (12). VZV pneumonitis, either directly or from associated complications, was the principal cause of death. Pneumonitis occurred in 32% of the subjects with acute leukemia as compared to 19% in those with solid tumors. In the preantiviral era the mortality from dissemination to the lungs was 25%.

Absolute lymphocyte counts (ALC) correlated with risk for virus dissemination and death. At ALC above $500/\mu l$, visceral dissemination and mortality rates were 21% and 7%, respectively. For ALC below $500/\mu l$, the respective rates were 48% and 10%; further rising to 71% and 29% at ALC less than $100/\mu l$. The interruption of chemotherapy during the incubation period did not lessen the risk for visceral dissemination. It is noteworthy that varicella was a self-limiting infection in the 25 children who completed anticancer therapy within the preceding 1-6 months. Thus, for children who have completed anticancer treatment, antiviral therapy is indicated only if infection occurs within the month after termination of immunosuppressive therapy.

Passive immunization with a high-titered anti-VZV globulin preparation substantially reduces the morbidity and mortality of varicella in the immunosuppressed host (23,24). Prophylaxis with varicella zoster immune globulin is indicated for the susceptible immunocompromised host following close exposure to the virus. However, despite passive immunization, visceral dissemination and deaths have been reported (23,24). Therefore, passively protected subjects who develop progressive cutaneous varicella, "toxicity," or evidence of visceral dissemination should receive antiviral chemotherapy.

Although principally an infection of childhood, chickenpox in adult cancer patients is associated with similar risks as their pediatric counterparts (25,27).

Organ Transplant

Bone marrow transplant (BMT) recipients are among the highest risk groups for fatal varicella. Locksley et al., from the Fred Hutchinson Cancer

Research Center in Seattle, reported 28% mortality (28). Of interest, 39% had a pretransplant history of the infection, which contrasts sharply with a 10% incidence of prior varicella in childhood cancer patients (22). Therefore, varicella in BMT may represent reactivation of the host's latent virus or infection with a wild strain to which there has been a loss of "memory."

Eighty percent of VZV infections occur during the first 9 months after transplantation, and it is during this period that fatalities have been reported. Specific antiviral therapy is warranted for varicella during the 9 months following transplantation. For subjects with onset of infection beyond 9 months, without evidence of graft versus host disease, not receiving immunosuppressive therapy (e.g., corticosteroids, antithymocyte globulin, cyclosporin, etc.) and with no other reasons for altered host defenses, expectant observation may be considered. However, if the cutaneous lesions are progressive, evidence of "toxicity" appears, or visceral dissemination occurs, then specific antiviral therapy should be instituted.

Bradley et al. reported 80% mortality for five adult renal transplant recipients with varicella (29), and Feldhoff et al. found 5% (1/19) mortality for pediatric renal transplants (30). The factors responsible for the differences in outcome in the two groups of patients was not apparent. In both series the subjects were receiving immunosuppressive therapy in the form of chemotherapy, antilymphocyte globulins, and/or total lymphoidal irradiation. Intensity and duration of the immunosuppressive therapy did not appear to be responsible for the differences in outcome.

Any organ transplant recipient in the months immediately following the procedure (length of risk not well characterized, other than for BMT) receiving immunosuppressive therapy or having other reasons for altered host defenses should receive specific antiviral treatment for varicella.

Cytotoxic Therapy

Soon after the introduction of steroids into clinical medicine in 1949 (31), a corticosteroid-treated patient with acute rheumatic fever developed fatal varicella (1953) (32). This drug and the other antimetabolites predispose to severe and fatal VZV infection (33,34). Subjects receiving these immunosuppressive agents, regardless of the underlying condition, will benefit from early antiviral therapy.

Other Immunodeficiencies

Children with congenital deficiencies of cell-mediated immunity are at risk for death from varicella (35,36). Subjects infected with human immunodeficiency virus (HIV), even in the absence of overt clinical disease, have demonstrated deficiencies in cell-mediated immunity and therefore are candidates for antiviral therapy for varicella. Studies to define the course in varicella in those infected with HIV are needed.

Adults

In 1942, Waring et al. reported the first cases of fatal disseminated pulmonary varicella in apparently otherwise healthy adults (16). The incidence of varicella pneumonia in adults is 16-34% (37,38). It has been postulated that if all adults with the infection had chest roentgenograms, the incidence might be as high as 50% (38). Triebwasser et al., in a review of 246 cases of pneumonia, reported that the mortality was 11% (39). A recent analysis from the Centers for Disease Control estimated the varicella fatality rate in adults at 30.9 per 100,000 infections (0.03%) (40). The available data suggest fatal infection is uncommon in adults; however, it would seem prudent that all adults with chickenpox should be observed closely for the earliest signs of pulmonary dissemination. Once the latter is evident or seems imminent, antiviral therapy should be instituted.

Harris and Rhoades found a 41% mortality for varicella pneumonia occurring during pregnancy (41), a rate comparable to that for children with cancer (23) and bone marrow recipients (28). However, the true risk for pneumonitis in pregnant women is not known. (See section on Acyclovir in Pregnancy for discussion of treatment.)

Miscellaneous

Fatal varicella has been reported from Third World countries in children with severe starvation and protein deprivation (42,43). While this degree of malnutrition is distinctly uncommon in the United States, there are associated medical conditions (e.g., chronic wasting diseases, short bowel syndrome, etc.) that can have sufficient malnutrition to suppress host defenses to increase the risk for fatal infection.

Subjects with extensive burns (44,45) or cystic fibrosis (46), while not at risk for dissemination, do have morbidity with varicella. For the burn victim in whom the area of injury is not grafted, the vesicular lesions of VZV provide foci for serious secondary bacterial infections. In cystic fibrosis patients, there appears to be a deterioration of pulmonary function.

Antiviral therapy is warranted for severely malnourished infants and those with extensive thermal injuries. Subjects with cystic fibrosis with moderate to severe pulmonary involvement would benefit from therapy to decrease the further lung deterioration associated with varicella.

ACYCLOVIR THERAPY

Intravenous

Efficacy for the treatment of VZV infections has been demonstrated for three antiviral drugs: leukocyte interferon (47), adenine arabinoside (Ara-A) (48), and acyclovir (49,50). ACV has emerged as the preferred treatment (23,51). It is administered intravenously at a dosage of 1500 mg/m^2/day divided into 8-h intervals. As will be discussed later, patients should be kept well hydrated. Duration of therapy is for a minimum of 7 days or at least until no new lesions or fever have occurred for 2 days, whichever is greater. Peak serum levels of 20-25 μg/ml (52-54), three- to fourfold or more greater than the IC$_{50}$ (50% inhibitory concentration) of <1-7 μg/ml for VZV isolates (55), can be expected.

When administered early in the course of infection, the drug substantially reduces the risk for pneumonitis (23). For the 16 children with cancer and varicella treated with ACV within 72 h of infection, none developed pneumonitis as compared to 29% in a historical control group prior to specific antiviral therapy. ACV has also reduced the duration of fever and the appearance of new lesions and accelerated healing (23,50,51,56-59). Shepp et al., in a comparison of ACV and Ara-A for treatment of herpes zoster in BMT recipients, found significantly less cutaneous dissemination in those receiving ACV (51). An important difference between ACV and Ara-A relates to risk of VZV pneumonitis developing during therapy. In one study, none of the 16 ACV-treated patients developed VZV pneumonitis as compared to 6 of 21 (29%) Ara-A-treated patients (23). The higher figure associated with Ara-A is comparable to the incidence of VZV pneumonitis in children with cancer in the era before the availability of antiviral therapy (23). It should be noted, however, that there were no deaths in the Ara-A-treated subjects who developed dissemination to the lungs. In this same series, the only death was in a child who presented with fulminating VZV pneumonitis and who failed to respond to both drugs (23).

The use of ACV rather than Ara-A is supported by decreased risk of pneumonitis, ease of administration (infusion over 1 h, three times a day vs. a 12-h continuous infusion for Ara-A), lesser amounts of intravenous fluid, especially important for critically ill patients (1 ml of fluid for 7 mg of drug vs. 2 ml of fluid for 1 mg Ara-A), and decreased risk for significant adverse reactions. Early therapy is the key to maximum benefit from ACV.

Oral

The role of oral ACV in the treatment of varicella has not been established. Oral absorption is limited to 15-20% of the ingested dose, producing peak serum levels one tenth that of a similar intravenous dose (53). After a standard oral adult dose of 200 mg, peak serum levels are usually slightly less than the IC_{50} for VZV. However, Novelli et al. reported satisfactory clinical responses with high-dose oral ACV in immunocompromised children with varicella (60,61). Dosages as high as 650 mg/m² per dose (compared to 115 mg/m² for an adult receiving a standard dose of 200 mg) were administered to children. Peak serum levels were equivalent to or slightly higher than the inhibitory concentrations of ACV for VZV. Until further data establish the efficacy and safety of high-dose oral ACV for varicella, this form of therapy should be considered experimental. As of this writing, the intravenous route of treatment is recommended.

Pregnancy

Teratogenicity has not been reported with ACV therapy in laboratory animals (62). Review of the literature reveals that ACV has been administered to 17 women in the second or third trimesters of pregnancy (Table 2) (63-73). All the women tolerated the drug well, and the 17 infants delivered were normal. In one instance, the infant's serum and CSF ACV levels were measured approximately 30 h after the last dose of drug to the mother. No drug was found in either body fluid. Urine sample obtained from the infant 38 h after the last maternal dose revealed ACV concentrations of 12.5 μM, substantiating transplacental passage of ACV. Although the number of treated pregnant women is small, to date it does appear that ACV has been administered to pregnant women safely and without adverse effects on the fetus. This suggests that a pregnant woman with disseminated infection or imminent dissemination can be considered for ACV therapy. To obtain more information on safety and efficacy, Burroughs

TABLE 2 Acyclovir Treatment During Pregnancy (63-73)

Trimester	No. treated	Route	Indication
Second	5	IV	VZV
Third	12		
	5	IV	VZV
	4	IV	HSV
	1	IV	Premature labor
	2	PO	VZV

Abbreviations: VZV, varicella zoster virus; HSV, herpes simplex virus; IV, intravenous; PO, oral.

Wellcome Company has established an Acyclovir in Pregnancy Registry (personal communication, E. B. Andrews, Burroughs Wellcome Co., Raleigh, NC).

ADVERSE EFFECTS

Acyclovir is well tolerated and appears to offer a wide margin of safety (74). Relatively minor adverse effects reported during short-term therapy are nausea and vomiting (2-3%), headache, diarrhea, dizziness, anorexia, and fatigue. Long-term suppressant therapy has been associated with vertigo, arthralgias, and insomnia. Allergic reactions in the form of a rash have also occurred. Phlebitis and local site irritation have been described in 3-5% of recipients of the intravenous drug. Whether this is due to direct drug effect (extravasation) or the unusually high pH (>9.0) of the solution is not known. ACV elimination is primarily renal and involves both tubular secretion and glomerular filtration (54). Increases in BUN or creatinine can be expected in 10% of adults receiving intravenous drugs. In children, rapid bolus of drug was associated with abnormalities of BUN and creatinine. However, the drug should be routinely infused over 1 h, thereby eliminating this cause of renal toxicity. Renal dysfunction seems to be transient. ACV crystalluria is also known to occur following bolus administration when hydration is inadequate, with intravenous dosing intervals more frequent than every 8 h and in the presence of diminished urinary output (74-76).

Twenty-two cases of ACV-related neurotoxicity have been reported (77). Manifestations include a combination of disorientation, hallucinations, delirium, tremors, ataxia, myoclonic jerks, slurred speech, and other motor or mental disturbances. These adverse effects have been reversible. Feldman and colleagues correlated neurotoxicity with markedly increased serum drug concentrations (77). Their patient, an adolescent with cancer, had a normal to minimally elevated BUN and creatinine. However, measured serum creatinine and ACV clearances were less than 30 ml/min/1.73 m^2. The authors proposed that the patient's extensive chemotherapy produced sufficient renal damage to decrease the creatinine and ACV clearances but insufficient damage to be reflected in the BUN and serum creatinine.

Bean and Aeppli, in a study of intravenous ACV in ambulatory patients, found that the minor adverse reactions correlated with elevated drug levels (78). These subjects had abnormal renal function. At present most clinical facilities do not have the capabilities of measuring ACV levels.

TABLE 3 Dosage Adjustment Recommended for Patients with Renal Impairment

Creatinine clearance (ml/min/1.73 m^2)	Percent usual dose	Dosing interval (h)
>50	100	8
25-50	100	12
10-25	100	24
0-10	50	24

Source: Reproduced with permission from Blum et al. (54).

Therefore, creatinine clearance should be performed in patients predisposed to renal dysfunction (e.g., organ transplant recipients, patients with cancer or structural abnormalities of the kidney, neonates, and the elderly). A measured creatinine clearance is preferable to a serum creatinine or calculated creatinine clearance, since abnormalities in the latter two parameters may be minimal and not reflect a decrease in ACV clearance. Table 3 indicates dosage adjustments for subjects with abnormal creatinine clearance (54).

REFERENCES

1. Elion, G. B., Furman, P. A., Fyfe, J. A., De Miranda, P., Beauchamp, L., and Schaeffer, H. J. (1977). Selectivity of action of an antiherpetic agent, 9-(2-hydroxyethoxymethyl) guanine. *Proc. Natl. Acad. Sci. USA* 74:5716-5720.
2. Elion, G. B. (1983). The biochemistry and mechanism of action of acyclovir. *J. Antimicrob. Chemother.* 12(Suppl.):9-17.
3. Almeida, J. D., Howatson, A. F., and Williams, M. G. (1962). Morphology of varicella (chicken pox) virus. *Virology* 16:353-355.
4. Schauf, V., and Tolpin, M. (1984). Varicella-zoster virus. In Belshe, R. B. (ed.): *Textbook of Human Virology*. Littleton, MA, PSG Publishing Co., pp. 829-851.
5. Weller, T. H. (1953). Serial propagation in vitro of agents producing inclusion bodies derived from varicella and herpes zoster. *Proc. Soc. Exp. Biol. Med.* 83:340-346.
6. Martin, J. H., Dohner, D. E., Wellinghoff, W. J., and Gelb, L. D. (1982). Restriction endonuclease analysis of varicella-zoster vaccine virus and wild-type DNA's. *J. Med. Virol.* 9:69-76.
7. Gordon, J. E. (1962). Chickenpox: An epidemiological review. *Am. J. Med. Sci.* 244:362-389.

8. Rolleston, J. D. (1937). The history of the acute exanthemata: The Fitzpatrick lectures for 1935 & 1936. Delivered before the Royal College of Physicians of London. London, William Heinemann, pp. 32-45.

9. Taylor-Robinson, D., and Caunt, A. E. (1972). Varicella virus. In: *Virology Monographs*. New York, Springer-Verlag, pp. 4-7.

10. Scott-Wilson, J. H. (1978). Why "chicken" pox? *Lancet* 1:1152.

11. Trousseau, A. (1882). Clinical medicine. Lectures delivered at the Hotel-Dieu, Paris, Ed. 3, McCormack, J. R., and Bazire, P. V. (translators). Philadelphia, P. Blakiston, p. 1:136.

12. Bullowa, J. G. M., and Wishik, S. M. (1935). Complications of varicella. *Am. J. Dis. Child.* 49:923-932.

13. Schleussing, H. (1927). Nekrosen in Leber, Milz und Nebennieren bei nicht vereiterten Varizellen. *Verh. Dtsch. Ges. Pathol.* 22:288-292.

14. Philadelphy, A., and Haslhofer, L. (1934). Varicellen bei leukamischer Lymphadenose. *Arch. Dermatol. Syph.* 169:512-518.

15. Baron, M. F. (1935). Un cas de varicella mortelle. *Nourrisson* 23:157-159.

16. Waring, J. J., Neubuerger, K., and Geever, E. F. (1942). Severe forms of chickenpox in adults. *Arch. Intern. Med.* 69:384-408.

17. Fish, S. A. (1960). Maternal death due to disseminated varicella. *JAMA* 173:978-981.

18. Cheatham, W. J., Weller, T. H., Dolan, T. F., Jr., and Dower, J. C. (1956). Varicella, report of two fatal cases with necropsy, virus isolation and serologic studies. *Am. J. Pathol.* 32:1015-1035.

19. Haggerty, R. J., and Eley, R. C. (1956). Varicella and cortisone. *Pediatrics* 18:160-162.

20. Meyers, J. D. (1974). Congenital varicella in term infants: Risk reconsidered. *J. Infect. Dis.* 129:215-217.

21. Brunell, P. A. (1960). Placental transfer of varicella-zoster antibody. *Pediatrics* 38:1034-1038.

22. Feldman, S., Hughes, W. T., and Daniel, C. B. (1975). Varicella in children with cancer: Seventy-seven cases. *Pediatrics* 56:388-397.

23. Feldman, S., and Lott, L. (1987). Varicella in children with cancer: Impact of antiviral therapy and prophylaxis. *Pediatrics* 80:465-472.

24. Zaia, J. A., Levin, M. J., Preblud, S. R., Leszczynski, J., Wright, G. G., Ellis, R. J., Curtis, A. C., Valerio, M. A., and LeGore, J. (1983). Evaluation of varicella-zoster immune globulin: Protection of immunosuppressed children after household exposure to varicella. *J. Infect. Dis.* 147:737-743.

25. Merselis, J. G., Kaye, D., and Hook, E. W. (1964). Disseminated herpes zoster. *Arch. Intern. Med.* 113:679-686.

26. Sokal, J. E., and Firat, D. (1965). Varicella-zoster infection in Hodgkin's disease. *Am. J. Med.* 39:452-463.

27. Schimpff, S., Serpick, A., Stoler, B., Rumack, B., Mellin, H., Joseph, J. M., and Block, J. (1972). Varicella-zoster infection in patients with cancer. *Ann. Intern. Med.* 76:241-254.

28. Locksley, R. M., Flournoy, N., Sullivan, K. M., and Meyers, J. D. (1985). Infection with varicella-zoster virus after marrow transplantation. *J. Infect. Dis.* 152:1172-1181.
29. Bradley, J. R., Wreghitt, T. G., and Evans, D. B. (1987). Chickenpox in adult renal transplant recipients. *Nephrol. Dial. Transplant.* 1:242-245.
30. Feldhoff, C. M., Balfour, H. H., Simmons, R. L., Najarian, J. S., and Mauer, S. M. (1981). Varicella in children with renal transplants. *Pediatrics* 98:25-31.
31. Hench, P. S., Kendall, E. C., Slocumb, C. H., and Polley, H. F. (1949). The effect of a hormone of the adrenal cortex (17-hydroxy-11-dehydrocorticosterone: compound E) and of pituitary adrenocorticotropic hormone on rheumatoid arthritis; preliminary report. *Mayo Clin. Proc.* 24:181-197.
32. Josserand, P., et al. (1953). Varicelle mortelle a forme hemorrhagique dans le decours d'un traitement par cortisone—A.C.T.H. *Pediatrie* 8:947-948.
33. Finkel, K. C. (1961). Mortality from varicella in children receiving adrenocorticosteroids and adrenocorticotropin. *Pediatrics* 18:436-441.
34. Etteldorf, J. N., Roy, S. III, Summitt, R. L., Sweeney, M. J., Wall, H. P., and Berton, W. M. (1967). Cyclophosphamide in the treatment of idiopathic lipoid nephrosis. *Pediatrics* 70:758-766.
35. Ammann, A. J. (1977). T-cell and T-B cell immunodeficiency disorders. *Pediatr. Clin. North Am.* 24:293-311.
36. Rosen, F. S. (1974). Primary immunodeficiency. *Pediatr. Clin. North Am.* 21:533-549.
37. Weber, D. M., and Pellecchia, J. A. (1965). Varicella pneumonia: Study of prevalence in adult men. *JAMA* 192:228-229.
38. Mermelstein, R. H., and Freireich, A. W. (1961). Varicella pneumonia. *Ann. Intern. Med.* 55:456-463.
39. Triebwasser, J. H., Harris, R. E., Bryant, R. E., and Rhoades, E. R. (1967). Varicella pneumonia in adults: Report of seven cases and a review of literature. *Medicine* 46:409-423.
40. Preblud, S. R. (1981). Age-specific risks of varicella complications. *Pediatrics* 68:14-17.
41. Harris, R. E., and Rhoades, E. R. (1965). Varicella pneumonia complicating pregnancy: Report of a case and review of literature. *Obstet. Gynecol.* 25:734-740.
42. Purtilo, D. T., and Connor, D. H. (1975). Fatal infections in protein-calorie malnourished children with thymolymphatic atrophy. *Arch. Dis. Child.* 50:149-152.
43. Salomon, J. B., Mata, L. J., and Gordon, M. D. (1968). Malnutrition and the common communicable diseases of childhood in rural Guatemala. *Am. J. Public Health* 58:505-516.
44. Weintraub, W. H., Lilly, J. R., and Randolph, J. G. (1974). A chickenpox epidemic in a pediatric burn unit. *Surgery* 76:490-494.

45. Smith, E. I., and DeWeese, M. S. (1969). The topical therapy of burns in children. *Arch. Surg.* 98:462-468.
46. Macdonald, N. E., Morris, R. F., and Beaudry, P. H. (1987). Varicella in children with cystic fibrosis. *Pediatr. Infect. Dis. J.* 6:414-416.
47. Arvin, A. M., Kushner, J. H., Feldman, S., Baehner, R. L., Hammond, D., and Merigan, T. C. (1982). Human leukocyte interferon for the treatment of varicella in children with cancer. *N. Engl. J. Med.* 306:761-765.
48. Whitley, R., Hilty, M., Haynes, R., Bryson, Y., Connor, J. D., Soong, S., Alford, C. A., and the National Institute of Allergy and Infectious Disease Collaborative Antiviral Study Group. (1982). Vidarabine therapy of varicella in immunosuppressed patients. *J. Pediatr.* 101:125-131.
49. Prober, C. G., Kirk, L. E., and Keeney, R. E. (1982). Acyclovir therapy of chickenpox in immunosuppressed children—a collaborative study. *J. Pediatr.* 101:622-625.
50. Balfour, H. H. Jr. (1984). Intravenous acyclovir therapy for varicella in immunocompromised children. *J. Pediatr.* 104:134-136.
51. Shepp, D. H., Dandliker, P. S., and Meyers, J. D. (1986). Treatment of varicella-zoster virus infection in severely immunocompromised patients: A randomized comparison of acyclovir and vidarabine. *N. Engl. J. Med.* 314:208-212.
52. Laskin, O. L., Longstreth, J. A., Saral, R., De Miranda, P., Keeney, R., and Lietman, P. S. (1982). Pharmacokinetics and tolerance of acyclovir, a new anti-herpesvirus agent, in humans. *Antimicrob. Agents Chemother.* 21:393-398.
53. De Miranda, P., and Blum, M. R. (1983). Pharmacokinetics of acyclovir after intravenous and oral administration. *J. Antimicrob. Chemother.* 12:29-37.
54. Blum, M. R., Liao, S. H. T., and De Miranda, P. (1982). Overview of acyclovir pharmacokinetic disposition in adults and children. *Am. J. Med.* 73 (Suppl.):186-192.
55. Biron, K. K., and Elion, G. B. (1980). In vitro susceptibility of varicella-zoster virus to acyclovir. *Antimicrob. Agents Chemother.* 18:443-447.
56. Meyers, J. D., Wade, J. C., Shepp, D. H., and Newton, B. (1984). Acyclovir treatment of varicella-zoster virus infection in the compromised host. *Transplantation* 37:571-574.
57. Al-Nakib, W., Al-Kandari, S., El-Khalik, D. M. A., and El-Shirbiny, A. M. (1983). A randomised controlled study of intravenous acyclovir (Zivirax) against placebo in adults with chickenpox. *J. Infect.* 6(Suppl.):49-56.
58. Boguslawska-Jaworska, J., Koscielniak, E., and Rodziewicz, B. (1984). Acyclovir therapy for chickenpox in children with hematological malignancies. *Eur. J. Pediatr.* 142:130-132.
59. Shulman, S. T. (1985). Acyclovir treatment of disseminated varicella in childhood malignant neoplasms. *Am. J. Dis. Child.* 139:137-140.

60. Novelli, V. M., Marshall, W. C., Yeo, J., and McKendrick, D. (1984). Acyclovir administered perorally in immunocompromised children with varicella-zoster infections. *J. Infect. Dis.* 149:478.

61. Novelli, V. M., Marshall, W. C., Yeo, J., and McKendrick, D. (1985). High-dose oral acyclovir for children at risk of disseminated herpesvirus infections. *J. Infect. Dis.* 151:372 (letter).

62. Tucker, W. E. Jr. (1982). Preclinical toxicology profile of acyclovir: An overview. *Am. J. Med.* 73(Suppl.):27-30.

63. Anderson, H., Sutton, R. N. P., and Scarffe, J. H. (1984). Cytotoxic chemotherapy and viral infections: The role of acyclovir. *J. R. Coll. Physicians Lond.* 18:51-55.

64. Lagrew, D. C. Jr., Terrance, G. F., Hager, W. D., and Yarrish, R. L. (1984). Disseminated herpes simplex virus infection in pregnancy: Successful treatment with acyclovir. *JAMA* 252:2058-2059.

65. Grover, L., Kane, J., Kravitz, J., and Cruz, A. (1985). Systemic acyclovir in pregnancy: A case report. *Obstet. Gynecol.* 65:284-287.

66. Glaser, J. B., Loftus, J., Ferragamo, V., Mootabar, H., and Castellano, M. (1986). Varicella-zoster infection in pregnancy. *N. Engl. J. Med.* 315:1416 (letter).

67. Cox, S. M., Phillips, L. E., DePaolo, H. D., and Faro, S. (1986). Treatment of disseminated herpes simplex virus in pregnancy with parenteral acyclovir: A case report. *J. Reprod. Med.* 31:105-107.

68. Greffe, B. S., Dooley, S. L., Deddish, R. B., and Krasny, H. C. (1986). Transplacental passage of acyclovir. *J. Pediatr.* 108:1020-1021.

69. Carter, P. E., Duffty, P., and Lloyd, D. J. (1986). Neonatal varicella infection. *Lancet* 2:1459 (letter).

70. Landsberger, E. J., Hager, W. D., and Grossman, J. H. III. (1986). Successful management of varicella pneumonia complicating pregnancy: A report of three cases. *J. Reprod. Med.* 31:311-314.

71. Hankins, G. D. V., Gilstrap, L. C. III, Patternson, A. R., and Hall, W. (1987). Acyclovir treatment of varicella pneumonia in pregnancy. *Crit. Care Med.* 15:336 (letter).

72. Leen, C. L. S., Mandal, B. K., and Ellis, M. E. (1987). Acyclovir and pregnancy. *Br. Med. J.* 294:308 (letter).

73. Hankey, G. J., Bucens, M. R., and Chambers, J. S. W. (1987). Herpes simplex encephalitis in third trimester of pregnancy: Successful outcome for mother and child. *Neurology* 37:1534-1537.

74. Keeney, R. E., Kirk, L. E., and Brigden, D. (1982). Acyclovir tolerance in humans. *Am. J. Med.* 73(Suppl.):176-181.

75. Brigden, D., Rosling, A. E., and Woods, N. C. (1982). Renal function after acyclovir intravenous injection. *Am. J. Med.* 73(Suppl.):182-185.

76. Potter, J. L., and Krill, C. E. (1986). Acyclovir crystalluria. *Pediatr. Infect. Dis.* 5:710-712.

77. Feldman, S., Rodman, J., and Gregory, B. (1988). Excessive acyclovir serum concentrations and neurotoxicity. *J. Infect. Dis.* (in press).
78. Bean, B., and Aeppli, D. (1985). Adverse effects of high-dose intravenous acyclovir in ambulatory patients with acute herpes zoster. *J. Infect. Dis.* 151: 362-364.
79. Feldman, S., and Stokes, D. C. (19??). Varicella zoster and herpes simplex pneumonias. *Semin. Respir. Infect.* 2:84-95.

14
Acyclovir for Herpes Zoster

J. Clark Huff   *University of Colorado School of Medicine, Denver, Colorado*

INTRODUCTION

Prevention and successful therapy of human infections with varicella zoster virus (VZV) have remained major challenges to public health physicians and clinicians. In the United States, over 90% of adults have antibodies to VZV as evidence of prior infection and thus may carry VZV in a latent state (1). Although most VZV infections do not cause mortality or serious morbidity, a viral infection of this prevalence is a matter of great public health significance. Even if serious or complicated illnesses occur in only a small percentage of cases, the absolute number of such significant infections is sizable.

Although effective public health measures for preventing infections with VZV are not yet a reality, the last decade has brought to the clinician improved modes of therapy for the more serious VZV infections. With the advent of the modern era of antiviral chemotherapy, in particular the availability of acyclovir for clinical use, prospects for more effective control of human VZV infections are finally encouraging.

CLINICAL CHARACTERISTICS OF VZV INFECTIONS

Varicella or chickenpox, the primary or initial infection of an individual with VZV, is a systemic illness associated with viremia. Typically, a prodromal phase of fever and malaise for 1 or 2 days is followed by the eruption of a vesicular rash over 3-5 days. Within about 5 days, vesicles progress to crusted lesions which subsequently heal, sometimes leaving behind small round scars. Resolution of the illness occurs as the host immune system, particularly cell-mediated immunity, responds to check the viral infection.

VZV, like herpes simplex virus (HSV), is capable of establishing itself in a latent state. Latency is thought to be established during the initial viremic phase, and latent VZV is not recognized and cleared by the host immune system. The site of latency is thought to be in nerve tissue, primarily ganglia. Although VZV has not been cultured from apparently normal ganglia, recent investigations by nucleic acid hybridization techniques have shown evidence of VZV in sensory ganglia (2,3).

The recurrent or reactivation variety of VZV infections, herpes zoster or shingles, occurs when latent VZV reactivates (4). Herpes zoster is a

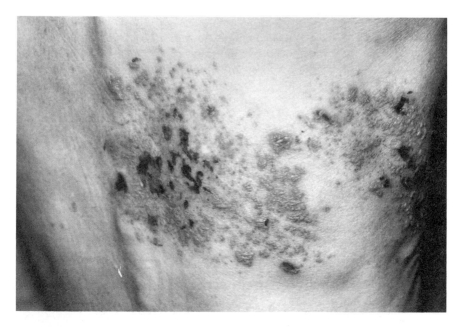

FIGURE 1 Thoracic herpes zoster in an elderly man. Grouped vesicles on erythematous bases are distributed in a dermatomal pattern. In some areas, the lesions have progressed to produce hemorrhagic scabs.

localized cutaneous eruption which usually is vesicular and which is associated with neurologic symptoms in the same area as the eruption, usually
hypesthesia, burning, and pain. The neurologic symptoms may precede
the cutaneous eruption by many days and present a diagnostic dilemma.
The skin lesions of zoster are typically distributed on the skin approxi-
mating the cutaneous innervation of the sensory nerves arising from a
single sensory ganglion (Fig. 1). Grouped vesicles on erythematous bases
appear for 3-5 days (Fig. 2), then new lesions cease to appear, and crusting and healing occur over 1-2 weeks. As with varicella, the host immune
defenses respond to the antigenic stimulation of the recurrent viral infection and control the productive viral infection.

The incidence of herpes zoster increases at least four- to five fold between young adulthood and the 70s (5). The explanation for the direct
relation between age and the occurrence of zoster is thought to be waning

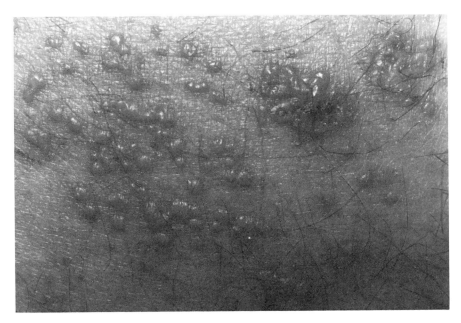

FIGURE 2 Vesicular herpes zoster. Vesicles are grouped on erythematous bases.

immune defenses to VZV that occur with age and with the time interval
from the initial infection (6).

   In many individuals, zoster causes no serious complications. However, the elderly and patients with abnormal cell-mediated immune defenses may experience more serious, complicated, or even fatal episodes
of zoster. In elderly patients, the most frequently recognized complication of zoster is postherpetic neuralgia. Severe, often life-disrupting pain
may follow zoster and persist for months to years (5). When the ophthalmic branch of the trigeminal nerve is involved, as occurs in about 20% of
zoster cases, the eye may be affected, and permanent visual impairment
may result (Fig. 3) (7,8). Less frequent complications include motor nerve
involvement, hearing loss, secondary bacterial infections, and encephalitis.

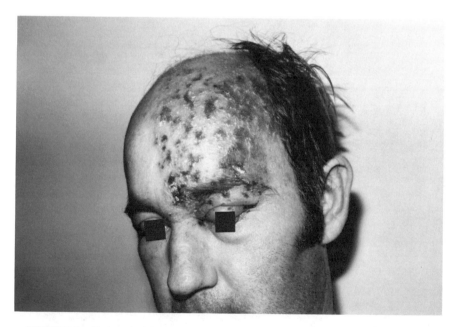

FIGURE 3   Ophthalmic herpes zoster in the scabbing stage. Herpes zoster in the
distribution of the ophthalmic branch of the trigeminal nerve (V1) may be complicated by eye involvement.

Patients with depressed cell-mediated immunity, such as patients with Hodgkin's disease or other lymphoreticular malignancies, bone marrow transplant patients, patients on chemotherapy or immunosuppressive drugs, or patients with infections due to the human immunodeficiency virus (HIV), not only may experience complications similar to those of elderly individuals, but may also suffer additional serious complications. Cutaneous zoster lesions may be hemorrhagic, gangrenous, or ulcerative; several dermatomes may be involved simultaneously; a widespread varicellalike rash representing viral dissemination (Fig. 4), occurs frequently; and visceral infections with VZV may occur. Hepatitis and pneumonitis due to VZV are bad prognostic signs and are often associated with mortality.

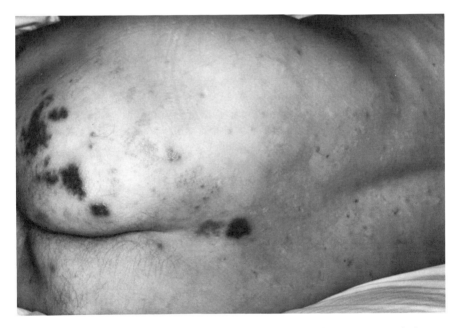

FIGURE 4 Lumbosacral herpes zoster in a lymphoma patient. The zoster lesions are necrotic, and discrete varicelliform lesions, representing dissemination, are present on the back.

Diagnosis of VZV infections is usually made on the clinical characteristics of the cutaneous eruption. A rapid, sometimes helpful, diagnostic test is a Tzanck prepration. Scrapings of cells from the base of a vesicle are placed on a microscope slide, dried, and stained for cell morphology, often with a Wright stain or Giemsa stain. With VZV, multinucleated epithelial giant cells are seen. HSV may mimic VZV infections clinically; unfortunately, HSV produces indistinguishable giant cells on a Tzanck preparation.

Viral culture is the most specific diagnostic procedure for VZV infections. Because viral cultures of VZV may not become positive for 5-7 days, they are rarely helpful in making therapeutic decisions.

PREVIOUS THERAPIES FOR VZV INFECTION

Prior to the advent of acyclovir, therapies for VZV infections were of questionable efficacy or were impractical (Table 1). The medical literature is filled with many "testimonial" reports of therapy for VZV infections, often without any controlled clinical trials. Because of the great variability of the course and severity of infections, it is essential that any therapy adopted for this common human illness have adequate documentation of its efficacy and safety.

One of the first drug therapies advocated for herpes zoster was systemic glucocorticosteroid administration. The rationale for such therapy derived from the widespread use of steroids for many diseases after such drugs became readily available in the 1950s and 1960s and from reports that such therapy prevented postherpetic neuralgia (9,10). Two controlled

TABLE 1 Previous Therapies for VZV Infections

Drug	Indication
Systemic steroids	Possible prevention of postherpetic neuralgia
Idoxuridine in dimethyl sulfoxide	Used topically for herpes zoster but not clearly effective or practical
Cytosine arabinoside	None (not effective or harmful)
Adenine arabinoside	Intravenous therapy of immunosuppressed patients with herpes zoster or varicella
Human leukocyte interferon	None (not approved or readily available although shown to be effective in both herpes zoster and varicella in cancer patients)

studies subsequently presented more objective evidence that use of systemic steroids for acute zoster lessened the frequency of postherpetic neuralgia (11,12), and such therapy was subsequently widely adopted. However, questions continue to be raised about these studies (13), and other controlled studies have shown no value of steroid therapy in preventing postherpetic neuralgia (14,15).

The question of the value of steroid therapy remains unanswered. Concern regarding the therapy is based primarily on the growing appreciation of the role of host cell-mediated immunity in controlling VZV infections and the known depression of such immunity by high-dose systemic steroid therapy. Nevertheless, immunocompetent patients seem to tolerate such therapy well and do not usually experience the more serious complications of zoster seen in immunosuppressed subjects.

When drugs with in vitro activity against herpesviruses emerged, attempts to treat VZV infections ensued. Idoxuridine, a thymidine analog, was applied topically on the skin for herpes zoster (16,17). Although the drug is toxic to cells and is highly insoluble, frequent topical applications of the drug dissolved in dimethyl sulfoxide, when started early in the illness, appeared to favorably alter the course of the disease. Additional studies to document the effectiveness of this approach have not been accomplished.

Another potential antiviral drug, thought to be potentially useful for VZV infections, was cytosine arabinoside. Even though there were reports of cases in which the drug appeared to be beneficial, controlled studies in herpes zoster subsequently showed no effect (18) or an adverse effect on the outcome (19). The experience with cytosine arabinoside ironically was a valuable one: it pointed out that drugs with in vitro antiviral activity may not work in the clinical disease and that careful controlled clinical studies are essential.

The next potential antiviral drug for VZV, vidarabine (adenine arabinoside), was the subject of careful clinical trials. A multicenter trial by the NIAID Collaborative Antiviral Study Group in immunosuppressed patients with herpes zoster demonstrated clearly the value of intravenous vidarabine (20). In this blind, controlled, crossover study, patients receiving the vidarabine first experienced accelerated clearance of virus from lesions, cessation of new vesicle formation, a shorter time to total pustulation, and reduced acute pain. Benefit was greatest in younger patients with lymphoreticular malignancies treated early in the course of zoster. In a follow-up double-blind, placebo-controlled study by the NIAID Collaborative Antiviral Study Group (21), 121 immunosuppressed patients with localized herpes zoster of 72 h duration or less were treated with intravenous vidarabine 10 mg/kg per day over 12 h for 5 days (n = 63) or placebo (n = 58). Drug recipients were found to have accelerated cutaneous healing, as evidenced by more rapid cessation of lesion formation and reduction in time to total pustulation and scabbing. Most importantly, therapy decreased cutaneous dissemination from 24% to 8% (p = .014) and zoster-related visceral complications from 19% to 5% (p = .015). The duration of postherpetic neuralgia was also decreased in drug recipients (p = .047). No serious drug toxicity was noted.

A similar careful study of intravenous vidarabine in 34 immunosuppressed patients with varicella of 72 h or less duration documented the value of this drug for VZV therapy (22). New vesicle formation and fever ceased sooner in vidarabine recipients. Most significantly, visceral complications (including pneumonitis) and mortality were less frequent in drug recipients than in placebo recipients. The value of intravenous vidarabine in immunosuppressed patients with varicella has been widely accepted in the 1980s (23).

Finally, studies have been undertaken to evaluate the effectiveness of human leukocyte interferon in the therapy of VZV infections in patients with cancer. Because VZV is inhibited in vitro by interferon (24) and interferon production appears to correlate with recovery in zoster (25), administration of human leukocyte interferon appeared rational. In a randomized, double-blind, placebo-controlled study in 90 cancer patients with zoster, high doses of intramuscular interferon produced a decrease in cutaneous dissemination, a shortened duration of new lesion formation, and diminished severity of postherpetic neuralgia (26). Likewise, in a similar study of human leukocyte interferon in 44 children with cancer who developed varicella, interferon recipients had decreased duration of new lesion formation and fewer episodes of life-threatening dissemination in survivors (27).

Although studies show efficacy of both vidarabine and human leukocyte interferon for VZV infections, there are practical limitations to these therapies. Vidarabine must be administered as a continuous intravenous infusion and thus is practical therapy only for hospitalized patients with the most serious infections. Human leukocyte interferon injections are given intramuscularly, usually every 12 h, and also are appropriate only for hospitalized patients with serious infections. In addition, human leukocyte interferon is not readily available. Whether other types of interferon preparations are equally effective for VZV infections is not yet clear.

ACYCLOVIR THERAPY FOR VZV INFECTIONS

Preclinical Studies

With the report of Schaeffer and colleagues that the nucleoside deriva-
tive 9-(2-hydroxyethoxymethyl) guanine or acycloguanosine had good activity in vitro against a number of herpesviruses, was effectve in vivo in
animal models of HSV infections, and had extremely low toxicity (28), a
new chapter in antiviral chemotherapy began. Acyclovir, as this new compound was named, is the prototype of antiviral compounds whose activities are dependent on specific interactions with virus-specific proteins but
whose interactions with normal cellular proteins are minimal.

Acyclovir was found to inhibit replication of VZV in vitro at concentrations (3.65-3.75 μM) considerably higher than those required for
inhibition of HSV (29,30) but easily obtainable in vivo (31,32). The explanation for the viral specificity of acyclovir against VZV, as with HSV,
was shown to be activation of the drug by phosphorylation in virus-infected
cells by viral thymidine kinase and the selectivity of acyclovir triphosphate
for viral DNA polymerase (33). Likewise, resistance by VZV to acyclovir
is determined by diminished activity of viral thymidine kinase or altered
affinity of the DNA polymerase for the triphosphate (34).

Intravenous Acyclovir Therapy

After appropriate preclinical studies of acyclovir, controlled studies of
intravenous acyclovir therapy of subjects with herpes zoster were undertaken. In a double-blind randomized trial of intravenous acyclovir 5 mg/kg
every 8 h for 5 days, in 56 nonimmunocompromised patients with zoster,
Peterslund and colleagues found that the 27 acyclovir patients had significantly improved cutaneous healing and shortened acute pain (35). Pain
3 months after zoster was not prevented by the acyclovir therapy (36).
Subsequently, Bean and colleagues in a double-blind placebo-controlled
study of 500 mg/m^2 three times a day for 5 days found similar encouraging improvement in acute pain and cutaneous lesions as well as a decreased
period of viral shedding in acyclovir recipients (37). Comparable results
were reported by McGill and colleagues in a double-blind, placebo-controlled randomized study of 5 mg/kg every 8 h for 5 days in 37 patients
with acute herpes zoster (38). Significantly more rapid improvement in
cutaneous involvement and a favorable effect on acute pain were noted
in acyclovir recipients. Neither eye involvement nor postherpetic neuralgia
was prevented in the acyclovir recipients. Juel-Jensen et al. found in a

randomized, double-blind, placebo-controlled trial of 10 mg/kg every 8 h for 5 days in 40 patients with zoster that acyclovir recipients fared better in pain and cutaneous parameters but not significantly so (39). Eye complications of ophthalmic zoster appeared to be fewer in the acyclovir group. A more recently reported study of intravenous acyclovir 10 mg/kg every 8 h for 5 days also demonstrated improvement in skin lesions and pain favoring acyclovir but not statistically significant differences. In this study complications (generalization of rash and keratitis) were seen only in the placebo group (40).

All controlled studies of intravenous acyclovir for therapy of herpes zoster in nonimmunocompromised patients have shown differences favoring acyclovir but have not shown clear value in preventing complications, such as postherpetic neuralgia. Not all patients in these studies were treated early in the course of zoster, and therapy was usually terminated after 5 days.

Studies in immunosuppressed patients with zoster have demonstrated a clear role of intravenous acyclovir therapy. Following the initial report of a favorable response of herpes zoster to acyclovir therapy by Selby et al. (41), Balfour et al. entered 94 immunosuppressed patients into a double-blind, placebo-controlled study of 500 mg/m^2 of acyclovir administered intravenously three times a day for 7 days (42). The progression of zoster was halted, including cutaneous dissemination and visceral involvement. Based on the clear results of this study, no additional placebo-controlled studies have been performed in immunosuppressed subjects. Meyers et al. noted favorable outcomes in 40 bone marrow transplant patients treated with 500 mg/m^2 every 8 h for 7 days (43). Results were superior to those usually seen in this group of patients at high risk of complications. In a comparison study of intravenous acyclovir (500 mg/m^2 every 8 h for 7 days) and intravenous vidaribine (10 mg/kg/day for 7 days) in 22 immunocompromised patients, Shepp et al. found acyclovir to be superior (44). The frequency of cutaneous dissemination; the periods of culture positivity and new lesion formation; the intervals to decreased pain, pustulation, crusting, and healing; and the incidence of fever were all significantly improved with acyclovir therapy. Some immunocompromised patients with zoster may require therapy longer than 7 days (45), and zoster may recur shortly following successful therapy in profoundly immunosuppressed patients (46).

As suggested by the initial favorable report of Selby et al. (41), intravenous acyclovir may also favorably alter the course of varicella. In the only controlled study published, Proper et al. administered acyclovir 500 mg/m² every 8 h for 7 days or placebo to immunosuppressed children (47). Of the 11 placebo patients without pneumonitis at entry, five developed pneumonitis, compared to none of the seven acyclovir recipients. In this study, other clinical parameters were not significantly different between the two groups. In a report of intravenous acyclovir therapy of eight immunosuppressed children with varicella, Balfour noted that patients treated before the third day of the rash recovered without complications, whereas many of those treated later did not (48). Other reports have concluded that intravenous acyclovir is beneficial for treatment of varicella in immunosuppressed children (49) and that such therapy is superior to intravenous vidarabine (50).

In only one instance has intravenous acyclovir therapy in normal individuals with varicella been studied. Al-Nakib et al. found that when normal adults were treated with acyclovir 10 mg/kg every 8 h for 5 days or placebo in a double-blind study, acyclovir recipients had more rapid resolution of vesicles and less fever on the third, fourth, and sixth days of therapy (51). Otherwise, no significant differences in clinical parameters between acyclovir and placebo recipients were noted.

A number of case reports of acyclovir therapy for complications of herpes zoster and varicella have also been published. Such reports have concluded that intravenous acyclovir may be valuable for therapy of encephalitis associated with herpes zoster (52-57), facial palsy associated with herpes zoster (58,59), and pneumonitis in adult varicella (60).

Adverse effects with intravenous acyclovir therapy have been few. Rises in serum creatinine have been noted in some studies, particularly in instances in which the drug has been infused rapidly (37), but this side effect is rare when the drug is infused slowly over 1 h and good hydration is maintained (61). This adverse effect is due to deposition of the drug in the kidneys and is usually transient and totally reversible. Nausea, vomiting, and abdominal pain are occasionally encountered and often resolve with lowering the dose or skipping a dose (62). If infiltration of acyclovir at a high concentration occurs in the skin, local side effects such as a vesicular reaction (63) may occur. Finally, in complicated patients receiving multiple other drugs as well as intravenous acyclovir, reversible neurologic symptoms such as lethargy, agitation, tremor, disorientation, and transient hemiparesis have been reported (64). In general, intravenous acyclovir therapy for zoster is exceedingly well tolerated and free of adverse reactions.

Oral Therapy

Most patients with VZV infections are not ill enough to warrant hospitalization, and intravenous acyclovir therapy is therefore inappropriate. Fortunately, acyclovir is available in oral formulations that are used for therapy of herpes simplex infections, and the possibility of outpatient oral acyclovir therapy of VZV infections interests many clinicians. Acyclovir capsules given at 200 mg five times a day early in the course of zoster may be helpful (65), but because of the higher drug levels needed to inhibit replication of VZV, compared to HSV, and the 20% absorption of oral acyclovir, most clinicians thought that higher doses would be needed. In a double-blind, placebo-controlled study of 400 mg by mouth five times a day for 5 days in 41 patients with acute herpes zoster, acyclovir recipients experienced reduced days of new lesion formation within the affected dermatome but no other significant differences (66). In a second study of a similar dosage given for 10 days, the outcome in acyclovir recipients was better than that in placebo recipients in almost all parameters, but statistically significant differences were not demonstrated (67). In a comparison of intravenous acyclovir 5 mg/kg three times a day and oral acyclovir 400 mg five times a day for 5 days, no differences were noted in the pain or cutaneous healing (68). The need for a higher oral dosage for successful therapy of zoster was anticipated (69), and studies of 600 and 800 mg five times a day were undertaken. In a double-blind, placebo-controlled study of 600 mg five times a day for 10 days in 71 patients with ophthalmic zoster, Cobo et al. noted that a beneficial effect of acyclovir therapy was seen primarily in patients treated within 72 h (70,71). While signs and symptoms of zoster resolved more promptly and viral shedding was decreased in acyclovir-treated patients, this study documented a striking difference in the incidence and severity of the eye complications of zoster. Dendritic keratopathy, stromal keratitis, and uveitis occurred significantly less frequently in acyclovir recipients. Although acute pain was less in acyclovir recipients, postherpetic neuralgia was unaffected.

In the United Kingdom, a large double-blind, placebo-controlled study was undertaken to evaluate the effectiveness of 800 mg of acyclovir administered five times a day for 7 days to nonimmunocompromised patients over age 60 with zoster of 72 h duration or less. A 1986 analysis of 205 cases in nonimmunocompromised patients (72) showed a significant effect of acyclovir in reducing times to arrest of new lesion formation, loss of vesicles, and full crusting in patients entered within 48 h of the onset of the rash. Acute pain was also reduced in acyclovir recipients. A subsequent report including 364 patients entered in this study confirmed the original observations and included an evaluation of postherpetic neuralgia (73). No effect of acyclovir on the occurrence of pain in the 6 months following the zoster was noted.

A similar study of the 800-mg five-times-a-day dosage was undertaken in the United States, except therapy was continued for 10 days and 187 adults of any age with zoster of 72 h duration or less were entered (67). Compared to placebo recipients, acyclovir recipients experienced significantly shortened times to cessation of viral shedding (2.3 vs. 3.1 days), to 50% scabbing (3.3 vs. 4.8 days), and to 50% healing (7.1 vs. 9.6 days). After 2 days of therapy, the frequency of new lesion formation (31.4% vs. 51.7%) and the severity of acute pain were reduced in acyclovir recipients. In a follow-up of patients for the occurrence of pain, acyclovir recipients experienced less pain than placebo recipients (37.5% vs. 52.6%), particularly a persistent pain (4.2% vs. 16.7%) in months 1-3 following the zoster. No differences in pain were noted beyond 3 months. Although this study does not show that acyclovir prevents the life-disrupting type of postherpetic neuralgia that persists for years, the results are at least encouraging that acyclovir therapy may favorably affect the occurrence of postherpetic neuralgia.

No controlled studies of oral acyclovir therapy of zoster in immunocompromised patients have been accomplished. However, oral acyclovir, taken continuously, in a prophylactic manner, may prevent VZV infections in immunocompromised subjects in a manner similar to its effect on HSV infections (74,75).

Careful studies of oral acyclovir for therapy of varicella have not been reported. Oral acyclovir has been given to immunocompromised children with varicella and appears to be well tolerated (76). Its effectiveness is not yet clear.

In controlled studies of oral acyclovir, with dosages up to 4 g a day, for therapy of herpes zoster, the drug has proved to be exceedingly well tolerated and safe. Although common complaints, such as nausea, vomiting, and headache, are occasionally seen in acyclovir recipients, such complaints are seen with equal frequency in placebo recipients. Hematologic studies and blood chemistry studies appear to be unaffected by oral acyclovir therapy.

Topical Acyclovir

Few studies of acyclovir used topically for VZV infections have been done. Levin et al. reported a double-blind study of 5% acyclovir in propylene glycol or vehicle alone in 43 immunocompromised patients with localized herpes zoster (77). Topical applications were made every 4h for 10 days. Patients treated with acyclovir healed the skin lesions significantly more rapidly and had a somewhat shorter duration of pain. The practical difficulty of frequent topical applications, as well as the greater ease of oral acyclovir therapy, makes it unlikely that topical acyclovir will be used widely for herpes zoster.

Topical acyclovir used in the eye has been compared to intraocular topical steroids for treatment of acute ophthalmic herpes zoster (78). Corneal epithelial disease resolved significantly more rapidly in acyclovir-treated patients. Steroid-treated patients required a significantly longer period of therapy than acyclovir recipients. A 63% recurrence rate occurred in the steroid group, compared to 0% in the acyclovir group. Either topical acyclovir favorably affected the outcome of ophthalmic zoster or topical steroids adversely affected the outcome. The precise role of topical intraocular acyclovir for ophthalmic zoster is not clear. Based on the excellent results with oral acyclovir, such therapy may not be necessary if appropriate oral acyclovir therapy is used.

CONCLUSIONS

Based on current information, it is clear that acyclovir has an important role in the treatment of VZV infections (Table 2). In immunocompromised patients with potentially serious herpes zoster, intravenous acyclovir should be administered at 500 mg/m^2 (approximately 10 mg/kg) every 8 h for 7 days, or longer if needed. Similar therapy may be employed for immunosuppressed patients with potentially serious varicella. For ambu-

TABLE 2 Uses of Acyclovir for VZV Infections

Route	Dosage	Indication
Intravenous	500 mg/m^2 (10 mg/kg) every 8 h in a 1-h infusion for 7 days	Potentially serious varicella or herpes zoster usually in immunosuppressed patients
Oral	600-800 mg every 4 h 5 times a day for 7-10 days	Potentially serious cases of herpes zoster in the elderly or cases of ophthalmic zoster

latory immunosuppressed patients with less serious VZV infections, perhaps oral acyclovir therapy will suffice, but studies have not yet been reported.

Information regarding the precise role of oral acyclovir for VZV infections is not clear. Most younger patients with zoster require only conservative symptomatic therapy. For elderly nonimmunosuppressed patients with potentially serious zoster, and patients with ophthalmic zoster, either intravenous acyclovir therapy or oral acyclovir 600-800 mg five times a day for 7-10 days would be appropriate. Perhaps, for some patients, several days of intravenous acyclovir, followed by oral acyclovir would also be of benefit. No data available to date document a role of oral acyclovir in therapy of varicella, although questions regarding its role in therapy of adults with varicella will continue to be asked.

No consensus exists as to whether combination acyclovir therapy and systemic steroid therapy might lessen the frequency or severity of postherpetic neuralgia. The efficacy of systemic steroids used along with acyclovir for prevention of postherpetic neuralgia has not been shown (15). Such combination therapy cannot be recommended at present.

Acyclovir appears to favorably alter the course of human VZV infections and to prevent certain serious complications. Because VZV infections are so common and most VZV infections have benign outcomes, acyclovir should not be used for most infections. However, when targeted to those cases in which varicella or zoster is likely to be serious, use of acyclovir is clearly appropriate. Because of the effectiveness and safety of acyclovir, it is unlikely that other antiviral agents will soon surpass this drug for control of VZV infections.

REFERENCES

1. Gershon, A. A., and Steinberg, S. P. (1981). Antibody responses to varicella-zoster virus and the role of antibody in host defense. *Am. J. Med. Sci.* 282: 12-17.
2. Hyman, R. W., Ecker, J. R., and Tenser, R. B. (1983). Varicella-zoster virus RNA in human trigeminal ganglia. *Lancet* 2:814-816.
3. Gilden, D. H., Vafai, A., Shtram, Y., Becker, Y., Devlin, M., and Wellish, M. (1983). Varicella-zoster virus DNA in human sensory ganglia. *Nature* 306: 478-801.
4. Hope-Simpson, R. E. (1965). The nature of herpes zoster: A long-term study and a new hypothesis. *Proc. R. Soc. Med.* 58:9-20.
5. Ragozzino, M. W., Melton, L. J., Kurland, L. T., Chu, C. P., and Perry, H. O. (1982). Population-based study of herpes zoster and its sequalae. *Medicine* 61:310-316.

6. Berger, R., Florent, G., and Just, M. (1981). Decrease of the lymphoproliferative response to varicella-zoster virus antigen in the aged. *Infect. Immun.*
32:24-27.

7. Liesegang, T. J. (1984). The varicella-zoster virus: Systemic and ocular features. *J. Am. Acad. Dermatol.* 11:165-191.

8. Cobo, M., Foulks, G. N., Liesegang, T., Lass, J., Sutphin, J., Wilhelmus,
K., and Jones, D. B. (1987). Observations on the natural history of herpes
zoster ophthalmicus. *Current Eye Res.* 6:195-199.

9. Sauer, G. C. (1955). Herpes zoster: Treatment of postherpetic neuralgia with
cortisone, corticotropin and placebos. *Arch. Dermatol.* 71:488-491.

10. Elliott, F. A. (1964). Treatment of herpes zoster with high doses of prednisone. *Lancet* 2:610-611.

11. Eaglstein, W. H., Katz, R., and Brown, J. A. (1970). The effects of early
corticosteroid therapy on the skin eruption and pain of herpes zoster. *JAMA*
211:1681-1683.

12. Keczkes, K., and Basheer, A. M. (1980). Do corticosteroids prevent postherpetic neuralgia? *Br. J. Derm.* 102:551-555.

13. Levinson, W., and Shaw, J. C. (1985). Treatment of herpes zoster with corticosteroids—fact or faith? *West. J. Med.* 142:117-118.

14. Clemmensen, O. J., and Andersen, K. E. (1984). ACTH versus prednisone
and placebo in herpes zoster treatment. *Clin. Exp. Dermatol.* 9:557-563.

15. Esmann, V., Geil, J. P., Kroon, S., Fogh, H., Peterslund, N. A., Petersen,
C. S., Ronne-Rasmussen, J. O., and Danielsen, L. (1987). Prednisolone does
not prevent post-herpetic neuralgia. *Lancet* 2:126-129.

16. Juel-Jensen, B. E., MacCallum, F. O., MacKenzie, A. M. R., and Pike, M.
C. (1970). Treatment of zoster with idoxuridine in dimethyl sulfoxide. Results of two double-blind controlled trials. *Br. Med. J.* 4:776-780.

17. Dawber, R. (1974). Idoxuridine in herpes zoster: Further evaluation of intermittent topical treatment. *Br. Med. J.* 2:526-527.

18. Davis, C. M., VanDersarl, J. V., and Coltman, C. A. (1973). Failure of cy-
tarabine in varicella-zoster infections. *JAMA* 224:122-123.

19. Stevens, D. A., Jordon, G. W., Waddell, T. F., and Merigan, T. C. (1973).
Adverse effect of cytosine arabinoside on disseminated zoster in a controlled
trial. *N. Engl. J. Med.* 289:873-878.

20. Whitley, R. J., Chien, L. T., Dolin, R., Galasso, G. J., Alford, C. A., and
Collaborative Study Group. (1976). Adenine arabinoside therapy of herpes
zoster in the immunosuppressed. *N. Engl. J. Med.* 294:1193-1199.

21. Whitley, R. J., Soong, S. J., Dolin, R., Betts, R., Linnemann, C., Alford,
C. A., and the NIAID Collaborative Antiviral Study Group. (1982). Early
vidarabine therapy to control the complications of herpes zoster in immunosuppressed patients. *N. Engl. J. Med.* 307:971-975.

22. Whitley, R., Hilty, M., Haynes, R., Bryson, Y., Connor, J. D., Soong, S.-J.,
Alford, C. A., and the NIAID Collaborative Study Group (1982). Vidarabine therapy of varicella in immunosuppressed patients. *J. Pediatr.* 101:125-131.

23. Wade, N. A., Lepow, M. L., Veazey, J., and Meuwissen, H. J. (1985). Progressive varicella in three patients with Wiskott-Aldrich syndrome: Treatment with adenine arabinoside. *Pediatrics* 75:672-675.

24. Rasmussen, L., Holmes, A. R., Hofmeister, B., and Merigan, T. C. (1977). Multiplicity-dependent replication of varicella-zoster virus in interferon-treated cells. *J. Gen. Virol.* 35:361-368.

25. Stevens, D. A., and Merigan, T. C. (1972). Interferon, antibody, and other host factors in herpes zoster. *J. Clin. Invest.* 51:1170-1178.

26. Merigan, T. C., Rand, K. H., Pollard, R. B., Abdallah, P. S., Jordon, G. W., and Fried, R. P. (1978). Human leukocyte interferon for the treatment of herpes zoster in patients with cancer. *N. Engl. J. Med.* 298:981-987.

27. Arvin, A. M., Kushner, J. H., Feldman, S., Baehner, R. L., Hammond, D., and Merigan, T. C. (1982). Human leukocyte interferon for the treatment of varicella in children with cancer. *N. Engl. J. Med.* 306:761-765.

28. Schaeffer, H. J., Beauchamp, L., De Miranda, P., Elion, G. B., Bauer, D. J., and Collins, P. (1978). 9-(2-Hydroxyethoxymethyl)guanine activity against viruses of the herpes group. *Nature* 272:583-585.

29. Crumpacker, C. S., Schnipper, L. E., and Zaia, J. A. (1979). Growth inhibition by acycloguanosine of herpes viruses isolated from human infections. *Antimicrob. Agents Chemother.* 15:642-645.

30. Biron, K. K., and Elion, G. B. (1980). In vitro susceptibility of varicella-zoster virus to acyclovir. *Antimicrob. Agents Chemother.* 18:443-447.

31. De Miranda, P., Whitley, R. J., Blum, M. R., Keeney, R. E., Barton, N., Cocchetto, D. M., Good, S., Hemstreet, G. P., Kirk, L. E., Page, D. A., and Elion, G. B. (1978). Acyclovir kinetics after intravenous infusion. *Clin. Pharmacol. Ther.* 26:718-728.

32. Blum, M. R., Liao, S. H. T., and De Miranda, P. (1982). Overview of acyclovir pharmacokinetic disposition in adults and children. *Am. J. Med.* 73 (1A):186-192.

33. Fyfe, J., and Biron, K. (1980). Phosphorylation of acyclovir by a thymidine kinase induced by varicella zoster virus. In Nelson, J. D., and Grassi, C. (eds.): *Current Chemotherapy and Infectious Disease.* Proceedings of the 11th International Congress on Chemotherapy. 19th Interscience Conference on Antimicrobial Agents and Chemotherapy. Boston, Vol. 2. Washington D.C., American Society of Microbiology, pp. 1378-1379.

34. Biron, K., Fyfe, J. A., Noblin, J. E., and Elion, G. B. (1982). Selection and preliminary characterization of acyclovir-resistant mutants of varicella zoster virus. *Am. J. Med.* 73(1A):383-386.

35. Peterslund, N. A., Seyer-Hansen, K., Ipsen, J., Esmann, V., Schonheyder, J., and Juhl, H. (1981). Acyclovir in herpes zoster. *Lancet* 2:827-830.

36. Esmann, V., Ipsen, J., Peterslund, N. A., Seyer-Hansen, K., Schonheyder, H., and Juhl, H. (1982). Therapy of acute herpes zoster with acyclovir in the non-immunocompromised host. *Am. J. Med.* 73(1A):320-325.

37. Bean, B., Braun, C., and Balfour, H. H. (1982). Acyclovir therapy for acute herpes zoster. *Lancet* 2:118-121.
38. McGill, J., MacDonald, D. R., Fall, C., McKendrick, G. D. W., and Copplestone, A. (1983). Intravenous acyclovir in acute herpes zoster infection. *J. Infect.* 6:157-161.
39. Juel-Jensen, B. E., Khan, J. A., and Pasvol, G. (1983). High-dose intravenous acyclovir in the treatment of zoster: A double-blind, placebo-controlled trial. *J. Infect.* 6(Suppl. 1):31-36.
40. VandeBroek, P. J., VanderMeer, J. W. M., Mulder, J. D., Versteeg, J., and Mattie, H. (1984). Limited value of acyclovir in the treatment of uncomplicated herpes zoster: A placebo-controlled study. *Infection* 12:338-341.
41. Selby, P. P., Powle, R. J., and Jameson, B. (1979). Parenteral acyclovir therapy for herpes virus infection in man. *Lancet* 2:1267-1270.
42. Balfour, H. H., Bean, B., Laskin, O. L., Ambinder, R. E., Meyers, J. D., Wade, J. C., Zaia, J. A., Aeppli, D., Kirk, L. E., Segreti, A. C., Keeney, R. E., and the Burroughs Wellcome Collaborative Acyclovir Study Group. (1983). Acyclovir halts progression of herpes zoster in immunocompromised patients. *N. Engl. J. Med.* 308:1448-1453.
43. Meyers, J. D., Wade, J. C., Shepp, D. H., and Newton, B. (1984). Acyclovir treatment of varicella zoster infection in the compromised host. *Transplantation* 37:571-574.
44. Shepp, D. H., Dandliker, P. S., and Meyers, J. D. (1986). Treatment of varicella-zoster virus infection in severely immunocompromised patients: A randomized comparison of acyclovir and vidaribine. *N. Engl. J. Med.* 314:208-212.
45. McMonigal, K. A., Balfour, H. H., and Bean, B. (1987). Response of immunocompromised patients with acute herpes zoster to intravenous acyclovir. *Minn. Med.* 70:333-335.
46. Oblon, D. J., Elfenbein, G. J., Rand, K., and Weiner, R. S. (1986). Recurrent varicella-zoster infection after acyclovir therapy in immunocompromised patients. *South. Med. J.* 79:256-257.
47. Prober, C. G., Kirk, L. E., and Keeney, R. E. (1982). Acyclovir therapy in chickenpox in immunosuppressed children—A collaborative study. *J. Pediatr.* 101:622-625.
48. Balfour, H. H. (1984). Intravenous acyclovir therapy for varicella in immunocompromised children. *J. Pediatr.* 104:134-136.
49. Dan, M., Michaeli, D., and Siegman-Igra, Y. (1985). Intravenous acyclovir for herpesvirus in immunocompromised patients. *Isr. J. Med.* 21:27-31.
50. Shulman, S. T. (1985). Acyclovir treatment of disseminated varicella in childhood malignant neoplasms. *Am. J. Dis. Child.* 139:137-140.
51. Al-Nakib, W., Al-Kandari, S., El-Khalik, D. M. A., and El-Shirbiny, A. M. (1983). A randomized controlled study of intravenous acyclovir (Zovirax) against placebo in adults with chickenpox. *J. Infect.* 6(Suppl.):49-56.

52. Steele, R. W., Keeney, R. E., Bradsher, R. W., Moses, E. B., and Soloff, B. L. (1983). Treatment of varicella-zoster meningoencephalitis with acyclovir-demonstration of virus in cerebrospinal fluid by electron microscopy. *Am. J. Clin. Pathol.* 80:57-60.

53. Ehrensaft, D. V., and Safani, M. M. (1985). Acyclovir and disseminated varicella zoster and encephalitis (Letter). *Ann. Intern. Med.* 102:421.

54. Bowman, R. V., Lythall, D. A., and DeWytt, C. N. (1985). A case of herpes zoster associated encephalitis treated with acyclovir. *Aust. N.Z. J. Med.* 15: 43-44.

55. Cheesbrough, J. S., Finch, R. G., and Ward, M. J. (1985). A case of herpes zoster associated encephalitis with rapid response to acyclovir. *Postgrad. Med. J.* 61:145-146.

56. Whyte, M. K. B., and Ind, P. W. (1986). Effectiveness of intravenous acyclovir in immunocompetent patient with herpes zoster encephalitis. *Br. Med. J.* 293:1536-1537.

57. Johns, D. R., and Gress, D. R. (1987). Rapid response to acyclovir in herpes zoster-associated encephalitis. *Am. J. Med.* 82:560-562.

58. Stafford, F. W., and Welch, A. R. (1986). The use of acyclovir in Ramsay Hunt Syndrome. *J. Laryngol. Otol.* 100:337-340.

59. Ivarsson, S., Andreasson, L., and Ahlfors, K. (1987). Acyclovir treatment in a case of facial paralysis caused by herpes zoster. *Pediatr. Infect. Dis. J.* 6:84.

60. Hankins, G. D. V., Gilstrap, L. C., and Patterson, A. R. (1987). Acyclovir treatment of varicella pneumonia in pregnancy (Letter). *Crit. Care Med.* 15: 336-337.

61. Bean, B., and Aeppli, D. (1985). Adverse effects of high-dose intravenous acyclovir in ambulatory patients with acute herpes zoster. *J. Infect. Dis.* 151: 362-365.

62. Balfour, H. H. (1986). Acyclovir therapy for herpes zoster: Advantages and adverse effects. *JAMA* 255:387-388.

63. Sylvester, R. K., Ogden, W. B., Draxier, C. A., and Lewis, F. B. (1986). Vesicular eruption: A local complication of concentrated acyclovir infusions. *JAMA* 255:385-386.

64. Wade, J. C., and Meyers, J. D. (1983). Neurologic symptoms associated with parenteral acyclovir treatment after bone marrow transplantation. *Ann. Intern. Med.* 98:922-925.

65. Finn, R., and Smith, M. A. (1984). Oral acyclovir for herpes zoster (Letter). *Lancet* 2:575.

66. McKendrick, M. W., Case, C., Burke, C., Hickmott, E., and McKendrick, G. D. W. (1984). Oral acyclovir in herpes zoster. *J. Antimicrob. Chemother.* 14:661-665.

67. Huff, J. C., Bean, B., Balfour, H. H., Laskin, O. L., Connor, J. D., Corey, L., Bryson, Y. J., McGuirt, P. (1988). Therapy of herpes zoster with oral acyclovir. *Am. J. Med.* 85(2A): 84-89.

68. Peterslund, N. A., Esmann, V., Ipsen, J., Dencker Christensen, K., and Munck Petersen, C. (1984). Oral and intravenous acyclovir are equally effective in herpes zoster. *J. Antimicrob. Chemother.* 14:185-189.
69. McKendrick, M. W., McGill, J. I., Bell, A. M., Hickmott, E., and Burke, C. (1984). Oral acyclovir for herpes zoster (Letter). *Lancet* 2:925.
70. Cobo, L. M., Foulks, G. N., Liesegang, T., Lass, J.. Sutphin, J., Wilhelmus, K., Jones, D. B., Chapman, S., and Segreti, A. (1985). Oral acyclovir in the therapy of acute herpes zoster ophthalmicus. *Ophthalmology* 92:1574-1583.
71. Cobo, L. M., Foulks, G. N., Liesegang, T., Lass, J., Sutphin, J. E., Wilhelmus, K., Jones, D. B., Chapman, S., Segreti, A. C., and King, D. H. (1986). Oral acyclovir in the treatment of acute herpes zoster ophthalmicus. *Ophthalmology* 93:763-770.
72. McKendrick, M. W., McGill, J. I., White, J. E., and Wood, M. J. (1986). Oral acyclovir in acute herpes zoster. *Br. Med. J.* 293:1529-1532.
73. Wood, M. J., Ogan, P. H., McKendrick, M. W., Care, C. D., McGill, J. I., and Webb, E. M. (1988). Efficacy of oral acyclovir treatment of acute herpes zoster. *Am. J. Med.* 85(2A): 79-83.
74. Pettersson, E., Hovi, T., Ahonen, J., Fiddian, A. P., Salmela, K., Hockerstedt, K., Eklund, B., Von Willebrand, E., and Hayry, P. (1985). Prophylactic oral acyclovir after renal transplantation. *Transplantation* 39:279-281.
75. Stoffel, M., Squifflet, J. P., Pirson, Y., Lamy, M., and Alexandre, G. P. J. (1987). Effectiveness of oral acyclovir prophylaxis in renal transplant recipients. *Transplant. Proc.* 19:2190-2193.
76. Novelli, V. M., Marshall, W. C., Yeo, J., and McKendrick, G. D. (1984). Acyclovir administered perorally in immunocompromised children with varicella-zoster infections. *J. Infect. Dis.* 149:478.
77. Levin, M. J., Zaia, J. A., Hershey, B. J., Davis, L. G., Robinson, G. V., and Segreti, A. C. (1985). Topical acyclovir treatment of herpes zoster in immunocompromised patients. *J. Am. Acad. Dermatol.* 13:590-596.
78. McGill, J., and Chapman, C. (1983). A comparison of topical acyclovir with steroids in the treatment of herpes zoster keratouveitis. *Br. J. Ophthalmol.* 67:746-750.

15
Acyclovir in Epstein-Barr Virus Infections

Stephen E. Straus *National Institute of Allergy and Infectious Diseases, National Institutes of Health, Bethesda, Maryland*

INTRODUCTION

Epstein-Barr virus (EBV) is a herpesvirus that is transmitted predominantly in saliva and infects most people (1). Throughout the world EBV infections typically occur before age 5 and lead to few or no symptoms. Persons who live in hygienic and uncrowded environments, however, commonly avoid exposure to EBV until they initiate intimate sexual behavior during adolescence or early adulthood. One third to one half of primary infections at that age result in acute infectious mononucleosis (IM), a syndrome characterized by fever, pharyngitis, adenopathy, an atypical lymphocytosis, and heterophile antibody responses. These features mainly reflect an excessive immune reaction to the virus.

There are numerous complications of IM, including massive splenomegaly at risk of rupture, hypertrophic tonsils which compromise the airway, encephalitis, hepatitis, hemolytic anemia, neutropenia, and thrombocytopenia (Table 1). In the setting of congenital or acquired cellular immunodeficiencies pneumonia, aplastic anemia, and profound lymphoproliferation, problems can be fatal.

EBV persists in salivary tissues and B lymphocytes for life. Virus reactivation is common, but only in immunocompromised persons such as transplant recipients and AIDS patients does it represent a substantial risk of reinitiating lymphoproliferation and other severe or chronic disorders (Table 1).

TABLE 1 Complications of EBV Infections

Acute	Chronic
Streptococcal pharyngitis	Chronic mononucleosis
Hepatitis	Hemophagocytic syndrome
Granulocytopenia	Aplastic anemia
Hemolytic anemia	Lymphocytic interstitial pneumonia
Thrombocytopenia	Hairy leukoplakia
Splenic rupture	Polyclonal lymphoproliferation
Airway obstruction	African Burkitt's lymphoma
Encephalitis	Nasopharyngeal carcinoma
Pneumonia	Thymic carcinoma
Myocarditis	

TREATMENT OF EBV INFECTIONS

General Considerations

Treatment of EBV infections is primarily supportive, consisting of rest, hydration, antipyretics, and analgesics (2). Admonitions to avoid activities that could lead to splenic rupture are appropriate. Occasionally, hospitalization is required for management of airway compromise, hemolysis, dehydration, splenic rupture, or encephalitis.

Corticosteroids play a controversial role in the medical management of IM. Despite a dearth of objective data, corticosteroids are widely regarded as speeding resolution of the symptoms and signs of IM, presumably through its ability to suppress excessive host reactions to EBV.

Antiviral Therapy

Chronic and grave complications of EBV infections urge us to seek specific and effective therapy. There are now numerous agents known to impair the replication of EBV in vitro or the outgrowth of EBV-infected B cell lines (3-13) (Table 2). The best characterized of these are inhibitors of the viral DNA polymerase, most of which are nucleoside analogs. These drugs differ widely in potency and duration of effect on EBV DNA replication in lymphoblastoid cell lines. Considering both the potency and toxicity of the compounds, the most promising ones should be bromo-vinyldeoxyuridine (BVdU) and ganciclovir (DHPG) (9-13). The former

TABLE 2 Agents Shown to Inhibit EBV Growth in Order of Relative Potency

Agent	Reference
Interferons	
Alpha	3,4
Beta	5
Gamma	3,5
DNA polymerase inhibitors	
Phosphonoacetate	6
Phosphonoformate	7
Acyclovir	8-10
Bromovinyldeoxyuridine	10-12
Ganciclovir	9,10,13
Fluoromethylarabinosyluridine	10
Fluoroiodoarabinosyluridine	10
Fluoroiodoarabinosylcytidine	10

suffers rapid degradation in man and thus is not a practical agent for systemic therapy. The latter compound is known from its extensive use in life-threatening cytomegalovirus infections to exhibit substantial bone marrow toxicity (14). There are anecdotal reports of its activity in severe EBV infection.

Acyclovir

As reviewed more extensively elsewhere in this volume, acyclovir's antiviral action depends on its conversion to a triphosphorylated form. This is facilitated by herpes simplex and varicella zoster viruses by virus-encoded thymidine kinase. EBV was recently found to contain a gene with significant sequence homology to other deoxypyrimidine kinases, but whether an enzymatically active gene product is synthesized is still unknown (15). Thus, the factors promoting phosphorylation of acyclovir in EBV-infected B cells are not yet understood. Nonetheless, acyclovir inhibits EBV DNA replication by 50% at concentrations ranging between 0.1 and 1 μg/ml (8-10). Although not strictly equivalent to the concentration necessary to arrest virus proliferation, this result does suggest that acyclovir possesses in vitro inhibitory activity in the range of drug concentrations that are readily achieved intravenously (5-15 μg/ml) and nearly attained orally (0.5-3 μg/ml) as well (16).

TABLE 3 Outcome of Controlled Trials of Acyclovir for Acute Infectious Mononucleosis

Route	Dose	Duration	Number of patients	Virus recovery rate relative to period of treatment					Clinical improvement	Ref.
				Before	During	Soon after[a]	Long after[b]			
IV	500 mg/m² q8h	5 days	10	4/6	0/6	3/13	4/13	None significant. Resolution of weight loss, pharyngitis?	17
	Placebo	5 days	10	1/5	2/4	4/13	0/2		
IV	10 mg/k q8h	7 days	15	14/15	1/29	12/14	8/15	None significant. Resolution of pharyngitis, tonsillor swelling, weight loss, fever?	18
	Placebo	7 days	16	15/16	30/32	13/15	9/16		
Oral	800 mg 5/day	7 days	28	16/16	18/29	22/22	12/16	None	19
	Placebo	7 days	28	19/20	38/38	29/29	16/20		

[a]Less than 1 month after infection.
[b]More than 1 month after infection.

Acyclovir Trials in Acute EBV Infection

There have been three reports of controlled trials of acyclovir in IM (Table 3). Two entailed the use of intravenous drug for 5 and 7 days, respectively. These studies revealed no conclusive impact of treatment on the duration or severity of symptoms, although there were trends to improvement in some features of the disease. The more rigorous trial of Andersson et al. showed acyclovir to significantly reduce the likelihood of recovering EBV in the saliva (18). This effect was restricted to the period of treatment. A controlled study of high-dose oral acyclovir showed treatment to be associated with a minimal virologic response and no symptomatic benefit (19).

Very recently Andersson et al. reported the results of an open trial of intravenous acyclovir (10 mg/kg three times daily) combined with prednisolone (0.7 mg/kg per day) for 10 days in 11 hospitalized patients with severe mononucleosis (20). Compared to historical controls, the treated patients appeared to have more rapid resolution of fever and adenopathy. Inhibition of virus shedding was not prevented by prednisolone.

Trials in Chronic EBV Infection

As indicated in Table 1, there is a wide range of chronic illness associated with EBV. Most uses of acyclovir in such patients have been on a compassionate basis. There are published reports of beneficial effects of intravenous treatments in polyclonal lymphoproliferative disorders in transplant recipients and in patients with severe chronic mononucleosis with uveitis, pneumonitis, and other visceral complications (21,22). Greenspan and his colleagues (personal communication) performed a placebo-controlled trial of oral desciclovir, an acyclovir pro-drug, in 14 patients with symptomatic infections with human immunodeficiency virus (16). Preliminary analysis indicates treatment to lead to resolution of lesions in drug-treated patients, a finding similar to that of Schofer et al., who used acyclovir itself for treatment (23). Acyclovir has not seemed to benefit boys with the X-linked lymphoproliferative syndrome and severe IM (24).

Recently, we completed a study of intravenous acyclovir (500 mg/m^2 surface area three times daily for 7 days) followed by oral acyclovir (800 mg four times daily for 30 days) in 27 patients with a syndrome of chronic fatigue and unusual EBV serologic profiles (25). There is substantial controversy regarding the role of EBV in this disorder (26). Preliminary analysis of our study indicated no beneficial effects of treatment on the symptoms or laboratory features of this syndrome.

CONCLUSION

Among the agents capable of inhibiting EBV growth (Table 2), acyclovir has been the best studied. Acyclovir levels achieved during intravenous treatment are adequate to transiently inhibit virus shedding in the oropharynx. High-dose oral acyclovir therapy has a more modest influence on virus shedding rates. Considering the pathogenesis of IM, it is not surprising that this virologic response was not accompanied by a clinical response. The features of IM are considered to be largely immunopathologic in nature. It is encouraging that initial data suggest beneficial effects of adding prednisolone, which could afford some symptomatic improvement while not impairing the activity of concomitant antiviral therapy. Controlled trials of corticosteroids alone or in combination with acyclovir for IM are now warranted.

Severe chronic EBV infections are sufficiently rare to make controlled trials difficult. Multicenter studies would need to be undertaken. Theoretically, acyclovir could prove more effective clinically in these disorders than in IM, both because the severity of the chronic infections affords a greater range for potential improvement and because the disease is less likely to resolve spontaneously, unlike IM.

REFERENCES

1. Fleisher, G. R. (1984). Epstein-Barr virus. In Belshe, R. B. (ed.): *Textbook of Human Virology*. Littleton, MA, PSG Publishing, pp. 853-886.
2. Straus, S. E. (1988). Infectious mononucleosis. In Rakel, R. E. (ed.): *Conn's Current Therapy*. Philadelphia, W. B. Saunders, pp. 80-81.
3. Kure, S., Tada, K., Wada, J., and Yoshie, O. (1986). Inhibition of Epstein-Barr virus infection in vitro by recombinant human interferons α and γ. *Virus Res.* 5:377-390.
4. Garner, J. G., Hirsch, M. S., and Schooley, R. T. (1985). Prevention of Epstein-Barr virus-induced B-cell outgrowth by interferon alpha. *Infect. Immun.* 43(3):920-924.
5. Lotz, M., Tsoukas, C. D., Fong, S., Carson, D. A., and Vaughan, J. H. (1985). Regulation of Epstein-Barr virus infection by recombinant interferons. Selected sensitivity to interferon-γ. *Eur. J. Immunol.* 15:520-525.
6. Manor, D., and Margalith, M. (1979). *Cancer Biochem. Biophys.* 3:157-162.
7. Margalith, M., Manor, D., Usieli, V., and Goldblum, N. (1980). Phosphonoformate inhibits synthesis of Eptein-Barr virus (EBV) capsid antigen and transformation of human cord blood lymphocytes by EBV. *Virology* 102:226-230.
8. Colby, B. M., Shaw, J. E., Elion, G. B., and Pagano, J. S. (1980). Effect of acyclovir [9-(2-hydroxyethoxymethyl)guanine] on Epstein-Barr virus DNA replication. *J. Virol.* 34(2):560-568.

9. Van der Horst, C. M., Lin, J.-C., Raab-Traub, N., Smith, M. C., and Pagano, J. S. (1987). Differential effects of acyclovir and 9-(1,3-dihydroxy-2-propoxymethyl) guanine on herpes simplex virus and Epstein-Barr virus in a dually infected human lymphoblastoid cell line. *J. Virol.* 61(2):607-610.

10. Lin, J.-C., Smith, M. C., and Pagano, J. S. (1985). Comparative efficacy and selectivity of some nucleoside analogs against Epstein-Barr virus. *Antimicrob. Agents Chemother.* 27(6):971-973.

11. Zhang, Z.-X., Liu, Y. X., Hong-Shen, C., Allaudeen, H. S., and De Clercq, E. (1984). Effect of (E)-5-(2-bromovinyl)-2'-deoxyuridine on several parameters of Epstein-Barr virus infection. *J. Gen. Virol.* 65:37-46.

12. Lin, J.-C., Smith, M. C., Choi, E. I., De Clercq, E., Verbruggen, A., and Pagano, J. S. (1985). Effect of (E)-5-(2-bromovinyl)-2'-deoxyuridine on replication of Epstein-Barr virus in human lymphoblastoid cell lines. *Antiviral Res.* (Suppl.) 1:121-126.

13. Lin, J.-C., Smith, M. C., and Pagano, J. S. (1984). Prolonged inhibitory effect of 9-(1,3-dihydroxy-2-propoxymethyl)guanine against replication of Epstein-Barr virus. *J. Virol.* 50(1):50-55.

14. Masur, H., Lane, H. C., Palestine, A., Smith, P. D., Manischewitz, J., Stevens, G., Fujikawa, L., Macher, A. M., Nussenblatt, R., Baird, B., Megill, M., Wittek, A., Quinnan, G. V., Parrillo, J. E., Rook, A. H., Eron, L. J., Poretz, D. M., Goldenberg, R. I., Fauci, A. S., and Gelmann, E. P. (1986). Effect of 9-(1,3-dihydroxy-2-propoxymethyl)guanine on serious cytomegalovirus disease in eight immunosuppressed homosexual men. *Ann. Intern. Med.* 104:41-44.

15. Littler, E., Zeuthen, J., McBride, A. A., Trost Sorensen, E., Powell, K. L., Walsh-Arrand, J. E., and Arrand, J. R. (1987). Identification of an Epstein-Barr virus-coded thymidine kinase. *EMBO J.* 5:1959-1966.

16. Brigden, D., and Whiteman, P. (1985). The clinical pharmacology of acyclovir and its prodrugs. *Scand. J. Infect. Dis.* (Suppl.) 47:33-39.

17. Pagano, J. S., Sixbey, J. W., and Lin, J.-C. (1983). Acyclovir and Epstein-Barr virus infection. *J. Antimicrob. Chemother.* 12(Suppl. B):113-121.

18. Andersson, J., Britton, S., Ernberg, I., Andersson, U., Henle, W., Sköldenberg, B., and Tisell, A. (1986). Effect of acyclovir on infectious mononucleosis: A double-blind, placebo-controlled study. *J. Infect. Dis.* 153:283-290.

19. Andersson, J., Sköldenberg, B., Henle, W., Giesecke, J., Ortqvist, A., Julander, I., Gustavsson, E., Akerlund, B., Britton, S., and Ernberg, I. (1987). Acyclovir treatment in infectious mononucleosis: A clinical and virological study. *Infection* 15(Suppl. 1):S14-S21.

20. Andersson, J., and Ernberg, I. (1988). The management of Epstein-Barr virus infections. *Amer. J. Med.* 85 (Suppl 2A):107-115.

21. Hanto, D. W., Frizzera, G., Gajl-Peczalska, K. J., Sakamoto, K., Purtilo, D. T., Balfour, H. H. Jr., Simmons, R. L., and Najarian, J. S. (1982). Epstein-Barr virus-induced B-cell lymphoma after renal transplantation. *N. Engl. J. Med.* 306:913-918.

22. Schooley, R. T., Carey, R. W., Miller, G., Henle, W., Eastman, R., Mark, E. J., Kenyon, K., Wheeler, E. O., and Rubin, R. H. (1986). Chronic Epstein-Barr virus infection associated with fever and interstitial pneumonitis: Clinical and serologic features and response to antiviral chemotherapy. *Ann. Intern. Med.* 104:636-643.
23. Schofer, H., Ochsendorf, F., Helm, F., and Milbrandt, R. (1987). Treatment of oral hairy leukoplasia in AIDS patients with vitamin A acid (topically) or acyclovir (systemically). *Dermatologica* 174:150-151.
24. Sullivan, J. L., Medveczky, P., Forman, S. J., Baker, S. M., Monroe, J. E., and Mulder, C. (1984). Epstein-Barr virus induced lymphoproliferation. *N. Engl. J. Med.* 311(18):1163-1167.
25. Straus, S. E., Dale, J. K., Armstrong, G., Preble, O., Lawley, T., and Henle, W. (1987). Acyclovir (ACV) treatment of a chronic fatigue syndrome with unusual EBV serologic profiles: Lack of efficacy in a controlled trial. *Clin. Res.* 35:618A.
26. Straus, S. E., Tosato, G., Armstrong, G., Lawley, T., Preble, O. T., Henle, W., Davey, R., Pearson, G., Epstein, J., Brus, I., and Blaese, R. M. (1985). Persisting illness and fatigue in adults with evidence of Epstein-Barr virus infection. *Ann. Intern. Med.* 102(1):7-16.

16
Use of Acyclovir in the Immunocompromised Host

Andria Langenberg* and Lawrence Corey   *University of Washington, Seattle, Washington*

INTRODUCTION

The selection of the patient for acyclovir use currently depends on assessment of the frequency, severity, and site of herpesvirus-related symptoms, the immunologic competence of the patient, and an individualized assessment of the risk of toxicity. Acyclovir (ACV) has been repeatedly demonstrated to be highly effective for the treatment of herpes simplex virus (HSV) infections, varicella zoster virus (VZV), and selected cases of Epstein-Barr virus (EBV) infections with low overall toxicity. In this chapter, we discuss the use of acyclovir in the immunocompromised host with HSV and VZV infections. The use of ACV in patients with acquired immunodeficiency syndrome (AIDS) is discussed in a separate chapter.

HERPES SIMPLEX VIRUS INFECTIONS

Herpes simplex virus (HSV) infections are becoming of increasing importance in the immunocompromised (IC) patient. More extensive and suppressive chemotherapeutic regimens for malignancy, immunosuppressive therapy for transplantation, longer survival of patients with extensive burns, and new therapies of primary immunodeficiency disorders such as common variable immunodeficiency have all contributed to longer survival and increased the prevalence of infectious complications among

---

*Present affiliation: University of California, San Francisco, California

these patients. As such, the opportunistic herpesviruses are a frequently recognized cause of clinical infection. Knowledge of their clinical manifestations, the diagnostic mechanisms needed to confirm their presence, and specific treatment recommendations have become the purview of all primary care physicians.

HSV is the most common clinically recognized herpesvirus infection. An awareness of the prevalence of HSV infection is important in identifying and managing the patient at risk of developing severe mucocutaneous and/or disseminated HSV infection. Seroepidemiologic studies have indicated that by age 30, 60% of the U.S. population has antibody to HSV-1, and 20% to HSV-2; by age 50, these prevalence figures increase to 80% and 35%, respectively (1,2). Many of these people appear to be asymptomatic but are at increased risk for reactivating HSV and manifesting clinical symptoms of infection in a setting of deficiency in cell-mediated immunity.

Clinical Manifestations and Complications of HSV Infection

Mucocutaneous infections, both orolabial and genital, are the most common manifestations of HSV. Several studies of the natural history of HSV infection have shown that the frequency and severity of mucocutaneous HSV infections are increased in immunocompromised persons and that the degree of the immunocompromise affects the clinical course. For example, in studies of bone marrow, renal, and cardiac transplantation recipients with HSV-1 antibody prior to transplantation, HSV will reactivate in the first 30 days posttransplant in 35-85% (3-9) of seropositives. Less is known about the frequency of reactivation of HSV-2, but as the seropositivity rate of HSV-2 increases in the population, the frequency of encountering clinically apparent genital HSV in the immunocompromised patient has also increased. Thirty percent of IC patients with symptomatic recurrent HSV have been reported to excrete HSV from multiple sites— i.e., mouth and genitalia, lip and face, etc. (9).

Reactivation of HSV is responsible for most morbidity and mortality in this population. In the normal host, recurrent herpes labialis lesions generally involve an area less than 100 mm², last a mean of 42 h from onset of lesions to resolution of the vesicle stage, have a median of 24 h of maximal viral shedding and pain, and have complete healing in 8 days (10,11). The course in the IC host often involves multiple anatomic sites and an area of greater than 100 mm². Pain may last for 13 days, and lesions may require 10 days for resolution of the vesicle stage and 20 days

TABLE 1   Comparisons of the Symptoms and Signs of Recurrent Orolabial HSV in Normal Versus Immunocompromised Patients

	Normal	IC
Mean lesion size	< 100 mm²	> 100 mm²
Mean time for vesicle stage	< 42 h	10 days
Mean duration of viral shedding	< 24-180 h	13-17 days
Mean duration of pain	24 h	13 days
Mean duration to crusting	8 days	20-30 days
Percent with HSV infection of multiple sites	< 1%	38%
Incidence of fungal superinfection	< 0.1%	20-30%

for complete healing. Viral shedding may persist for 13-17 days. Many patients have lesions that last more than 1 month, with associated secondary infection and disfigurement (Table 1) (4,12,13). The size of the lesions and presence of secondary bacterial or fungal infection are major factors in the rapidity of healing. Particularly severe cases may require skin grafting (5).

HSV reactivation most commonly occurs within 2-4 weeks of induction chemotherapy or transplantation, at the time of maximal immunosuppression (3-5). Dissemination of HSV via viremic spread is a relatively infrequent complication, in that autopsy series demonstrate HSV in visceral tissue in only 0.13-3.1% of patients with malignancies. Visceral involvement is found most frequently in the esophagus and in the pulmonary, hepatic, and central nervous systems (14,15). While cutaneous lesions are often present with disseminated HSV, they may not occur until late in the course, and isolated visceral infection may occur without cutaneous lesions. This is especially true of HSV infection of the esophagus and lung, which often result from contiguous spread of infection from the pharynx (16,17). Table 2 lists visceral anatomic sites clinically affected by HSV infection.

Diagnosis

While many mucocutaneous HSV lesions can be diagnosed clinically, the diversity of the clinical manifestations of HSV, the presence of concomitant superinfection with *Candida*, and the difficulty of discerning HSV infection from lesions due to cytotoxic agents have made laboratory confirmation of the diagnosis useful (26,27).

TABLE 2 Visceral Anatomic Sites and Clinical Syndromes Associated with HSV in the IC Host

Anatomic site	Clinical syndrome
Gastrointestinal	
Esophagus	Occurs weeks (mean 72 days) after bone marrow transplant with dysphagia, nausea and vomiting, fever, and occasional hematemesis. Distal esophagus most commonly involved. Endoscopy with biopsy and brushings is optimal diagnostic procedure. Superinfection with *Candida* common (16,18)
Liver	Occasional cases, presenting with fever, leukopenia, rapid increase in ALT and AST, and occasionally DIC. Distinctive histology with patchy coagulation necrosis with nuclear inclusions (15,19)
Stomach, colon, pancreas	Acute hemorrhagic pancreatitis; gastric or colonic ulcerations with bleeding (20)
Pulmonary	Fever and interstitial infiltrates; focal or diffuse hemorrhagic pneumonitis with a predominance of pathology in the tracheobronchial tree. Associated with ARDS (17,21,22)
Other	Epiglottitis, adrenal necrosis, glomerulonephritis, bone marrow involvement, monoarticular arthritis, encephalitis (rare) (20,23-25)

While typical clustered vesicles on an erythematous base are often the presenting signs of HSV, lesions often ulcerate quickly and are "atypical" in appearance (Table 1; Fig. 1, before page 47). Herpetic mucosal lesions may be indistinguishable from radiation-induced mucositis or confused with fungal or bacterial infections.

Viral isolation in cell culture remains the gold standard for the laboratory confirmation of HSV infection. HSV can be isolated with varying sensitivity and efficacy from a variety of human and nonhuman cell lines. Characteristically, cytopathic effect due to HSV develops within 1-7 days after inoculation. Ninety percent of cultures are positive by 3-4 days after inoculation. Relative to the normal host, in the immunocompromised patient the time period during which virus is excreted from mucocutaneous sites is prolonged and the amount of virus increased (27). In general, dacron or cotton swabs placed into a protein medium containing antibiotics, held at 4 °C, and inoculated within 24 h after collection yield the best sensitivity.

Detection of HSV antigen or DNA from mucosal sites or tissue is being utilized with increasing frequency. Monoclonal antibodies in immunofluorescent or immunoperoxidase assays are useful for type and subtype identification and confirmation. Cytologic examination of lesion scrapings for the presence of giant cells via Tzanck (Giemsa) or Papanicolaou staining is also a rapid and at times clinically useful test with a sensitivity of 50-60% in comparison with cell culture. These cytologic tests, although rapid and inexpensive, do not differentiate HSV from VZV.

Treatment

Acyclovir is the only therapy proven effective in immunocompromised patients for mucocutaneous HSV disease. Few controlled studies exist for treatment of visceral or disseminated HSV in the immunocompromised. However, because of its proven effectiveness in mucocutaneous disease, most authorities recommend the use of systemic acyclovir for the treatment of visceral or disseminated HSV in the IC patient.

Prophylaxis

Fifty to eighty percent of bone marrow transplant patients will reactivate HSV within the first 30 days after induction. Reactivation rates in renal transplant recipients and adults undergoing induction chemotherapy for leukemia approach 25-60%. Several trials have demonstrated continuous systemic ACV to be helpful in HSV-seropositive patients to reduce the risk and severity of reactivation (7,8,28-36). This has been achieved with both IV and oral formulations of acyclovir (Tables 3, 4). Patients treated with prophylactic ACV demonstrated an incidence of HSV recurrence of 0-10% versus 50-80% incidence in placebo-treated patients (Table 3) (7, 8,28,29,37). Approximately 50% of breakthrough recurrences in ACV-treated patients are asymptomatic rather than clinically apparent lesions.

Detailed dosage regimens are outlined in Table 5. The usual IV dose of acyclovir is 250 mg/m^2/8 h. The most commonly utilized oral regimen is 400 mg three times daily. The effectiveness of oral therapy as compared to intravenous (IV) therapy has not been directly evaluated. However, results from a randomized, placebo-controlled study involving bone marrow transplant recipients with an oral regimen of 400 mg five times a day were similar to a previously reported IV dosing study (38). Oral regimens have been associated with an increased incidence of breakthrough recurrences relative to IV regimens perhaps due to the inability of severely ill

TABLE 3 Studies Evaluating Intravenous Acyclovir for Suppression of HSV in Immunocompromised Patients

Author	Condition/ disease	Dose	Frequency (×/day)	Duration (days)	No. of patients on placebo/ acyclovir	HSV infections (%) Placebo	HSV infections (%) Acyclovir	P value
Saral (8)	Bone marrow transplant	250 mg/m²	3	18	10/10	70	0	<.01
Saral (7)	Acute leukemia	250 mg/m²	3	32	15/14	73	0	<.001
Lundgren (28)	Bone marrow transplant	250 mg/m²	2	33	17/16	47 (78)[a]	0	<.05
Hann (29)	Bone marrow transplant	5 mg/kg	2	30	10/10	50	0	<.05
Hann (29)	Acute leukemia	5 mg/kg	2	30	20/19	50	11	<.05
Shepp (38)	Bone marrow	250 mg/m²	1	28	13/14	69	29 (43)[b]	<.05

[a]Patients with high pretransplant HSV titers.
[b]Including asymptomatic viral shedders.
Source: Reproduced, with modifications, with permission from Fiddian (131).

TABLE 4 Studies Evaluating Oral Acyclovir for Suppression of HSV in Immunocompromised Patients

Author	Condition/disease	Dose	Frequency (×/day)	Duration (days)	No. of patients on placebo/acyclovir	HSV infections (%)		P value
						Placebo	Acyclovir	
Wade (16)	Bone marrow transplant	400 mg	5	35	24/24	68	21 (4)[a]	<.01
Prentice (30)	Bone marrow transplant	400 mg	4	42[b]	(10)[c]/20	(50)[c]	25 (20)[a]	NA[d]
Schuch (31)	Bone marrow transplant	400 mg	4	96	–/20	—	25 (10)[a]	NA
Gluckman (32)	Bone marrow transplant	200 mg	4	43	19/20	68	0	<.001
	Non-Hodgkin lymphoma	200 mg	4	42	20/20	70	5	<.001
Anderson (33)	Acute lymphoblastic leukemia							
Fiddian (37)	Cardiac transplant	200 mg	4	84[b]	(10)[c]/10	(80)[c]	0	NA
Griffin (34)	Renal transplant	200 mg	4	84[b]	41/40	55	5	<.001
Pettersson (35)	Renal transplant	200 mg	4	28[b]	17/18	53	0	<.001
Seale (36)	Renal transplant	200 mg	3	30[b]	21/19	67	5	<.001

[a]Percent HSV infections in "compliant" patients.
[b]Prophylaxis commenced after transplantation.
[c]Historical controls.
[d]Not analyzed.
Source: Reproduced, with modifications, from Fiddian (131).

TABLE 5   Current Status of Antiviral Chemotherapy of HSV and VZV Infections in the Immunocompromised Patient

Type of infection	Treatment and benefits
Mucocutaneous HSV infections	
Acute symptomatic first or recurrent episodes	IV or oral acyclovir relieves pain and speeds healing; with localized external lesions, topical acyclovir may be beneficial
Suppression of reactivation of disease	IV or oral acyclovir taken daily prevents recurrences during high-risk periods (e.g., immediately after transplant); lesions will recur when therapy is discontinued
Visceral HSV infections	
HSV esophagitis, pneumonitis, and disseminated HSV infections	No controlled studies have been performed; systemic acyclovir or vidarabine should be considered
Varicella (primary VZV) infections	
Immunosuppressed patients	Acyclovir or vidarabine reduces complications, acyclovir less toxic; immunoprophylaxis with ZIG administration in incubation period is recommended
Varicella zoster infections	
Mucocutaneous infections	Acyclovir, vidarabine, and high-dose leukocyte interferon reduce duration of lesions and complications; acyclovir is the preferred agent
Antiviral dosages	
HSV infection in immunosuppressed patients	IV acyclovir 5 mg/kg q8h × 7-14 days, depending on the response; oral ACV 200-400 mg PO 5 ×/day for 7-14 days; topical ACV 4-6 ×/day for 7-10 days
Suppression of HSV infection	400 mg PO tid (higher dosages can be utilized if clinically necessary)
Varicella zoster infections	IV ACV 500 mg/m^2 or 8-10 mg/kg q8h. Oral not recommended if high risk for dissemination

patients to comply with the oral regimen (39). Protection has been associated with intake of >40% of this dose (40), and complete protection has been reported with 800 mg/day in four divided doses (32).

Single daily dosing of 250 mg/m² IV was ineffective in suppressing HSV recurrences in bone marrow transplant setting, suggesting that relatively constant suppressive levels of acyclovir are needed to provide effective therapy (41). In selected patients, prolonged long-term suppression with doses of 200-400 mg bid may be beneficial (42,43). Once short-term suppression is completed and medication discontinued, patients will often develop recurrences within 7-21 days. These may either be left untreated (if mild) or treated early with topical therapy or systemic therapy as discussed below.

Treatment of Established Infection

Multiple studies have demonstrated the efficacy of acyclovir for the therapy of established HSV in IC patients. In general, oral or systemic acyclovir will produce a 60-80% reduction in viral shedding, a 30-60% decrease in local symptoms, and a 25-65% decrease in duration to complete healing of lesions as compared to placebo-treated patients (9,12,13,37, 44-46). With the intravenous preparation, the most commonly utilized dose is 250 mg/m²/8 h. Orally, 400 mg five times a day is most commonly used. Topical application of 5% ointment six times a day has also demonstrated some benefit, albeit with the disadvantage of treatment only of visible, external lesions (9). Consideration should also be given to treating minor oral symptoms prior to bronchoscopy or minor genital symptoms if urinary catheterization is necessary. Insertion of these instruments through an HSV-infected area may provide a portal for further extension of disease (47).

Detailed treatment regimens are outlined in Table 5. The choice between IV or oral regimens in an individual patient depends on ease of administration. In general, we recommend IV therapy for the severely ill patient and oral therapy for those able to comply with an oral regimen comfortably.

Toxicity

At the doses described above, acyclovir has demonstrated few toxicities. In general, ACV has not been associated with hematologic or hepatic toxicity. Occasionally, neurologic side effects have been reported with high-dose use of ACV in IC patients at doses of 500 mg/m². This dose is usually utilized for the treatment of varicella zoster virus infection (see below) and may cause side effects especially in the setting of renal insufficiency (33). In the setting of dehydration, or preexistent renal disease, transient renal insufficiency has been noted with delivery of more than 5 mg/kg/m² per infusion. Transient tubular insufficiency has been a complication of rapid intravenous infusion in early studies, but slow administration therapy (1 L of fluid per gram of drug), and slower infusion (over 1 h) appears to avoid these renal complications (48).

Occasional increases in liver function tests have been described in ACV recipients, but a causal relationship has not been demonstrated by rechallenge. The confounding variables of multiple drugs and other possible etiologies of hepatic injury in the IC patient obviously often coexist (49). Neither renal function in renal transplant patients (36) nor bone marrow engraftment in bone marrow transplant recipients (32,40) has been adversely affected by ACV administration. Indeed, a decreased incidence and severity of graft vs. host disease has been reported in bone marrow transplant recipients receiving ACV and increased engraftment in those receiving methotrexate (40). Other anecdotal toxicities include rash, severe headache, and dizziness.

Side effects of oral ACV has been minimal. Occasional nausea and vomiting are reported, often apparently related to the lactose in the capsule preparation. Of interest, in patients on suppressive therapy some of these side effects appear to decrease with continued use of the drug.

Drug Resistance

HSV isolates that are resistant in vitro to ACV have been recognized (50). In vitro resistance to ACV may occur in three possible mechanisms: viruses that are deficient in the thymidine kinase (TK) enzyme that phosphorylates acyclovir, viruses with an altered TK enzyme that is inefficient in phosphorylating ACV, or viruses that have a DNA polymerase that is resistant to acyclovir triphosphate. Acyclovir-resistant strains have been isolated from patients who have never received acyclovir (51,52). Clinically, the TK-deficient form is the most common mechanism of in vitro resistance to acyclovir. It is of interest to note that TK-deficient HSV viruses are generally less neurovirulent and less efficient at establishing latency in vitro (53-56). However, some neurovirulent TK strains have been described. Strains that are TK altered or DNA polymerase resistant are in general fully neurovirulent and hence may be of more clinical and epidemiologic concern.

Correlation of clinical response with isolation of resistant strains has not been consistent, and both sensitive and resistant isolates of HSV-1 and

HSV-2 have been obtained from IC patients on prophylactic or suppressive therapeutic regimens who have breakthrough recurrences (29,55,57, 58). It appears that most patients are infected with a heterogeneous population of herpes simplex viruses—some ACV sensitive and some more resistant. Continued ACV use may select out the resistant isolates. Stopping ACV is often associated with "recolonization of the lesions with ACV-sensitive strains" (59). See Chapter 17 for a review of ACV resistance.

The most frequent clinical situation in which ACV-resistant strains are encountered is the IC patient with multiple recurrences of HSV and to whom multiple courses of ACV have been administered (40). Prophylaxis may reduce the chance for emergence by reducing viral multiplicity (60), although formal investigation of the relative risk of emergence of resistance with continuous versus intermittent therapy is needed. Higher doses of acyclovir or use of another antiviral agent such as vidarabine, ganciclovir, or foscarnet may be necessary. In selected cases, evaluation of the in vitro sensitivity of isolates from nonresponding lesions may be useful. The use of alternative antivirals may be necessary to achieve healing.

In summary, we currently recommend that all candiates for bone marrow, renal, heart, heart-lung, and liver transplantation and those with hematologic malignancy (prior to induction of chemotherapy) undergo routine HSV serology. If the patient is seropositive, prophylaxis with systemic ACV as outlined in Figure 2 is recommended. If the patient is seronegative to HSV, no prophylactic intervention is necessary. For established disease, we generally recommend prompt therapy with systemic acyclovir. This will help reduce the morbidity and rate of visceral spread of infection. If virus persists from lesions for extended periods of time, testing for in vitro resistance to acyclovir in a reference laboratory is recommended.

VARICELLA ZOSTER VIRUS INFECTIONS

Recent reviews have detailed the significant morbidity and occasional mortality of varicella zoster virus (VZV) infections in immunocompetent and immunocompromised patients (47,61-63). The increasing number of immunocompromised patients and their longer survival have increased the frequency of VZV infections in this patient group. In addition VZV is a frequent complication of HIV infection (64). While generally self-limited in normal children, primary varicella in susceptible IC children, particularly those with acute lymphocytic leukemia, has been shown to result in visceral dissemination and pneumonia in one third of cases with an attendant mortality of 7% (65).

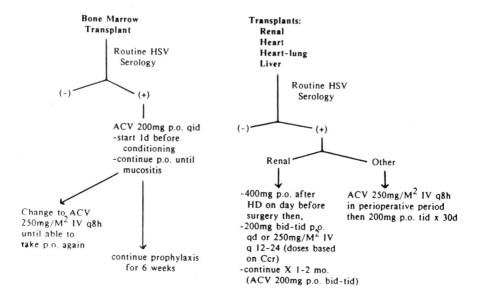

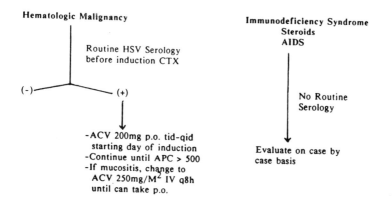

FIGURE 2 Strategy for use of prophylactic ACV in IC patients. Abbreviations: qid, 4 times daily; q8h, every 8h; HD, hemodialysis; bid, twice a day; tid, 3 times a day; qd, daily; Ccr, creatinine clearance; CTX, chemotherapy; APC, absolute poly count. [Source: Reproduced, with modifications, with permission from Gold, D. and Corey, L. (44).]

In general, antiviral chemotherapy is warranted in all cases of varicella and in most cases of herpes zoster in IC patients. Acyclovir is an important antiviral agent with low toxicity for the treatment of these VZV
infections in the immunocompromised patient. In addition, in selected
patients, vidarabine and/or leukocyte interferon may be useful therapeutic drugs.

Clinical Manifestations

In temperate regions, 85% of varicella infections occur before age 10. In
tropical and semitropical countries varicella infection occurs at an older
age, and the frequency of susceptible women of childbearing age is higher
(61,63). The incubation period of varicella varies from 11 to 21 days. After
exposure, virus replicates locally in the nasopharynx; a primary leukocyte-
associated viremia then occurs with seeding of reticuloendothelial cells,
followed by a secondary viremia with dissemination to the skin and vis-
cera. The clinical manifestations of varicella consist of fever and the development of a papulovesicular rash beginning on the face and trunk that
then extends peripherally over the next 2-5 days and lasts 5-7 days. Complications in the immunocompetent patient are uncommon but include
pneumonitis, hepatitis, or clinical encephalitis.

In immunocompromised patients, the severity of the cutaneous disease and the frequency of visceral dissemination are markedly increased.
The degree of impairment of cell-mediated immunity has been correlated
with clinical severity of illness (66,67). Prolonged new lesion formation
with an increased number and duration of large vesicular lesions is noted,
and hemorrhage into the lesions is common. Fever may persist for up to
2 weeks. Visceral disease occurs in one third of patients, and the overall
untreated mortality is about 7%. Mortality rates of greater than 20% have
been reported in some untreated populations (65). Pneumonitis, hepatitis,
encephalitis, myelitis, Guillain-Barré, and coagulopathy can be manifestations of dissemination. Another complication often encountered is secondary bacterial infection usually due to staphylococci or Group A strepto-
cocci.

Diagnosis

Seroepidemiologic studies indicate that less than 5% of cases are subclinical, and thus the diagnosis of varicella infection can usually be made
clinically (68). Laboratory diagnosis can be useful in differentiating VZV
from HSV and from other vesiculobullous diseases. VZV grows in human

fibroblast cell lines, usually requiring 7-10 days for identification by its characteristic cytopathic effect. As VZV is quite cell associated, the scraping of lesions for the detection of VZV antigen by direct immunofluorescent assay (IFA) detection has increased sensitivity over cell culture. The smear for IFA can be prepared from the base of a lesion at the time of swabbing for culture, or prepared in the clinical laboratory from the culture swab. Staining with polyclonal or monoclonal antibodies is the method used in most clinical virology labs. These assays have excellent specificity (69,70).

In addition, lesion scraping may be stained by Wright-Giemsa (Tzanck preparation) to visualize multinucleated giant cells characteristic of herpesvirus cytopathology. The Tzanck prep is 50-70% sensitive in comparison to viral isolation. Although rapid, inexpensive, and confirmatory if positive, the Tzanck test does not distinguish HSV from VZV, and a negative result does not reliably exclude a herpesvirus etiology (71). Antibodies to VZV rise within 2-20 days after onset of lesions and will with most assays (ELISA and IFA) persist for life (72,73). The Western blot assay may distinguish primary from secondary antibody responses to VZV (74). A positive antibody titer indicates past exposure to VZV and is an excellent indicator of who is susceptible and hence a candidate for passive immunoprophylaxis (see below).

Prevention

Prevention of visceral dissemination is the most important goal for the treatment of varicella in the immunocompromised host. Studies in the 1970s indicated that passive immunoprophylaxis with high-titered human immune globulin (ZIG), if given early in the incubation period, will prevent 50% and/or ameliorate up to 80% of varicella infection (75). ZIG is most effective in prevention of infection if given within 72 h of onset of exposure. It will diminish disease signs (i.e., decrease number of lesions) and decrease fever if given up to 10 days after exposure. As such, all susceptible immunocompromised persons should be given VZIG at a dose of 1 vial (2 cc IM) per 40 lb. of body weight (76). If lesions develop despite the use of VZIG, then antiviral chemotherapy may be administered.

The recent development of a live attenuated varicella vaccine will have a large impact on the clinical management of varicella infection in IC patients. Developed in Japan over 15 years ago (77), a live attenuated VZ vaccine has been shown to be immunogenic, safe, and protective in normal (78,79) as well as immunocompromised children (80-84). The vaccine is given IM, replicates locally, and may occasionally produce cutaneous local or even disseminated lesions. However, no cases of severe varicella have occurred in leukemic children after immunization. Low-grade fever has been reported 10-14 days after inoculation, and mild rashes may occasionally occur (84,86). Eight percent of leukemic vaccinees with household exposure to VZ virus remained free of illness after vaccination. Mild disease with an average of 50 lesions developed in the remainder (82). Thus, despite the occasional vaccine breakthrough, varicella after vaccination in leukemic children appears mild (82,84). The vaccine strain can become latent in dorsal nerve root ganglia and reactivate to cause zoster. The frequency of the development of zoster after vaccination appears to be one third of the frequency after naturally acquired varicella (85).

Immunocompromised children are to be vaccinated while in remission. The duration of protection conferred by the vaccine is unclear, with loss of detectable serum antibody in some leukemic children 1 year after vaccination. A booster response to revaccination has been noted (82). While this vaccine is not yet available in the United States, it is likely that licensure will result in its use as a means of preventing varicella infection in immunocompromised children.

Treatment of Established Varicella

Intravenous acyclovir effectively prevents dissemination (86-88) and is the treatment of choice for varicella in the IC patient. Details of the approach to the treatment of varicella are included in Chapter 00 on the use of acyclovir in children. Double-blind, placebo-controlled studies have also demonstrated that interferon and vidarabine are effective in ameliorating varicella. However, significant side effects limit their clinical usefulness.

Leukocyte interferon at intramuscular dosages of 3.5×10^5 units per kg per day for 48 h followed by 1.75×10^5 units per kg per day for 72 h decreased the incidence of life-threatening dissemination and increased the rate of healing in IC children with varicella. One fatal case of recurrent viremia occurred after therapy (89). Flulike side effects of fever, myalgia, nausea, and headache are associated with intravenous interferon and, although well tolerated, are greater in incidence than side effects seen with intravenous acyclovir.

Intravenous vidarabine has also been shown to reduce morbidity and mortality and to speed healing in immunocompromised patients with varicella. Toxicity in the form of neurologic sequelae, bone marrow suppression, and hepatic dysfunction have been reported in 0-50% of patients (72,88,90).

IV vidarabine treatment may cause neurotoxicity which rarely has resulted in chronic encephalopathy (90). In a direct comparison of the efficacy and toxicity of vidarabine versus acyclovir in IC children with varicella, acyclovir exhibited significantly fewer side effects (90). In fact, a retrospective review of intravenous vidarabine use in children revealed neurotoxicity in 6 of 34 cases versus none of 24 treated with acyclovir. Intrathecal methotrexate and acute lymphocytic leukemia (ALL) were associated risk factors in these six children.

Controlled studies have revealed the effectiveness of IV acyclovir for the therapy of varicella. In one trial 7 of 11 placebo-treated patients developed visceral dissemination or pneumonitis as compared to 0 of 7 ACV-treated patients (86). In another trial, 12 of 25 placebo versus 1 of 25 ACV-treated patients deteriorated clinically during the treatment period (91).

Because of its efficacy, availability, and reduced toxicity, acyclovir appears to be the drug of choice for the therapy of varicella in both immunocompromised children and adults. The dosage is either 24-30 mg/kg/day or 500 mg/m^2, given as 8-10 mg/kg every 8 h. Patients should be well hydrated, and intravenous acyclovir should be given by slow infusion over 1 h. A controlled trial of the effectiveness of a high-dose oral regimen of acyclovir treatment for primary varicella has not been performed, though preliminary case reports suggest efficacy (92,93).

In summary, if known exposure to VZV occurs, prophylaxis with ZIG should be instituted within 72 h for maximum benefit but can be administered within 10 days. If clinical disease develops, ACV should be administered (Table 5). Vaccination is likely to play an important role in improving prevention, control, and management of primary varicella.

ZOSTER

Reactivation of VZV with the subsequent development of zoster is a common occurrence in the IC patient, particularly those with lymphoproliferative malignancies (94,95). The overall incidence of zoster in the general population is 1.3-5 per 1000 persons per year (96-98) and increases with age, level of immunosuppression, and depressed cell-mediated immunity to VZV antigen. More than two thirds of reported cases of zoster occur in persons over the age of 50, whereas less than 10% occur in individuals under 20 years of age (98,99). The incidence of zoster in persons over 80 years of age is 10 per 1000 per year (96).

Individuals who have already experienced a recurrence are at about an equal statistical risk of a second recurrence. Repeat episodes of zoster have been reported in up to 22% of IC patients (100). In almost all instances the strain of VZ virus in recurrences is similar to that of the original varicella isolate. Rarely, zoster has been reported as an apparent reinfection (68,101). Multiple (more than three) episodes are likely to be dermatomal HSV recurrences, however.

Depression of cell-mediated immunity correlates clinically with onset of herpes zoster (67,102,103). In a recent study of the risk of zoster in children with leukemia, zoster occurred in 3.1 cases per 100 person-years of follow-up (85). Up to 24% of Hodgkin's disease and 50% of bone marrow transplant patients develop VZV within 24 months after onset of chemotherapy. Sequential sampling of sera from these patients has revealed increases in VZV antibody (IgM and IgG), often without overt clinical manifestation of disease, suggesting asymptomatic reactivation of infection (104,105). Radiation therapy may influence the frequency and site of reactivation by its immunosuppressive and local radiation energy effects on the sensory ganglion.

Bone marrow transplant patients typically develop herpes zoster 4-5 months after transplant; 30% will reactivate in the first year of follow-up (106). Renal and cardiac transplant patients develop zoster less often (3% and 10%, respectively) probably reflecting their less intensive immunosuppression (107,108). Patients receiving long-term corticosteroid drugs do not appear to be at increased risk for zoster, and alternate day prednisone therapy appears to confer no significant risk in increasing the incidence of disease (62). Hodgkin's disease, non-Hodgkin's lymphoma, head and neck cancer, bone marrow transplantation, and lack of complete tumor remission are risk factors for dissemination. Mortality from zoster in IC patients is uncommon, averaging less than 3% (62).

Clinical Manifestations

Clinically, a vesicular dermatomal rash preceded by local burning, pruritus, pain, characteristic herpes zoster, or shingles occurs in areas in which the rash of varicella previously predominated: 10-15% of cases present along the ophthalmic division of the trigeminal nerve, and more than 50% from T3 to L2. The individual lesions of zoster are not distinguishable from HSV or varicella, but they develop over a more prolonged course than that of varicella. In the normal host, vesicles develop in 12-24 h, forming pustules by the third day and developing crusts in 7-10 days that usually last for 2-3 weeks. New lesions may appear for 1-7 days, with recovery of virus for as long as 1 week (109,110).

TABLE 6

Zoster and complications	Normal host	IC host
Occurrence	1.5-5/1000/yr	22-50%
Cutaneous dissemination	17-35%	15-50%
Postherpetic neuralgia	9%	18-32%
Mortality	<0.5%	<5%

Manifestations of zoster in the immunocompromised patient include persistent infection with lesions lasting weeks to months (102), cutaneous dissemination (>2 dermatomes distant from the initial crop of lesions), and visceral dissemination. Evidence of cutaneous dissemination with 10-25 vesicles in areas remote from the involved dermatome are noted in 17-35% of unselected persons with zoster (15-50% of IC patients) (Table 6). These generally develop within a week of onset and can be easily missed on examination if few in number. Visceral dissemination, predominantly involving the liver, lungs, and brain, develops in 10-38% of IC persons manifesting cutaneous dissemination (94,100,103,107,108,111). Bone marrow transplant patients experience a 45% risk of dissemination, with a mortality of 38% if untreated (106).

Postherpetic neuralgia (PHN), which is the persistence of dermatomal pain after lesions have healed, is a common complication of zoster. In general, PHN occurs in 10-15% of persons developing zoster and is associated with age and lesion location (98,112). PHN is uncommon in patients with zoster below age 40, whereas 50% of the general population over age 60 and 20-60% of immunosuppressed persons develop PHN (106, 113,114). PHN decreases in most persons over time, but in a small number of persons it may persist for >6 months (Table 6). Anesthesia of the involved dermatome may also occur. The pathogenesis of this neuralgia has been correlated with alteration of central pain pathways due to peripheral nerve damage and loss of central nervous system pain-inhibiting fibers (115).

Other complications of VZV reactivation are also more common in IC patients. These may include motor neuropathies (0.5-2.3%), transverse myelitis, cranial nerve involvement, ophthalmologic zoster with contralateral hemiplegia (116), and, rarely, zoster encephalitis (0.2-0.5%) (117). Ophthalmic zoster occurs in 20-70% of patients (101). Cervical spinal VZV infections may result in keratitis, uveitis, and oculomotor palsies.

Lymphocytic pleocytosis is a common finding in patients with VZV infection, independent of clinical signs of CNS involvement. When clinical VZV encephalitis occurs, it may precede the rash by 7-10 days or present up to 2 months afterward. Fever, headache, altered mental status, and palsies of cranial or extracranial nerves, usually at the level of the rash, occur. Limited pathologic and virologic studies suggest that VZV encephalitis is due to direct infection by VZV and hence antiviral chemotherapy should be considered (117).

Bacterial superinfection of the involved skin is common in zoster, chiefly with *Staphylococcus aureus* and *Streptococcus*, and necessitates excellent local care with drying agents such as Burrow's solution and early treatment for clinical evidence of purulent secondary infection.

Diagnosis

Rapid diagnosis is important, as early institution of therapy with antivirals such as acyclovir has been shown to result in reduced morbidity and mortality (118). Diagnostic methods for herpes zoster are similar to those for varicella. Patients will also manifest a rise in antibody titer over the course of infection, and antibody assays on acute and convalescent sera may be useful retrospectively. The most commonly utilized assays are the fluorescent antimembrane antibody (FAMA) and enzyme-linked immunosorbent assay (ELISA) methods.

Treatment

Vidarabine, acyclovir, and high doses of systemic interferon have been shown to decrease the frequency of dissemination and complications of VZV infection in IC hosts. In bone marrow transplant patients with zoster, acyclovir has been shown to be effective and superior to vidarabine (88,118,119). In one trial (88), intravenous acyclovir shortened the duration of viral shedding, new lesion formation, interval to decreased pain, and period to complete healing. No cases of dissemination occurred in the acyclovir group, whereas vidarabine was associated with dissemination in 4 of 11 cases and neurotoxicity (tremors and seizures). Comparable hematologic, gastrointestinal, and hepatic toxicities occurred. Acyclovir was associated with increased risk of renal insufficiency in the setting of concomitant administration of cyclosporine.

Leukocyte interferon has also been shown to be an effective therapy of VZV infection in IC patients. In doses of 30-40 $\times$ 10^6 units daily, leukocyte interferon increased the healing time and decreased the duration of lesions. It also appeared to decrease the incidence of postherpetic neuralgia. ACV has not demonstrated a clinically documented effect on postherpetic neuralgia in IC patients (119,120).

All antivirals show maximum benefit if initiated within 3 days of onset of rash, although those treated at a later stage still derived benefit from acyclovir in the setting of zoster (118). Prophylactic acyclovir for the prevention of HSV infection has been shown to decrease the number of clinical and subclinical reactivation events of VZV during treatment of bone marrow transplant recipients (105,121).

The concentration of acyclovir that inhibits VZV is 10-fold higher than that for HSV (122,123); e.g., the ID_{50} of HSV is 0.1 μg/ml, whereas that of VZV is 1 μg/ml. Following a 1-h infusion of acyclovir at 10 mg/kg, adults demonstrate peak levels of average 10.7 μg/ml and trough 2.3 μg/ml. As only 20% of oral acyclovir is bioavailable, plasma concentrations achieved with oral ACV are much lower. With 1 g and 4 g per day in divided doses, peak levels are 0.7 and 1.8 μg/ml, and trough levels are 0.4 and 0.9 μg/ml, respectively. Thus, plasma levels barely exceed the ID_{50} of VZV with oral dosing (62,123). Oral treatment regimens of acyclovir for the therapy of VZV in the IC patient have not been formally compared to intravenous treatment.

Topical acyclovir has been utilized in one study, and though it improved the rate of cutaneous healing by 40% (9-10 days), no effect on dissemination, viral shedding, or pain was noted, resulting in marginal utility overall (124).

Acyclovir Resistance in VZV

Although in vitro resistance has been described (125-128) for VZ, clinical reports of resistant strains or decreased sensitivity associated with prolonged administration of acyclovir are rare (129,130). As with HSV, viruses with altered viral thymidine kinase or viral DNA polymerases appear to be mechanisms of in vitro resistance. Paired isolates from 20 patients before and after acyclovir treatment for zoster revealed no apparent in vivo development of VZV resistance (130). While VZV resistance has not yet been well recognized as a reason for clinical failure, only limited isolates have been evaluated to date.

Summary

Currently, the IC individual should be treated with acyclovir for manifestations of zoster, with the route determined by the severity of clinical involvement. Intravenous acyclovir arrests the progression and decreases the complications of zoster in these persons. The dose is 8-10 mg/kg every 8 h for 7-10 days. Renal complications of drug delivery are reduced with adequate hydration of the patient and slow infusion over 1 h per dose.

If disease manifestations are mild, oral regimen of 4 g acyclovir per day may be initiated with close follow-up. If disease progresses, patients should be switched to the intravenous route.

REFERENCES

1. Nahmias, A. J., Josey, W. E., Naib, Z. M., Luce, C. F., and Duffey, A. (1979). Antibodies to herpesvirus hominis types 1 and 2 in humans. *Am. J. Epidemiol.* 91:531-546.
2. Nahmias, A. J., Keyserling, H., Bain, R., et al. (1985). Prevalence of herpes simplex virus (HSV) type-specific antibodies in a U.S.A. prepaid group medical practice population. Presented at the 6th International Meeting of the International Society for STD Research, Brighton, England, July 32-Aug. 2, 1985 (abstract).
3. Korsager, B., Spencer, E. S., Mordhorst, C.-H., and Andersen, H. K. (1975). Herpesvirus hominis infections in renal transplant recipients. *Scand. J. Infect. Dis.* 7:11-19.
4. Meyers, J. D., Flournoy, N., and Thomas, E. D. (1980). Infection with herpes simplex virus and cell-mediated immunity after marrow transplant. *J. Infect. Dis.* 142:338-346.
5. Pass, R. F., Whitley, R. J., Whelchel, J. D., Diethelm, A. G., Reynolds, D. W., and Alford, C. A. (1979). Identification of patients with increased risk of infection with herpes simplex virus after renal transplantation. *J. Infect. Dis.* 140:487-492.
6. Lam, M. T., Pazin, G. J., Armstrong, J. A., and Ho, M. (1981). Herpes simplex infection in acute myelogenous leukemia and other hematologic malignancies: A prospective study. *Cancer* 48:2168-2172.
7. Saral, R., Ambinder, R. F., Burns, W. H., Angelopulos, C. M., Griffin, D. E., Burke, P. J., and Leitman, P. S. (1983). Acyclovir prophylaxis against herpes simplex virus infection in patients with leukemia. *Ann. Intern. Med.* 99:773-776.
8. Saral, R., Burns, W. H., Laskin, O. L., Santos, G. W., and Leitman, P. S. (1981). Acyclovir prophylaxis of herpes simplex virus infections: A randomized, double-blind, controlled trial in bone marrow transplant recipients. *N. Engl. J. Med.* 305:63-67.
9. Whitley, R. J., Levin, M., Barton, N., Hershey, B. J., Davis, G., Keeney, R. E., Whelchel, J., Diethelm, A. G., Kartus, P., and Soong, S. J. (1984). Infections caused by the herpes simplex virus in the immunocompromised host: Natural history and topical acyclovir therapy. *J. Infect. Dis.* 150:323-329.

10. Bader, C., Crumpacker, C. S., Schnipper, L. E., Ransil, B., Clark, J. E., Arndt, K., and Freedberg, I. M. (1978). The natural history of recurrent facial-oral infection with herpes simplex virus. *J. Infect. Dis.* 138:897.

11. Spruance, S. L., Overall, J. C. Jr., Kern, E. R., Krueger, G. G., Plian, V., and Miller, W. (1977). The natural history of recurrent herpes simplex labialis: Implications for antiviral therapy. *N. Engl. J. Med.* 297:69-75.

12. Meyers, J. D., Wade, J. C., Mitchell, C. D., Saral, R., Leitman, P. S., Durack, D. T., Levin, M. J., Segreti, A. C., and Balfour, H. H. (1982). Multicenter collaborative trial of intravenous acyclovir for treatment of mucocutaneous herpes simplex virus infection in the immunocompromised host. *Am. J. Med.* 73:229-235.

13. Wade, J. C., Newton, B., McLaren, C., Flournoy, N., Keeney, R. E., and Meyers, J. D. (1982). Intravenous acyclovir to treat mucocutaneous herpes simplex virus infection after marrow transplantation: A double-blind trial. *Ann. Intern. Med.* 96:265-269.

14. Buss, D. H., and Scharyj, M. (1971). Herpesvirus infection of the esophagus and other visceral organs in adults. *Am. J. Med.* 66:457.

15. Rosen, P., and Hajdu, S. I. (1971). Visceral herpesvirus infections in patients with cancer. *Am. J. Clin. Pathol.* 56:459-465.

16. McDonald, G. B., Sharma, P., Hackman, R. C., Meyers, J. D., and Thomas, E. D. (1984). Esophageal infections in immunosuppressed patients after marrow transplantation. *Gastroenterology* 88:1111-1117.

17. Ramsey, P. G., Fife, K. H., Hackman, R. C., Meyers, J. D., and Corey, L. (1981). Herpes simplex virus pneumonia: Clinical, virologic, and pathologic features in 20 patients. *Ann. Intern. Med.* 97:813-820.

18. Shortsleeve, M. J., Gauvin, G. P., Gardner, R. C., and Greenberg, M. S. (1981). Herpetic esophagitis. *Radiology* 141:611-617.

19. Flewett, T. H., Parker, R. G. F., and Phillip, W. M. (1969). Acute hepatitis due to herpes simplex virus in an adult. *J. Clin. Pathol.* 22:60-66.

20. Foley, F. D., Greenawald, K. A., Nash, G., and Pruitt, B. A. Jr. (1979). Herpesvirus infection in burned patients. *N. Engl. J. Med.* 282:652-656.

21. Graham, B. S., and Snell, J. D. (1983). Herpes simplex virus infection of the adult lower respiratory tract. *Medicine* (*Baltimore*) 62:384-393.

22. Tuxen, D. V., Cade, J. F., McDonald, M. I., Buchanan, M. R. C., Clark, R. J., and Pain, M. C. F. (1983). Herpes simplex virus from the lower respiratory tract in adult respiratory distress syndrome. *Am. Rev. Respir. Dis.* 126: 416-419.

23. Streitman, K., Beregi, E., Hallos, I., and Turi, S. (1977). Herpes nephropathy. *Clin. Nephrol.* 7:106-111.

24. Schlesinger, J. J., Gandara, D., and Bensch, K. G. (1978). Myoglobinuria associated with herpes-group viral infections. *Arch. Intern. Med.* 138:422-424.

25. Friedman, H. M., Pincus, T., Bigilisco, P., et al. (1980). Acute monoarticular arthritis caused by herpes simplex virus and cytomegalovirus. *Am. J. Med.* 69:241-247.

26. Greenberg, M. S., Cohan, S. G., Boosz, B., and Friedman, H. (1987). Oral herpes simplex infections in patients with leukemia. *J. Am. Dent. Assoc.* 114:483.
27. Corey, L. (1986). Laboratory diagnosis of herpes simplex. *Diagn. Microbiol. Infect. Dis.* 4:111S-119S.
28. Lundgren, G., Wilczek, H., Lonnqvist, B., Linholm, A., Wahren, B., and Ringden, O. (1985). Acyclovir prophylaxis in bone marrow transplant recipients. *Scand. J. Infect. Dis.* (Suppl.) 47:137-144.
29. Hann, I. M., Prentice, H. G., Blacklock, H. A., Ross, M. G. R., Brigden, D., Rosling, A. E., Burke, C., Crawford, D. H., Brumfitt, W., and Hoffbrand, A. V. (1983). Acyclovir prophylaxis against herpes virus infections in severely immunocompromised patients: Randomised double blind trial. *Br. Med. J.* 287:384-388.
30. Prentice, H. G. (1983). Use of acyclovir for prophylaxis of herpes infections in severely immunocompromised patients. *J. Antimicrob. Chemother.* 12B: 153-159.
31. Schuch, K., Ehninger, G., Vallbracht, A., Kumbier, L., and Ostendorf, P. (1985). Oral prophylaxis of herpes infections with acyclovir (ACV) after BMR. *Exp. Haematol.* 13/17:106.
32. Gluckman, E., Lotsberg, J., Devergie, A., Zhao, X. M., Melo, R., Gomez-Morales, M., Nebout, T., Mazeron, M. C., and Perol, Y. (1983). Prophylaxis of herpes infections after bone marrow transplantation by oral acyclovir. *Lancet* 2:706-708.
33. Anderson, H., Scarffe, J. H., Sutton, R. N. P., Hickmott, E., Brigden, D., and Burke, C. (1984). Oral acyclovir prophylaxis against herpes simplex virus in non-Hodgkin lymphoma and acute lymphoblastic leukaemia patients receiving remission induction chemotherapy. A randomised double-blind, placebo controlled trial. *Br. J. Cancer* 50:45-49.
34. Griffin, P. J. A., Clobert, J. W., Williamson, E. P. M., Fiddian, A. P., Hickmott, E., Sells, R. A., and Salaman, J. R. (1985). Oral acyclovir prophylaxis of herpes infections in renal transplant recipients. *Transplant. Proc.* 17:84-85.
35. Pettersson, E., Hovi, T., Ahonen, J., Fiddian, A. P., Salmela, K., Hockerstedt, K., Eklund, B., Von Willebrand, E., and Hayry, P. (1984). Prophylactic oral acyclovir after renal transplantation. *Transplantation* 39:279-281.
36. Seale, L., Jones, C. J., Kathpalia, S., Jackson, G. G., Mozed, M., Maddux, M. S., and Packham, D. (1985). Prevention of herpes virus infection in renal allograft recipients by low-dose oral acyclovir. *JAMA* 254:3435-3438.
37. Fiddian, A. P. (1987). Acyclovir prophylaxis of herpes simplex virus infection after transplantation, a brief review. In Touraine, J. L., Traeger, J., Betvel, H., Brochier, J., Dubernard, J. M., Revillard, J. P., and Triau, R. (eds.): *Transplantation and Clinical Immunology*, Vol. XIV. Amsterdam, Excerpta Medica, pp. 130-134.

38. Shepp, D. H., Newton, B. A., Dandliker, P. S., Flournoy, N., and Meyers, J. D. (1985). Oral acyclovir therapy for mucocutaneous herpes simplex virus infections in immunocompromised marrow transplant recipients. *Ann. Intern. Med.* 102:783-785.

39. Ehninger, G., Vallbracht, A., Schuch, K., Kumbier, I., Dopfer, R., Schmidt, H., and Ostendorf, P. (1986). Oral Prophylaxe von Herpes-infektionen mit Acyclovir nach Knochenmarktransplantation: Eine klinische und klinishpharmakologische Untersuchung. *Klin. Wochenschr.* 64:570-574.

40. Wade, J. C., Newton, B., Flournoy, N., and Meyers, J. D. (1984). Oral acyclovir for prevention of herpes simplex virus reactivation after marrow transplantation. *Ann. Intern. Med.* 100:823-828.

41. Shepp, D. H., Dandliker, P. S., Flournoy, N., and Meyers, J. D. (1985). Once-daily intravenous acyclovir for prophylaxis of herpes simplex virus reactivation after marrow transplantation. *J. Antimicrob. Chemother.* 16: 389-395.

42. Dan, M., Siegman-Igra, Y., Weinberg, M., and Michaeli, D. (1986). Long-term suppression of recurrent herpes labialis by low-dose oral acyclovir in an immunocompromised patient. *Arch. Intern. Med.* 146:1438-1440.

43. Straus, S. E., Seidlin, M., Takiff, H., Jacobs, D., Bowen, D., and Smith, H. A. (1984). Oral acyclovir to suppress recurring herpes simplex virus infection in immunodeficient patients. *Ann. Intern. Med.* 100:522-524.

44. Gold, D., and Corey, L. (1987). Acyclovir prophylaxis for herpes simplex virus infection. *Antimicrob. Agents Chemother.* 31:361-367.

45. Chou, S., Gallagher, J. G., and Merigan, T. C. (1981). Controlled clinical trial of intravenous acyclovir in heart-transplant patients with mucocutaneous herpes simplex infections. *Lancet* 1:1392-1394.

46. Mitchell, C. D., Gentry, S. R., Boen, J. R., Bean, B., Groth, K. E., and Balfour, H. H. (1981). Acyclovir therapy for mucocutaneous herpes simplex infections in immunocompromised patients. *Lancet* 1:1389-1394.

47. Meyers, J. D. (1985). Treatment of herpesvirus infections in the immunocompromised host. *Scand. Infect. Dis.* (Suppl.) 47:128-136.

48. Balfour, H. H. (1986). Acyclovir therapy for herpes zoster: Advantages and adverse effects. *JAMA* 255:387-388.

49. Douglas, J. M., Critchlow, C., Benedetti, J., Mertz, G. J., Conner, J. D., Hintz, M. A., Fahnlander, A., Remington, M., Winter, C., and Corey, L. (1984). A double-blind study of oral acyclovir for suppression of recurrences of genital herpes simplex virus infection. *N. Engl. J. Med.* 310:1551-1556.

50. Barry, D. W., Lehrman, S. N., and Ellis, M. N. (1986). Clinical and laboratory experience with acyclovir-resistant herpesviruses. *J. Antimicrob. Chemother.* 18(Suppl. B):75-84.

51. Dekker, C., Ellis, M. N., McLaren, S., Hunter, G., Rogers, J., and Barry, D. W. (1983). Virus resistance in clinical practice. *J. Antimicrob. Chemother.* 12(Suppl. B):137-152.

52. Parris, D. S., and Harrington, J. E. (1982). Herpes simplex virus variants re-
    sistant to high concentrations of acyclovir exist in clinical isolates. *Antimi-
    crob. Agents Chemother.* 222:71-77.
53. Coen, D. M., and Schaffer, P. A. (1980). Two distinct loci confer resistance
    to acycloguanosine in herpes simplex virus type 1. *Proc. Natl. Acad. Sci.
    USA* 77:2265-2269.
54. Crumpacker, C. S., Schnipper, L. E., Marlow, S. I., Kowalsky, P. N., Her-
    shey, B. J., and Levin, M. D. (1982). Resistance to antiviral drugs of herpes
    simplex virus isolated from a patient treated with acyclovir. *N. Engl. J. Med.*
    306:343-346.
55. Christophers, J., Sutton, R. N. P., Noble, R. V., and Anderson, H. (1986).
    Clinical resistance to acyclovir of herpes simplex virus infections in immuno-
    compromised patients. *J. Antimicrob. Chemother.* 18(Suppl. B):121-125.
56. Crumpacker, C. S. (1988). Significance of resistance of herpes simplex virus
    to acyclovir. *J. Am. Acad. Dermatol.* 18(1 pt. 2):190-195.
57. Wade, J. C., McLaren, C., and Meyers, J. D. (1983). Frequency and signifi-
    cance of acyclovir-resistant herpes simplex virus isolated from marrow trans-
    plant patients receiving multiple course of treatment with acyclovir. *J. Infect.
    Dis.* 148:1077-1082.
58. Burns, W. H., Santos, G. W., Saral, R., Laskin, O. L., and Lietman, P. S.
    (1982). Isolation and characterisation of resistant herpes simplex virus after
    acyclovir therapy. *Lancet* 1:421-423.
59. Straus, S. E., Takiff, H. E., Mindell, S., Seidlin, M., Bachrach, S., Lininger,
    L., DiGiovanna, J. J., Western, K. A., Smith, H. A., Lehrman, S. N., Creagh-
    Kirk, T., and Alling, D. W. (1984). Suppression of frequently recurring geni-
    tal herpes: A placebo-controlled double blind trial of oral acyclovir. *N. Engl.
    J. Med.* 310:1545-1550.
60. Ambinder, R. F., Letiman, P. S., Burns, H., and Saral, R. (1984). Prophy-
    laxis: A strategy to minimize antiviral resistance. *Lancet* 1:1154-1155.
61. Weller, T. H. (1983). Varicella and herpes zoster: Changing concepts of the
    natural history, control, and importance of a not-so-benign virus. *N. Engl.
    J. Med.* 209:1362-1366, 1434-1440.
62. Bean, B., and Englund, J. A. (1987). Treatment of varicella-zoster virus in-
    fection. *Clin. Lab. Med.* 7:853-868.
63. Gershon, A. A., Raker, R., Steinberg, S., et al. (1976). Antibody to varicella-
    zoster virus in parturient women and their offspring during the first year of
    life. *Pediatrics* 58:692.
64. Colebunders, R., Mann, J. M., Francis, H., Bila, K., Izaley, L., Ilwaya, M.,
    Kakonde, N., Quinn, T., Curran, J. W., and Piot, P. (1988). Herpes zoster
    in African patients: A clinical predictor of human immunodeficiency virus
    infection. *J. Infect. Dis.* 157(2):314-318.
65. Feldman, S., Hughes, W. T., and Daniel, C. B. (1975). Varicella in children
    with cancer: Seventy-seven cases. *J. Pediatr.* 56:383.

66. Arvin, A. M., Pollard, R. B., Rasmussen, L. E., and Merigan, T. C. (1978). Selective impairment of lymphocyte reactivity to varicella-zoster virus antigen among untreated patients with lymphoma. *J. Infect. Dis.* 137:531-540.

67. Arvin, A. M., Pollard, R. B., Rasmussen, L. E., and Merigan, T. C. (1980). Cellular and humoral immunity in the pathogenesis of recurrent herpes viral infections in patients with lymphoma. *J. Clin. Invest.* 65:869-878.

68. Ross, A. H. (1962). Modification of chickenpox in family contacts by administration of gamma globulin. *N. Engl. J. Med.* 267:369.

69. Weller, T. H. (1979). Varicella and herpes zoster. In Lennette, E. H., and Schmidt, N. J. (eds.): *Diagnostic Procedures for Viral, Rickettsial and Chlamydial Infections*, 5th Ed. Washington, D.C., American Public Health Association, pp. 375-398.

70. Drew, W. L., and Mintz, L. (1979). Rapid diagnosis of varicella-zoster virus infection by direct immunofluorescence. *Am. J. Clin. Pathol.* 73:699-701.

71. Solomon, A. R. (1986). The Tzanck smear: Viable and valuable in the diagnosis of herpes simplex, zoster and varicella. *Int. J. Dermatol.* 25(3):169-170.

72. Whitley, R. J., Hilty, M., Haynes, R., Bryson, Y., Connor, J. D., Soong, S. J., Alford, C. A. Jr., and the NIAID Collaborative Antiviral Study Group. (1982). Vidarabine therapy of varicella in immunosuppressed patients. *J. Pediatr.* 101:125-131.

73. Cradock-Watson, J. E., Ridehalgh, M. K. S., and Bourne, M. S. (1979). Specific immunoglobulin responses after varicella and herpes zoster. *J. Hyg. (Lond.)* 82:319-336.

74. Dubey, L., Steinberg, S. P., LaRussa, P., Oh, P., and Gershon, A. A. (1988). Western blot assay of antibody to varicella zoster virus. *J. Infect. Dis.* 157(5): 882-888.

75. Gershon, A. (1974). Zoster immune globulin: A further assessment. *N. Engl. J. Med.* 290:243-245.

76. Centers for Disease Control. (1984). Varicella-zoster immune globulin for the prevention of chickenpox. *MMWR* 33:84.

77. Takahashi, M., Otsuka, T., Okuno, Y., et al. (1974). Live vaccine to prevent the spread of varicella in children in hospital. *Lancet* 2:1288-1290.

78. Arbeter, A. M., Starr, S. E., Preblud, S. R., et al. (1984). Varicella vaccine trial in healthy children: A summary of comparative and follow-up studies. *Am. J. Dis. Child.* 138:434-438.

79. Creibel, R. E., Neff, B. J., Kuter, B. J., et al. (1984). Live attenuated varicella virus vaccine: Efficacy trial in healthy children. *N. Engl. J. Med.* 310: 1409-1415.

80. Izawa, T., Ihara, I., Hattoi, A., et al. (1977). Application of a live varicella vaccine in children with acute leukemia or other malignant disease. *Pediatrics* 60:805-809.

81. Brunell, P., Shebob, Z., Geisu, C., and Waugh, J. E. (1982). Administration of live varicella vaccine to children with leukemia. *Lancet* 2:1069-1072.

82. Gershon, A. A., Steinberg, S. P., Gelb, L., and the National Institute of Allergy and Infectious Diseases Varicella Vaccine Collaborative Study Group. (1986). Current status of varicella vaccine: Live attenuated varicella vaccine use in immunocompromised children and adults. *Pediatrics* (Suppl.) 78(4): 757-762.

83. Sakurai, N., Ihara, T., Ho, M., et al. (1982). Application of a live varicella vaccine in children with acute leukemia. In Shiota, H., Cheng, Y.-C., and Prussoff, W. H. (eds.): *Herpesvirus: Clinical, Pharmacological and Basic Aspects.* Amsterdam, Exerpta Medica, pp. 87-93.

84. Gershon, A., Steinberg, S., Belb, L., et al. (1984). Efficacy of live attenuated varicella vaccine in children with acute leukemia in remission. *JAMA* 252: 355-362.

85. Lawrence, L., Gershon, A. A., Holzman, R., Steinberg, S. P., and the NIAID Varicella Vaccine Collaborative Study Group. (1988). The risk of zoster after varicella vaccination in children with leukemia. *N. Engl. J. Med.* 318:543-548.

86. Prober, C. G., Kirk, L. E., and Keeney, R. E. (1982). Acyclovir therapy of chickenpox in immunosuppressed children—a collaborative study. *J. Pediatr.* 202:622.

87. Balfour, H. H. (1982). Intravenous acyclovir therapy for varicella in immunocompromised children. *J. Pediatr.* 104:134.

88. Shepp, D. H., Dandliker, P. S., and Meyers, J. D. (1986). Treatment of varicella-zoster virus infection in severely immunocompromised patients: A randomized comparison of acyclovir and vidarabine. *N. Engl. J. Med.* 314:208-212.

89. Arvin, A. N., Kushner, J. H., Feldman, S., Baehner, R. L., Hammond, D., and Merigan, T. C. (1981). Human leukocyte interferon for the treatment of varicella in children with cancer. *N. Engl. J. Med.* 306:761-765.

90. Feldman, S., Robertson, P. K., Lott, L., and Thornton, D. (1986). Neurotoxicity due to adenine arabinoside therapy during VZV infection in immunocompromised children. *J. Infect. Dis.* 154(5):889-893.

91. Nyerges, G., Meszner, Z., Gyarmati, E., and Kerpel-Fronius, S. (1988). Acyclovir prevents dissemination of varicella in immunocompromised children. *J. Infect. Dis.* 157(2):309-313.

92. Novelli, V. M., Marshall, W. C., Yeo, J., and McKendrick, G. D. (1984). Acyclovir administered perorally in immunocompromised children with varicella-zoster infections. *J. Infect. Dis.* 149:478.

93. Novelli, V. M., Marshall, W. C., Yeo, J., and McKendrick, G. D. (1985). High-dose oral acyclovir for children at risk of disseminated herpes virus infections. *J. Infect. Dis.* 151:372.

94. Mazur, M. H., and Dolin, R. (1978). Herpes zoster at the NIH: A 20 year experience. *Am. J. Med.* 75:738-743.

95. Pieblud, S. R. (1981). Age specific risks of varicella complications. *Pediatrics* 68:14-17.

96. Hope-Simpson, R. E. (1965). The nature of herpes zoster: A long term study and a new hypothesis. *Proc. Soc. Med.* 58:9-20.
97. Ragozzino, M. W., Melton, L. J. III, Kurland, L. T., Chu, C. P., and Perry, H. O. (1982). Risk of cancer after herpes zoster: A population based study. *N. Engl. J. Med.* 307:397-399.
98. Ragozzino, M. W., et al. (1982). Population-based study of herpes zoster and its sequelae. *Medicine (Baltimore)* 62:310.
99. Burgoon, C. F., et al. (1957). The natural history of herpes zoster. *JAMA* 264:265.
100. Schmipf, S., Serpick, A., Stoler, B., et al. (1972). Varicella-zoster infection in patients with cancer. *Ann. Intern. Med.* 76:241-254.
101. Berlin, B. S., and Campbell, T. (1979). Hospital-acquired herpes zoster following exposure to chickenpox. *JAMA* 211:1831-1833.
102. Gallagher, J. G., and Merigan, T. C. (1979). Prolonged herpes zoster infection associated with immunosuppressive therapy. *Ann. Intern. Med.* 92: 842-846.
103. Meyers, J. D., Fluornoy, N., and Thomas, E. D. (1980). Cell mediated immunity to varicella-zoster virus after allogenic marrow transplant. *J. Infect. Dis.* 141:479-487.
104. Skinhoj, P. (1985). Herpes virus infections in the immunocompromised patient. *Scand. J. Infect. Dis.* (Suppl. 47):121-127.
105. Ljungman, P., Lonnqvist, B., Bahrton, G., et al. (1986). Clinical and subclinical reactivations of varicella-zoster virus in immunocompromised patients. *J. Infect. Dis.* 153:840-847.
106. Locksley, R. M., Flournoy, N., Sullivan, K. M., and Meyers, J. D. (1985). Infections with varicella-zoster virus after marrow transplantation. *J. Infect. Dis.* 152(6):1172-1181.
107. Luby, J. P., Ramirez-Ronda, C., Rinner, S., Jull, A., and Vergne-Marini, P. (1977). A longitudinal study of varicella-zoster virus infections in renal transplant recipients. *J. Infect. Dis.* 135:659-663.
108. Rand, K. H., Rasmussen, L. E., Polard, R. B., Arvin, A., and Merigan, T. C. (1976). Cellular immunity and herpes virus infections in cardiac-transplant patients. *N. Engl. J. Med.* 296:1372-1377.
109. Oberg, G., and Svedmyr, A. (1969). Varicellaform eruptions in herpes zoster—some clinical and serological observations. *Scand. J. Infect. Dis.* 1:47.
110. Juel-Hensen, B. E., and MacCallum, F. O. (1972). *Herpes Simplex, Varicella and Zoster.* Philadelphia, J.B. Lippincott.
111. Gold, E. (1966). Serologic and virus-isolation studies of patients with varicella or herpes-zoster infection. *N. Engl. J. Med.* 274:181.
112. Hope-Simpson, R. E. (1975). Post herpetic neuralgia. *J. R. Coll. Gen. Prac.* 25:571.
113. Rogers, R. S. 3d, and Tindall, J. P. (1971). Herpes zoster in the elderly. *Postgrad. Med.* 50:153-157.

114. Stanfrom, E., Miller, S., and Haar, H. (1960). Herpes zoster in hematologic neoplasia: Some unusual manifestations. *Ann. Intern. Med.* 53:523-533.
115. Portenoy, R. K., Duma, C., and Foley, K. M. (1986). Acute herpetic and postherpetic neuralgia: Clinical review and current management. *Ann. Neurol.* 20:651.
116. Womack, L. W., and Liesegang, T. J. (1983). Complication of herpes zoster ophthalmia. *Arch. Ophthalmol.* 101:42.
117. Jemsek, J., Greenberg, S. B., Taber, L., Harvey, D., Gershon, A., and Couch, R. B. (1983). Herpes zoster-associated encephalitis: Clinicopathologic report of 12 cases and review of the literature. *Medicine (Baltimore)* 62:81.
118. Balfour, H. H. Jr., Bean, B., Laskin, O. L., Ambinder, R. F., Meyers, J. D., Wade, J. D., Zaia, J. A., Aeppli, D., Kirk, L. E., Segreti, A. C., Keeney, R. E., and the Burroughs Wellcome Collaborative Acyclovir Study Group. (1983). Acyclovir halts progression of herpes zoster in immunocompromised patients. *N. Engl. J. Med.* 308:1448-1453.
119. Winston, D., Eron, L., Ho, M., et al. (1985). Treatment of herpes zoster in immunocompromised cancer patients with recombinant leukocyte interferon. Presented at the 25th Interscience Conference on Antimicrobial Agents and Chemotherapy, Minneapolis, October 1985.
120. Merigan, T. C., Rand, K. H., Pollard, R. B., et al. (1978). Human leukocyte interferon for the treatment of herpes zoster in patients with cancer. *N. Engl. J. Med.* 298:981.
121. Jeffries, D. J. (1986). Acyclovir update. *Br. Med. J.* 293:1523.
122. Laskin, O. L. (1984). Acyclovir. Pharmacology and clinical experience. *Arch. Intern. Med.* 144:1241-1246.
123. Brigden, D., and Whiteman, P. (1985). The clinical pharmacology of acyclovir and its prodrugs. *Scand. J. Infect. Dis.* (Suppl. 47):33-39.
124. Levin, M. J., Zaia, J. A., Hershey, B. J., et al. (1985). Topical acyclovir treatment of herpes zoster in immunocompromised patients. *J. Am. Acad. Dermatol.* 13:590.
125. Crumpacker, C. S., Schnipper, L. E., Zaia, J. A., and Levin, M. J. (1979). Growth inhibition by acycloguanosine of herpesviruses isolated from human infections. *Antimicrob. Agents Chemother.* 15:642-645.
126. Biron, K. K., and Elion, G. B. (1980). In vitro susceptibility of varicella-zoster virus to acyclovir. *Antimicrob. Agents Chemother.* 18:443-447.
127. Shiraki, K., Yamanishi, K., and Takahashi, M. (1984). Susceptibility to acyclovir or Oka-strain varicella vaccine and vaccine-derived virus isolated from immunocompromised patients. *J. Infect. Dis.* 150:306-307.
128. Biron, K. K., Fyfe, J. A., Nobin, J. E., and Elion, G. B. (1982). Selection and preliminary characterization of acyclovir-resistant mutants of varicella-zoster virus. Proceedings of a symposium on acyclovir. *Am. J. Med.* 73 (Suppl.):383-386.

129. Barry, D. W., Nusinoff-Lehrman, S., Ellis, M. N., Biron, K. K., and Fur-
      man, P. A. (1985). Viral resistance, clinical experience. *Scand. J. Infect.
      Dis.* 47(Suppl.):155-168.
130. Cole, N. L., and Balfour, H. H. Jr. Varicella-zoster virus does not become
      more resistant to acyclovir during therapy. *J. Infect. Dis.* 153:605-608.
131. Fiddian, A. P. (1987). Prevention of herpes simplex virus infections in sus-
      ceptible patients. *Infection* 15(Suppl. 1):S21-25.

17
Use of Acyclovir in HIV-Positive Patients

Marcus A. Conant *University of California, San Francisco, California*

The epidemic of the acquired immunodeficiency syndrome (AIDS), a new sexually transmitted blood-borne disease caused by the human immunodeficiency virus (HIV), first appeared in the United States in 1978 and was recognized as a new syndrome by clinicians in early 1981.

The virus infects helper-T lymphocytes (CD4 cells) and monocytes. The resulting cellular dysfunction and death of helper-T lymphocytes leads to profound immunodeficiency with the subsequent appearance of a variety of opportunistic infections and malignancies. The most notable infections have been *Pneumocystis carinii* pneumonia (PCP), *Mycobacterium avium-intracellulare* (MAI), candidiasis, toxoplasmosis, and cryptococcosis.

Kaposi's sarcoma (KS), long thought to be a malignancy, may in fact be a reactive vascular hyperplasia caused directly by the HIV virus or by some other, yet unidentified infection or cofactor that becomes operational when the individual is infected with HIV. It is noteworthy that KS is seen almost exclusively in white men who acquire AIDS as a consequence of having sex with other men and is astonishingly rare among IV drug users, transfusion recipients, and children infected with HIV.

Common infections that are the bane of individuals with normal immune systems occur with greater frequency and greater severity and are more refractory to therapy in the HIV-infected immunocompromised patient. The infections most commonly seen are yeast and latent viral infections. These include oral and genital monilia and pruritis ani, all caused by *Candida albicans*, seborrheic dermatitis caused by the yeast *Pityrosporon ovale*, herpes simplex, and herpes zoster.

Bacterial infections, particularly folliculitis and occasionally bullous impetigo, are seen and respond readily to topical antibiotics. Tinea infections of the feet and onychomycosis of the nails are also common problems in the HIV-infected patient and are generally difficult to treat and rapidly recurrent if treatment is discontinued.

Acyclovir became available for investigational and clinical use at about the same time that the AIDS epidemic appeared in the United States. The HIV virus was not isolated until 1984, and early attempts to determine if acyclovir had any clinical efficacy in the treatment of patients with AIDS had to be done purely on a clinical and empirical basis. As so often happens, there were early enthusiastic reports that acyclovir was beneficial in the treatment of HIV-infected individuals. Unfortunately, these observations have proved to be spurious, and acyclovir appears to have no direct antiviral effect on HIV.

Acyclovir has proven to be extremely useful in the management of recurrent herpes simplex in HIV-infected immunosuppressed individuals. No studies have been done to estimate the incidence of perianal and intergluteal herpes simplex, but before the onset of the AIDS epidemic, the number of men presenting for treatment of perianal herpes was extremely low. In a practice caring for large numbers of HIV-infected men, a history of recurrent perianal herpes is now extremely common, suggesting that the immunosuppression attendant to HIV infection is in some way responsible for an increased frequency of recurrence of genital and perianal herpes.

While penile herpes in the HIV-infected individual is clinically identical to the same disease in the nonimmunocompromised host, perianal herpes is often difficult to diagnose. The most useful clinical clue is the history that the problem has been recurrent at periodic intervals, usually in the same location. On physical examination, one often observes nothing more than a painful linear fissure extending from the anal verge onto the glaborous skin of the buttocks. Occasionaly there may be nothing but a superficial erosion, and the patient often has concomitant pruritis ani with both monilia and tinea, and the entire area is so inflamed that a precise diagnosis by inspection alone is impossible.

A few patients have been seen with herpes of the gastrointestinal tract and rectum. Lesions of the pharynx have been noted, and rarely patients are seen where recurrent herpes can be recovered from the esophagus, stomach, and colon. In this group, endoscopy and colonoscopy is usually necessary to establish a definitive diagnosis (1).

Even if the diagnosis cannot be established, the clinician caring for a patient who has periodic recurrences of excruciating abdominal or intestinal pain should consider an empirical trial with high-dose oral acyclovir in an effort to rule out recurrent intestinal herpes as the cause of the patient's discomfort.

Studies have not yet been published on the optimal dose of acyclovir in the treatment of recurrent genital or perianal herpes in the HIV-infected individual. In our practice, patients are treated with acyclovir 400 mg qid until the lesion is healed, and then they are placed on suppressive therapy with 400 mg bid indefinitely. The number of patients who experience breakthrough on this dose is approximtely 20%, which is about the same breakthrough rate as that seen individuals not infected with HIV and not immunosuppressed.

Disseminated herpes simplex, while life-threatening, is extremely rare in the HIV-infected host. These patients should be hospitalized and managed aggressively with high-dose intravenous acyclovir.

Clinically significant resistance of herpes simplex to thymidine kinase (TK)-negative mutants have been described, but given the number of HIV-positive patients treated with acyclovir for recurrent herpes, the frequency of such resistance is astonishingly low. Patients with TK-negative results can be treated with intravenous foscarnet (2).

Herpes zoster was recognized early in the epidemic as a manifestation of immunosuppression from HIV infection. The patient generally presents with typical lesions characterized by grouped vesicles on an erythematous base involving one or two dermatomes on the same side of the body. Not infrequently, the erythematous base so commonly seen in the immunocompetent patient is absent in this population. Untreated, the disease may take 3 weeks or longer to heal. There may be considerable pain and discomfort, and scarring is common.

Prior to the time when we had oral acyclovir, dissemination of varicella with varicella pneumonia was a dreaded complication. Such patients needed hospitalization and treatment with high-dose systemic acyclovir. Aggressive therapy with oral acyclovir has virtually eliminated this problem. Recurrent episodes of herpes zoster have been seen in bone marrow transplant recipients and HIV-infected individuals, but this is decidedly rare.

Occasionally, HIV-infected patients are seen with small, scattered tense vessicles involving primarily the face, shoulders, and upper arms, though lesions can occur anywhere. Some of these lesions may show an erythematous halo, but the classic picture of a dewdrop on a rose petal, so typical of chickenpox, is often absent in the HIV-infected patient. Chickenpox of this type is seen most commonly in the HIV-infected patient who has no prior history of varicella, but it has been seen in patients with a clearly documented history of childhood chickenpox, and a few recurrent cases have been seen.

A study by Friedman-Kien and co-workers (3) found that 35-48 consecutive patients who presented with herpes zoster were positive for HIV. In this study, 7 of 33 patients developed full-blown AIDS in 2 years. The appearance of herpes zoster should alert the physician to the possibility that the patient is immunosuppressed, and an antibody test for HIV should be included in the clinical evaluation (3).

In a large study of 112 gay men from a New York practice, zoster was found to be associated with progression to AIDS in a substantial number of HIV infected men. A total of 22.8% of patients presenting with herpes zoster developed AIDS within 2 years, 45.5% within 4 years, and the authors estimated that 72.8% would develop AIDS in 6 years. In this study, clinically severe zoster and painful zoster involving facial dermatomes were associated with a higher incidence of progression to AIDS (4).

Paradoxically, physicians caring for large numbers of HIV-infected individuals have noted that while zoster is common in individuals before they develop full-blown CDC-defined AIDS, it is extremely rare in individuals who are profoundly immunosuppressed and who have developed one of the opportunistic infections pathognomonic of the AIDS diagnosis. This is particularly astounding since these patients are undoubtedly more severely immunosuppressed than those presenting with zoster early in the course of their disease (5).

A few patients have been seen with well-circumscribed, 3- to 6-mm, punched-out ecthymatous lesions surmounted by a thick serosanguinous eschar. Culture of the base of these lesions has demonstrated varicella. A typical history recounts that the patient experienced the appearance of two or three of these lesions simultaneously, and then over the next 4-6 weeks, one or two new lesions would appear each week, and the old lesions would heal slowly if at all. This condition also responds quickly to oral acyclovir (6).

Balfour et al. (7) showed in 1983 that acyclovir halted the progression of herpes zoster in immunocompromised patients. The effective dose, however, was appreciably higher than the dose of acyclovir necessary to control herpes simplex. Significantly fewer patients treated with acyclovir within the first 3 days after the onset of zoster had complications as compared to patients treated with placebo, but acyclovir also stopped progression of zoster in patients treated after 3 days (7).

HIV-infected patients presenting with herpes zoster should be treated aggressively with oral acyclovir at the earliest possible moment. Even in those patients in whom there is little or no herpetic neuralgia and dissemination appears unlikely, early treatment substantially shortens the course of the disease and prevents the extensive scarring, atrophy, and hypopigmentation so commonly seen in HIV-infected patients prior to the FDA approval of acyclovir in 1984.

The HIV-infected patient suffering from zoster or varicella is treated with acyclovir 800 mg five times a day for 5 days. On the fifth day the patient is reevaluated, and if there has been no new vessicle formation in the previous 48 h, acyclovir is discontinued. If there has been new vessicle formation, the acyclovir is continued for an additional 5 days.

Unhappily, a case of acyclovir-resistant varicella-zoster has been described in a 4-year-old child congenitally infected with HIV. This infant presented with the continuous recurrence of varicella and zoster over a 14-month period until her death. A single isolate revealed that this strain was clearly resistant to acyclovir in vitro.

In 1984, investigators at the University of California, San Francisco, described a new clinical condition in patients infected with HIV. Clinically, these patients presented with white plaques on the lateral borders of the tongue. Because of the lacy papillomatous nature of the lesion, it was dubbed "hairy" leukoplakia (8). Histologically, the lesion resembled a flat wart, but subsequent studies showed that the lesion was caused by the replication of Epstein-Barr virus on the lingual mucosa (9).

In one series of patients infected with HIV, 83% who developed hairy leukoplakia developed full-blown AIDS within 31 months, suggesting that this lesion has grave prognostic implications. Interestingly, the lesion appears and disappears spontaneously, and its clinical appearance does not seem to be related to the presence of ARC symptoms or to the patient's absolute number of helper-T cells. Treatment of hairy leukoplakia is undertaken for cosmetic and emotional reasons.

Hairy leukoplakia responds promptly to treatment with oral acyclovir in a dose of 800 mg qid for 3 weeks (10). Topical acyclovir is also effective in the treatment of this condition, and the lesion can be simply peeled off with 0.1% vitamin A acid applied once or twice a day (11).

One of the most unfortunate and devastating opportunistic infections to afflict individuals immunosuppressed by HIV is cytomegalovirus

(CMV) retinitis. The condition usually presents with retinal necrosis, hemorrhages, and exudates. Patients often consult their physician because of the sudden appearance of central scotomata, and cotton wool spots either in the area of the macula or in the peripheral areas of the retina are noted. The condition is steadily progressive and leads rapidly to complete retinal destruction and blindness.

A new antiviral chemotherapeutic agent, gangciclovir (9-[2-hydroxy-1-(hydroxymethyl)ethoxymethyl] guanine (BWB759U)) (DHPG), an analog of acyclovir, is very effective in the treatment of CMV retinitis. Most patients treated with DHPG have received the drug on a compassionate-plea basis because of impending blindness, and as a consequence good double-blind, placebo-controlled studies have not been possible. In a recent study of six patients with virologically confirmed CMV retinitis, treatment with gangciclovir universally arrested the progression of the retinitis and produced improvement in measurements of visual function. However, 3 weeks after the gangciclovir was discontinued, CMV activity recurred and worsening of visual function was observed (12). Clinical observations on patients receiving gangciclovir on a compassionate-plea basis suggest that the drug is very effective for 12-18 months. Then, without apparent explanation, the efficacy diminishes, and the CMV retinitis progresses even in the face of continued therapy. Gangciclovir has also been used successfully in the treatment of other CMV infections including CMV colitis and CMV pneumonitis (13).

The dideoxynucleoside analog 3′azido-2′,3′dideoxythymidine (azidothymidine, AZT), now called zidovudine, was found in 1985 to inhibit the newly isolated human retrovirus HIV (14). An initial multicenter, placebo-controlled, double-blind study was terminated early when it was demonstrated that zidovudine substantially increased the survival and decreased the frequency of opportunistic infections in patients who had had one episode of PCP (16). Surprisingly, acyclovir, another nucleocide analog that has no activity against HIV in vitro, appears to potentiate the anti-HIV activity of zidovudine in cell cultures without potentiating its toxicity (17). If this synergistic action could be translated to humans it would be extremely useful, since toxicity to zidovudine is the factor that limits its clinical usefulness. Unfortunately, early trials comparing zidovudine alone to the combination of zidovudine and acyclovir have been disappointing.

Work was presented as the Fourth International Conference on AIDS in Stockholm suggesting that the combination of zidovudine and acyclovir may be beneficial in the long-term management of HIV-infected patients.

Sigelmann reported on a multicenter, double-blind, placebo-controlled trial of zidovudine in combination with acyclovir performed at various centers in Europe and Australia. For the first 24-week period the occurrence of tumors, the Karnofsky scores, body weight, and T-cell counts were similar in patients receiving zodivudine alone and in groups receiving zidovudine and acyclovir. At 48 weeks, however, there were a significant improvement in survival and a reduction in the incidence and severity of opportunistic infections in patients receiving the combination of zidovudine and acyclovir. Further studies are under way to evaluate the significance of this observation (18).

From the beginning of the AIDS epidemic it was realized that some individuals infected with HIV quickly became ill with profound immunodeficiency, developed an opportunistic infection, and often died, while the sexual partner of that individual, presumably infected with the same strain of virus, would remain in an asymptomatic state for many years, and indeed a small percent of these patients have shown little or no immunosuppression after many years. Clearly, some cofactors must be involved in determining which patients become ill and die and which patients can coexist with their infection for prolonged periods of time. Work by Anthony Fauci and others has clearly shown that in vitro antigenic stimulation from a variety of unrelated antigens produces profound HIV augmentation with increased replication of the virus ande accelerated cell death of infected cells. Herpes simplex is an antigen that has been demonstrated as producing this effect.

Wainberg et al. demonstrated in 1986 that if lymphocytes derived from patients with a history of herpes simplex were stimulated with a herpes antigen, they could demonstrate proliferation in 6 out of 10 cases studied (19). It follows, but has not been demonstrated, that suppression of recurrent herpes simplex in the HIV-infected patient may decrease the antigenic stimulation of the AIDS virus by herpes and eliminates this cofactor as one of the events that accelerate the progression of the disease. For this reason many clinicians caring for HIV-infected patients are currently treating those individuals with suppressive acyclovir on a regular basis. On the other hand, Holmberg et al. could find no serological evidence that herpesviruses are cofactors in the development of AIDS and other HIV-associated conditions (20).

Acyclovir, one of the first truly effective antiviral chemotherapeutic agents, became commercially available shortly after the emergence of the AIDS epidemic. The research that led to a chain-terminating nucleoside analog such as acyclovir had already produced zidovudine, which has proved effective in prolonging the lives of people infected with HIV. Hopefully, this same technology will soon provide other chemotherapeutic agents useful in the management of herpes, AIDS, and other latent viral diseases.

REFERENCES

1. Smith, P., Lane, C., Gill, V., et al. (1988). Intestinal infections in patients with the acquired immunodeficiency syndrome (AIDS). *Ann. Intern. Med.* 108:328-333.
2. Youle, M., Hawkins, D., Collins, P., et al. (1988). Acyclovir-resistant herpes in AIDS treated with foscarnet. *Lancet* 2(8606):341-342.
3. Friedman-Kien, A. E., Lafleur, F. L., Gendler, E., et al. (1986). Herpes zoster: A possible early clinical sign for development of acquired immunodeficiency syndrome in high risk individuals. *J. Am. Acad. Dermatol.* 14:1023-1028.
4. Melbye, M., Grossman, R. J., Goedert, J. J., et al. (1987). Risk of AIDS after herpes zoster. *Lancet* 1:728-731.
5. Mandal, B. K. (1987). Herpes zoster in the immunocompromised. *J. Infect.* 14:1-5.
6. Gilson, I., Barnett, J. H., Jones, P. G., et al. (1989). Disseminated ecthymatous varicella zoster in AIDS. (Submitted.)
7. Balfour, H. H., Bean, B., Laskin, O. L., et al. (1983). Acyclovir halts progression of herpes zoster in immunocompromised patients. *N. Engl. J. Med.* 16:1448-1453.
8. Greenspan, D., Conant, M., and Silverman, S. (1984). Oral hairy leukoplakia in male homosexuals: Evidence of association with both papillomavirus and a herpes group. *Lancet* 2:831-834.
9. Greenspan, D., Greenspan, J., and Lennette, E. (1985). Replication of Epstein-Barr virus within the epithelial cells of oral "hairy" leukoplakia, an AIDS-associated lesion. *N. Engl. J. Med.* 313:1564-1571.
10. Resnick, L., Herbst, J., and Ablashi, D. (1988). Regression of oral hairy leukoplakia after orally administered acyclovir therapy. *JAMA* 259:000-000.
11. Schofer, H. (1987). Letter. *Dermatologica* 174:150-153.
12. Orellana, J., Teich, S., Winterkorn, J., et al. (0000). Treatment of cytomegalovirus retinitis with ganciclovir (9-[2-hydroxy-1-(hydroxymethyl)ethoxymethyl] guanine (BW B759U).
13. Laskin, O. L., Cederberg, D. M., Mills, J., et al. (1987). Gangciclovir for the treatment and suppression of serious infections caused by cytomegalovirus. *Am. J. Med.* 83:201-207.
14. Mitsuya, H., Weinhold, K. J., Furman, P. A., et al. (0000). 3'-Azido-3'deoxythymidine.

15. Mitsuya, H., and Broder, S. (1987). Strategies for antiviral therapy in AIDS. *Nature* 325:773-778.
16. Fischl, M. A., Richman, D. D., Grieco, H. M., et al. (1987). The efficacy of azidothymidine (AZT) in the treatment of patients with AIDS and AIDS-related complex: A double-blind, placebo-controlled trial. *N. Engl. J. Med.* 317:185-191.
17. Mitsuya, H., and Broder, S. (1987). Strategies for antiviral therapy in AIDS. *Nature* 325:773-778.
18. Sigelmann, M. (1988). Zidovudine plus or minus acyclovir in the treatment of AIDS patients' post-opportunistic infection. Fourth International Conference on AIDS, Stockholm.
19. Wainberg, M. A., Portnoy, J., Tsoukas, C., et al. (1987). Specific stimulation of lymphocytes from patients with AIDS by herpes simplex virus antigens. *Immunology* 60:275-280.
20. Holmberg, S., Stuart, J., Gerber, R., et al. (1988). Lack of serological evidence that herpes viruses are cofactors in the development of AIDS and other HIV-associated conditions. Fourth International Conference on AIDS, Stockholm.

Index

About the Editor

DAVID A. BAKER is Director, Division of Maternal-Fetal Medicine, and Associate Professor of Obstetrics and Gynecology, Oral Biology and Pathology at the State University of New York Health Sciences Center, Stony Brook. Dr. Baker is the author or coauthor of more than 100 technical articles, book chapters, reviews, and abstracts, a Fellow of the American College of Obstetricians and Gynecologists, and a member of the Society for Gynecologic Investigation, Infectious Disease Society for Obstetrics and Gynecology, International Society for Antiviral Research, and American Society for the Immunology of Reproduction, among other prestigious societies. He received the B.S. degree (1967) from Brooklyn College, New York, M.S. degree (1969) from the University of Rochester Medical Center, New York, and M.D. degree (1973) from the State University of New York Downstate, Brooklyn.